Also by Elizabeth Somer
──────────────

Age-Proof Your Body

Nutrition for Women

The Nutrition Desk Reference

The Essential Guide to Vitamins & Minerals

Food & Mood

The Origin Diet

Nutrition for a Healthy Pregnancy

NUTRITION
for a Healthy Pregnancy

THE COMPLETE GUIDE TO

EATING BEFORE, DURING, AND

AFTER YOUR PREGNANCY

SECOND EDITION

Elizabeth Somer, M.A., R.D.

An Owl Book

HENRY HOLT AND COMPANY   •   NEW YORK

Henry Holt and Company, LLC
Publishers since 1866
115 West 18th Street
New York, New York 10011

Henry Holt® is a registered trademark
of Henry Holt and Company, LLC.

Library of Congress Cataloging-in-Publication Data
Somer, Elizabeth.
    Nutrition for a healthy pregnancy : the complete guide to eating
before, during, and after your pregnancy / Elizabeth Somer.—2nd ed.
        p.   cm.
    "An Owl book."
    Includes bibliographical references and index.
    ISBN 0-8050-6998-4 (pbk.)
    1. Pregnancy—Nutritional aspects.   2. Pregnant women—
Nutrition.   I. Title.

RG559 .S66 2002   2002017239
618.2'4—dc21

Henry Holt books are available for special promotions
and premiums. For details contact: Director, Special Markets.

First Edition 1995
Second Edition 2002

Designed by Victoria Hartman

Printed in the United States of America
1   3   5   7   9   10   8   6   4   2

To my two sweet children,

Lauren and William,

who have taught me so much about

life, love, wonder, joy, and purpose

Contents

Foreword

Congratulations on your decision to have a baby! There will be some exciting times ahead of you. Eating properly is an everyday event that can have a profound influence on both you and your developing baby. Helping you to build the best baby you possibly can is the goal of *Nutrition for a Healthy Pregnancy*. In this book you will find recommendations for eating good food rich in nutrients and a commonsense approach to eating healthfully during this most critical period in your and your baby's life. Much of what you choose to do, or not do, will leave a legacy for your child that will last a lifetime.

Elizabeth Somer has done all the homework for you! Hundreds of scientific articles support the information she has packed between these two covers. She has covered pregnancy from "thinking about it" through postpartum, giving you the nuts and bolts of why proper nutrition is so important. *Nutrition for a Healthy Pregnancy* makes it easy to eat right, without overspending at the supermarket or living in the kitchen. Step by step, the menus provided deliver those critical nutrients that will take your baby from a few tiny cells to a whopping eight pounds (we hope!) within nine short months.

In these pages you will find a comprehensive view of the links between nutrition and pregnancy. This is the first book of its kind to present sound dietary guidelines on all aspects of pregnancy, including high-risk pregnancies such as teen pregnancy, multiple births, and over-forty pregnancy. Keeping up with the latest scientific data by reading hundreds of studies each month enables Elizabeth to consistently present the most current information available.

I hope you enjoy this insider's look at the growth and development of your soon-to-be new child. When you stop and consider how amazing life really is, the Baby-wise Diet makes all the sense in the world. Use this guide throughout your pregnancy—from the planning stages through your recovery—and good luck in working toward having the healthiest possible baby!

Miriam Erick, M.S., R.D.
Department of Nutrition,
Brigham and Women's Hospital, Boston,
and author of *No More Morning Sickness*

Preface

I've always been happy and generally satisfied, if not occasionally ecstatic, about life. But, in looking back from my vantage point as a well-seasoned mother of two children, I now realize that I didn't have a clue about how good life could be until I had kids.

For one thing, kids bring out a side of you that you probably never even knew was there—your mother-bear side, which makes you capable of superwoman-caliber love and protectiveness. Even before your baby has a face or a name (or even a recognizable gender, for that matter!), you want the very best for that little tyke.

The Magic Pill

If I were to tell you I had a pill that would boost your chances of having a perfect baby, would you take it? Not only would she have all her perfect little toes and fingers, but she'd reach full term at a perfect weight to guarantee health in the early months. If you took this pill, your baby would be exceptionally smart, emotionally well-adjusted, and would possibly sidestep most serious illness later in life, such as heart disease, cancer, diabetes, hypertension, and asthma. She might even be programmed to maintain a desirable weight.

This pill also would help you through your pregnancy. You'd gain the right amount of weight at the proper rate, so you would lower your risk for many pregnancy complications, such as gestational diabetes, hypertension, and preeclampsia. You'd also have an easier time regaining your figure after the baby was born. You'd feel great through your pregnancy, have the energy to "have a life" for the next nine months, avoid many pregnancy nuisances such as constipation and heartburn, and you might even keep a smile on your face rather than feeling moody and irritable like some of your other pregnant friends. In short, you would have the emotional and physical energy to enjoy this miraculous moment in your life and the peace of mind knowing you were doing everything you needed to do—just by taking that pill—to give your baby the best start on a full life of health and happiness.

Wouldn't you take that pill!? You'd be crazy not to! Well, it's not a pill, but it is a few simple guidelines for how to eat, move, and live that could make a huge difference in your pregnancy and your baby. You see, for the next nine months (and longer if you breast-feed), your baby will be totally dependent on you for all the nutrients she needs, including essential ones like water, protein, calcium, and folic acid. Those nutrients come either from your current diet or from the stores you stockpiled prior to pregnancy. So, use that mother-bear desire to protect your baby to your advantage by making a few simple changes in what you eat, when you move, and how you live. Never before in your life have the rewards for healthy living been so great!

The Ultimate Nutrition Book for Pregnancy

Nutrition for a Healthy Pregnancy is more than just a "how to eat" book. There are lots of books on the market that tell you how many glasses of milk you need and why you need folic acid. If you are like me, you want more than that. When I was pregnant with my first child, I scoured the shelves for a book that would give me the details, the latest research, the answers to all my questions. I wanted to know:

- What were researchers finding about how my diet during pregnancy would affect my baby's health when she was an adult?
- What herbs were safe during pregnancy?
- What levels of vitamin supplements were optimal, yet safe, and why?
- What tests should I request from my physician to monitor my nutritional status during pregnancy?
- Were some nutrients more important at different stages of pregnancy?

- I'd heard that some calcium supplements contained lead. Was that a danger during pregnancy and how could I avoid the risk, yet make sure I was getting enough of this vital mineral?
- How could I make sure I was getting everything I needed from my diet before, during, and after pregnancy?

No books existed that had the details I wanted, so I wrote *Nutrition for a Healthy Pregnancy*. Because so much new research has been uncovered since the first edition, it was time to update this book to stay true to my promise that *Nutrition for a Healthy Pregnancy* remain the very best source of easy-to-read, practical information for pregnancy based on a thorough review of the scientific literature. Literally thousands of studies, as well as numerous well-respected researchers, contributed to this guide.

In the following pages you'll find all the basics: what to eat, how to shop, healthy snacks, yummy recipes, a month-by-month checklist of nutritional needs, and quick-fix healthy menus. You'll also find much more than that. The following pages are chock-full of state-of-the-art findings on everything from how nutrition can improve fertility and prevent birth defects to how diet can help you avoid postpartum depression and strengthen the mother-child bond. This second edition includes the latest research on:

- How and why your diet can program your child's health for life.
- Why iron is so important for you and your baby, and what is the best test to check if you're iron deficient.
- What supplements you should take, how much, and when you should start.
- How Dad's diet affects when, and if, you conceive, as well as the health of your baby.
- Vegetarian diets and pregnancy.
- The "good fats" in fish that improve your baby's mental health and intellect.
- Organic versus conventional produce during pregnancy.
- New discoveries for a safe delivery, including what researchers are finding out about acupuncture in the delivery room.
- Optimal, not just adequate, nutrition during pregnancy and breast-feeding.
- How diet can prevent common problems, from morning sickness and food cravings to heartburn and muscle cramps.

- Nutritional guidelines for women carrying twins, triplets, and more.
- New discoveries on the benefits of breast-feeding.
- The more than 12,000 health-enhancing compounds, called phytochemicals, in fruits, vegetables, and whole grains.
- Which foods the nursing mom should avoid for a colicky baby.
- How to regain your figure after the baby is born.

What's New?

While the basic information in *Nutrition for a Healthy Pregnancy* is timeless, this book has had a face-lift. Along with a thorough update of the references and information, you'll find a new layout that helps you locate information in a snap. I've also reorganized the Baby-wise plan to include *Six Steps for a Healthy Pregnancy*. The steps are summarized at the beginnings of relevant chapters.

Six Steps for a Healthy Pregnancy

1. Eat well.
2. Pace the gain (how to manage your weight before, during, and after the baby is born).
3. Supplement responsibly.
4. Be safe (including information on alcohol, medications, seat belts, and more).
5. Exercise daily.
6. Get medical checkups.

You also will find a wealth of new tips, charts, and worksheets to help you put know-how into practice, including four weeks of new menus, twenty delicious new recipes, lots of snack ideas, hundreds of new diet tips and tricks to eat well, tips on how to eat better on a budget, super foods during pregnancy, healthy sweet treats, a detailed vitamin and mineral chart, and self-assessments and quizzes to monitor your progress.

Nutrition and Love

The dietary and nutrition guidelines in this book can help you design a personal and realistic plan that will maximize your chances of having a beautiful, healthy baby and a low-risk pregnancy. They are not intended to add further stress, higher expectations, or more guilt when not followed. The most important job you have in life is to produce, nurse, and raise a healthy child—one who makes the world a slightly better place because she is in it. That goal is always the guiding light for a good parent. Nutrition plays a key role in that goal, both for you and your baby, but it is valuable only if combined with love, dedication to the job of parenting, and respect for the individual who also happens to be your child.

Giving birth to and raising an emotionally and physically healthy child is one of the—if not THE most—important accomplishments of your life. My sincerest hope is that the information in this book contributes, even in a small way, to that wonder-filled life experience.

Acknowledgments

Thank you, dear friends and helpers who made the second edition of this book possible. A great big hug and thank-you to Jeanette Williams, who always has been a dear friend, but has evolved over the years into my recipe guru. What would I do without your willingness to create the recipes, share your thoughts, and give up your precious time to develop the yummy dishes in this book. The best part of writing a book has become the taste-testing parties!

Thank-yous also to David Smith, the best agent a writer can have; Martha Kaufman, my sweet friend and assistant who willingly checks references, types, files, runs errands, and keeps the office running smoothly; and Deborah Brody, my dear editor and mutual bike-enthusiast friend. Each of you helps remove the hassles, so I can get down to the daily business of loving my job.

I'm also deeply grateful to all the researchers around the world on whose work I have depended for the past twenty years to write my articles and books. A special thank-you to those researchers and experts who took time out of their busy schedules to answer my never-ending questions on the topic of nutrition and pregnancy, including: Lindsay Allen, Ph.D., at the University of California, Davis; Richard Anderson, Ph.D., at USDA Vitamin and Mineral Nutrition Laboratory in Beltsville, Maryland; Carol Archie, M.D., at the University of California in Los Angeles Medical Center; Steven Blair, Ph.D., at the Cooper Institute for Aerobics Research in Dallas; Wayne C. Callaway, M.D., at George Washington University in Washington, D.C.; Susan Carmichael, Ph.D., at the California Birth

Defects Monitoring in Emeryville; Larry Christensen, Ph.D., at the University of Southern Alabama in Mobile; Fergus Clydesdale, Ph.D., at the University of Massachusetts in Amherst; William Connor, M.D., at Oregon Health Sciences University in Portland; Andrew Czeizel, M.D., Director at the National Institute of Hygiene in Budapest; Bess Dawson-Hughes, at Tufts University in Boston; Johanna Dwyer, D.Sc., R.D., Tufts University School of Medicine in Boston; Irvin Emanuel, M.D., at the University of Washington in Seattle; Miriam Erick, M.S., R.D., at Brigham and Women's Hospital in Boston; Brenda Eskenazi, Ph.D., at the University of California, Berkeley; John Foreyt, Ph.D., at Baylor College of Medicine in Houston; Robert Heaney, M.D., at Creighton University in Omaha, Nebraska; Douglas Heimburger, M.D., at the University of Alabama in Birmingham; Richard B. Johnston, Jr., M.D., at the March of Dimes; Janet King, Ph.D., R.D., at the University of California, Berkeley; Susan Krebs-Smith, Ph.D., at the National Cancer Institute in Bethesda, Maryland; Maureen Murtaugh, Ph.D., R.D., at Rush-Presbyterian–St. Luke's Medical Center in Chicago; Judith Putnam at U.S. Department of Agriculture in Washington, D.C.; Barbara Rolls, Ph.D., at Pennsylvania State University in University Park; Robert Sack, Ph.D., at the Oregon Health Sciences University in Portland; Amy Subar, Ph.D., R.D., at the National Cancer Institute in Bethesda, Maryland; the late Varro Tyler, Ph.D., Sc.D.; Debra Waterhouse, M.P.H., R.D.; Walter Willett, M.D., Dr.P.H., at the Harvard School of Public Health in Boston; David Williamson, Ph.D., at the Centers for Disease Control in Atlanta; Bonnie Worthington-Roberts, Ph.D., previously at the University of Washington in Seattle; and Gary Zammit, Ph.D., at St. Luke's Hospital in New York City.

More than anything else, I'm grateful for two perfect children—Lauren and William—who have graced every day of my life since their births with more joy, pride, and hope than a mother could wish for. And, for Patrick Vance, the man who made it all possible.

Introduction

If you're reading this book, you are probably either pregnant or thinking seriously about it. That means you are contemplating the most miraculous experience of your life. It is a decision that will change you forever. But, if you are ready to commit yourself to the responsibility of parenthood, I guarantee pregnancy will be the start of the most rich and joyous experience of your life.

You probably have spent many moments pondering the new baby and how your life will change. What will the baby look like? What funny little mannerisms will he have? You probably are filled with hopes, dreams, and expectations. Will the baby have your red hair or Daddy's blue eyes? Will she inherit her granddad's wit or her grandma's gentleness? At the end of each daydream, however, is the first and foremost wish—please, just let my baby be healthy.

The Genetic Blueprint

Many factors influence the health of your baby and your pregnancy experience. For one, your genetic blueprint and your partner's, handed down from one generation to another, will have the first and final say on many physical and personality traits, from eye color to temperament. Every genetic blueprint has a flaw or two that might or might not become part of your baby's legacy. For example, diabetes or heart disease are prevalent in some families partially because of the genetic blueprint. On the other hand, your baby might have a genetic blueprint for longevity if your parents and other family members have lived to "ripe and healthy old ages."

You can't change your genetics, but you do make choices every day that increase or decrease either the seriousness of the consequences or your chances that those "weak links" in your blueprint will break. Your baby might inherit a high risk for developing hypertension, but with a healthy beginning and a lifetime of exercise and good diet that weak link might never develop or might result in only minor increases in blood pressure.

What You Eat = Your Baby

In the "old days," people thought of a baby as the "perfect parasite." Regardless of the mother's nutritional status prior to conception or dietary habits during pregnancy, the baby would draw all necessary nutrients from the mother's nutrient "stores." It didn't matter if the mother's diet was protein-poor, the baby would steal protein from her tissues. Her diet could be iron-depleted and the baby still would obtain ample iron by draining iron "reserves" somewhere in the mother's body. The mother should, but didn't have to, drink milk because the baby would siphon calcium from the mother's bones and teeth (thus, the old wives' tale that you loose a tooth for each child). This myth perpetuated a generally careless attitude toward the pregnant woman's diet, her weight gain, and how nutrition affected the baby's development.

That belief has taken a 180-degree turn. We now know that what you eat, or don't eat, during pregnancy has a profound effect on your baby's development and health at birth and later in life. According to researchers at the University of California, Davis, "when [nutrient] intakes fall below the threshold, fetal growth and development [are] affected more than . . . maternal health." That puts an even greater pressure on the mother to ensure optimal nutritional status before, during, and following pregnancy (if she plans to breast-feed).

Every Sprig of Broccoli

If you have been pregnant, are pregnant, or have talked to pregnant friends, you know there is no other life experience as miraculous or unique as producing a baby. Whether you have danced through life insensitive to your body's signals or have paid close attention to caring for your body, the changes that occur as a result of pregnancy cannot be ignored.

You feel different, you look different, you are more emotional or insecure, you may feel more loving or irritable. You cry at commercials or become angry at things that never bothered you before. Your sleep is affected or you experience heartburn for the first time in your life. All your physical and mental signals may be scrambled, so you don't know what to expect from yourself from one moment to another.

On top of all that, your body is changing and growing to nurture the developing little human being inside you. And, of course, the baby is growing from two cells to a highly diversified and complex miracle of life. It is no wonder your dietary needs change and your nutrient requirements are greater than at any other time in your adult life.

Coupled with your body's increasing demands for nutrients is your baby's absolute dependence on you during the next nine months for all the vitamins, minerals, protein, calories, and other essential food factors necessary to produce life. You are your baby's sole source of nutrition during the most critical period of development. Every choice you make, from the cereal you select to the supplements you take, to whether or not you drink coffee, directly affects your baby. Every gram of protein, every microgram of folic acid, every drop of water, every trace of copper comes from you. Every sprig of broccoli, every bite of pizza, every gulp of milk is an opportunity taken or missed to nourish your baby.

Some essential nutrients come from the limited stores you have stockpiled in your tissues if your diet was optimal prior to pregnancy. Other nutrients are not stored in your body or are stored in such limited amounts that the diet is virtually the only place your baby can get what is needed. Consequently, your baby is a product of what you have eaten before and during pregnancy. If this is your second or third child, this baby also is a product of what you have eaten after your last pregnancy to replenish lost stores. A baby grown on a diet composed mostly of refined, processed foods or inadequate calories is very different from a baby nourished on a variety of wholesome, nutritious foods.

Granted, some of the differences are subtle and a baby grown on a diet of Snickers and soda pop can arrive on the scheduled due date and appear "fine." However, how much healthier could that baby have been if the mother had snacked on carrots and milk instead? What long-term consequences will result? How will memory, concentration, IQ, health in later years, or even your grandchildren be affected? Why take the risk when eating right is so easy?

How Your Diet Affects Your Baby

Developing from two cells into a human being is a complicated process that requires a wide array of nutrients in varying amounts at different times. Your diet determines if those nutritional building blocks will be there when they are needed for your baby.

Growth is not just getting bigger. From conception to birth and beyond, all your baby's organs and tissues form, grow, and mature at different speeds, rates, and times—each with its own schedule, time line, and characteristic pattern. The following three general growth levels are operating simultaneously during the baby-making process:

1. the entire body is growing;
2. the organs and tissues are forming and increasing in size; and
3. the cells within each organ and tissue are differentiating, increasing in number, and expanding in size.

This symphony of growth processes is different every day, week, month, and trimester of your pregnancy. Each stage serves as a "critical period" where growth of a certain tissue or organ depends on the right mix and amount of forty-plus nutrients in your diet to ensure all nutritional building blocks are present when they are needed.

This close tie between your diet and your baby's development begins at the very beginning. The nutritional health of the uterus at the time of conception is critical to whether or not the fertilized egg successfully implants in the uterine wall and begins to develop. During the first few weeks following fertilization—called the implantation stage—the egg cell divides into many cells and these rudimentary cells sort themselves into three layers: the outer, middle, and inner layers. Diet is critical at this stage to ensure a healthy beginning, while inadequate nutrient intake at this stage can result in failure of the fertilized egg to implant or other conditions that result in the loss of the egg.

Nutrient needs during pregnancy reflect the rapid and dramatic growth that occurs in each of the three trimesters. You need more protein, calcium, phosphorus, and magnesium for the rapidly dividing cells and for bone formation. You need more iron, vitamin B_{12}, copper, and vitamin B_6 to produce hemoglobin in red blood cells for your rapidly expanding blood volume. You need twice as much folic acid for each of the billions of new cells to divide properly. Your nutritional state prior to becoming pregnant will determine how "packed" your vitamin and mineral stores are, and your diet during every stage of pregnancy will determine whether or not you have the nutritional "what it takes" to build every cell, tissue, and organ that makes up your child.

Programming Your Baby for Life

You are nourishing your baby to be born healthy *and* you are setting the stage for your baby's health throughout life. Recent research shows that the developing baby is much more sensitive to the mother's diet than previously thought, and some health consequences don't show up until much later in life. Poor intake of one or more essential nutrients during a critical period in an organ's growth can alter the structure or function of that organ for life.

A dramatic example of this occurs with folic acid, a B vitamin essential for normal cell division and growth. Inadequate amounts of this B vitamin early in pregnancy cause cells to divide wrong, resulting in malformation of the spinal cord, such as spina bifida and other neural tube defects. Inadequate nutrition at other critical periods during pregnancy contributes to an individual's risk later in life for heart disease, high blood pressure, diabetes, reduced intellectual ability, impaired immunity, and even obesity. If, for example, you are not eating well when your baby's pancreas is forming and its size, structure, or function is affected, he could be at a greater risk for diabetes later in life.

Research also shows that mothers who were underweight at birth are more apt to bear low-birth-weight babies themselves. Even the growth status of our grandmothers has affected our health by influencing our mothers' development in the womb. The changes are subtle, but they accumulate over time. Your diet is the nutritional legacy that your baby will live with forever. The responsibility is great, but not daunting; just use a little nutritional common sense by following the Baby-wise Diet outlined in this book.

Food, Love, and Your Baby's Personality

We know an infant's earliest impressions of the world form attitudes that continue to affect behavior into adulthood. For example, if food and love are there when the baby cries, that baby grows into an adult who views the world as a safe and trustworthy place to live. It is possible these attitudes begin even earlier, before your baby is born. Small babies born to malnourished mothers smile less and are more drowsy and passive compared to babies born to a well-nourished mother. The effects last into childhood, where children who were malnourished during development also perform less well in school.

Nutritious, wholesome food throughout pregnancy and the first years of life fuels more than just the physical health of your baby; it also nurtures trust, autonomy, feelings of safety and security, and other psychological and social needs. Before your baby can cry out for food, she or he must trust you to supply all the essential nutrients, when they are needed, so that your baby may grow into all the hopes and dreams of health you have for your child.

What You Eat = Your Pregnancy, Delivery, and Recovery

Besides your baby's immediate and lifelong health, what you eat before and during your pregnancy could be one of the most important considerations for your health and happiness during those nine months. Fortunately, most women do not develop serious complications during pregnancy, but it is the minor nuisances that turn a wonderful nine months into an ordeal. Fatigue, morning sickness, constipation, hemorrhoids, varicose veins, tooth and gum problems, leg cramps, nosebleeds, skin problems, colds and infections, mild depression, and mood swings are only a few of the nutritionally related side effects of pregnancy that might be avoided or at least lessened by proper diet.

For example, a diet and supplement program that guarantees optimal iron intake reduces your likelihood of experiencing fatigue, irritability, and mood swings. Ample intake of protein, carbohydrate, and vitamin B_6 can reduce some of the discomfort of morning sickness. Including a variety of fibrous foods in the daily fare reduces your risk for developing constipation and hemorrhoids.

What you eat prior to and during pregnancy also can affect your childbirthing experience. For one, an optimal diet helps prevent the onset of premature labor. Second, you will need all the strength and endurance you can muster to help bring that baby into the world and a well-nourished body is the foundation and source of that energy and resiliency. I can't promise you that following the Baby-wise Diet will guarantee a pain-free, one-hour labor, but you will be more able to cope and draw on your well-stocked energy reserves for any labor experience as compared to a woman whose body enters labor already fatigued and depleted of essential nutrients.

Think of yourself as a highly trained, competition athlete entering a marathon. You are most likely to run your best, experience minimal fatigue and damage to your body, and have the fortitude and reserves to push your hardest during the final stretch if your body is fueled for the event. In contrast, you are more likely to injure yourself, experience overexhaustion, or run out of energy if you have not taken the effort to nourish your body ahead of time.

The physical and emotional stresses of childbirth are enormous, regardless of whether your labor is three hours or thirty hours, you have a planned cesarean, or a long labor ends in cesarean. Your body will require optimal fuel and resources to mend and revitalize itself. There are stretches, tears, incisions, sutures, blood loss, lost sleep, and numerous other physical tolls on your body that must be tended. Nutrition is important in this mending process. In addition, your diet is essential for the health of your baby if you plan to breast-feed.

Now Is the Best Time to Be Born

Never before have babies had a better chance of being born alive and well. In the past, little was known about "birthing babies" and the survival of both the mother and the baby was mostly chance. Today, having a healthy baby is mostly up to you —not chance.

You can minimize the risks and maximize the likelihood of having a healthy baby, a smooth and enjoyable pregnancy, an uncomplicated delivery, and a quick recovery to your "old" (or an even better) self if you take the time to follow the *Six Steps for a Healthy Pregnancy* outlined in this book.

Nutrition for a
Healthy Pregnancy

❦

Chapter 1

The Prepregnancy Diet

Things to do for the three months to one year prior to conception:

1. **Nutrition:** Follow the guidelines outlined in the Baby-wise Diet (see Chapter 2).
2. **Weight:** If you are 20 percent above your desirable weight, gradually lose weight prior to conception. If you are more than 10 percent below your desirable weight, gradually gain weight before conception.
3. **Supplement:** Take a multiple vitamin and mineral that contains 100 to 200 percent of the Daily Value for all vitamins and minerals plus at least 400 mcg of folic acid and 18 mg of iron each day.
4. **Safety:** If you smoke, drink alcohol, or take any medication/drug not approved by your physician as safe during pregnancy, quit. Avoid secondhand smoke.
5. **Exercise:** If you are not already exercising regularly, begin a low-impact sport, such as walking, bicycling, or swimming at least three days a week.

Gearing Up for Pregnancy

The first "big day" may be when your pregnancy test comes back positive, but, in reality, you have been pregnant for weeks prior to this day and, in fact, nearly all cells have divided and begun organizing to form your baby's brain, heart, and other organs. Your baby's rapid growth demands a constant and hefty supply of all the essential nutrients, all of which will come from both your nutrient stores accumulated prior to conception and your dietary intake during those first few weeks before you know you're pregnant.

If you think of the nine months of pregnancy as an endurance event, such as running a marathon, then the months prior to conception are your training time where you prepare your body for one of the most strenuous and demanding events it will ever experience. For example, optimal nutrition before conception is critical to the prevention of many birth defects. One expert on prenatal care concluded that "the *preconception* visit may be the single most important health-care visit when viewed in the context of its effect on pregnancy." Put another way, babies *born* during a time when mothers don't eat perfectly are less affected healthwise compared to babies *conceived* when mothers are eating subperfect diets. Ideally you should be preparing for pregnancy at least one year before conception or one year and four to six weeks before that pregnancy test.

Programming Baby's Health

In the past, newborns were "healthy" if they looked and acted normal at birth. They also were pictured as "parasites," adjusting their intakes or robbing mom's nutrient stores when dietary intake was poor. Recent research shows that the developing baby is much more sensitive to the mother's nutritional status prior to and during pregnancy than previously thought, with the consequences not always showing up until much later in life.

The phenomenon is called "programming," which means that poor intake of one or more essential nutrients during critical periods in a developing organ's growth can permanently alter or program the structure, size, or function of that organ. The best example of this is folic acid, the B vitamin needed for normal development of the spinal cord. If folic acid is lacking during this early period, the neural tube does not form properly and the baby is born with spina bifida or other neural tube defects. (See Box 1.1.) Another example is poor nutrition during a critical period early in pregnancy when the pancreas and heart are forming, which may predispose the child to diabetes or heart disease later in life. The critical period for the kidney is later in pregnancy, and the critical period for the brain, nervous system, and lungs extends from early pregnancy through the first two years of life.

"There are very good data to support that fetal growth affects adult

BOX 1.1   WHAT ARE NEURAL TUBE DEFECTS?

Roughly one in every one thousand babies born in the United States has a neural tube defect (NTD). These defects occur within the first few days to weeks after conception, when the tube that should eventually become the baby's spinal cord and brain does not close properly, leaving an open seam. If the opening occurs in the spine, the baby is born with a portion of the spinal cord exposed or, less commonly, covered only with skin. This neural tube defect is called spina bifida. Two-thirds of these babies survive into childhood and suffer from lack of bladder or bowel control, paralysis below the waist, and/or fluid accumulation in the brain leading to mental retardation. If the open seam occurs at the top of the neural tube, as is the case with anencephalic babies, the brain never develops and the baby dies within a few hours of birth.

disease risks," says Irvin Emanuel, M.D., professor of epidemiology and pediatrics at the University of Washington in Seattle. Inadequate nutrition during fetal development increases the child's risk later in life for

- heart disease
- high blood pressure
- glucose intolerance and diabetes
- reduced intellectual ability
- impaired immunity
- lung disease
- schizophrenia
- brain cancer
- obesity
- shortened life expectancy

The child's increased risk for these and other diseases can lay dormant for years or decades until some negative lifestyle habit, such as sedentary living or obesity, triggers the flaw. According to Dr. Emanuel, even the nutritional status of our grandmothers affects our health by influencing how well our mothers developed in the womb. "The changes are subtle, but accumulate over generations," says Dr. Emanuel.

The responsibility is great, but not daunting, and even then you only need a little nutritional common sense. "Quality is the key when it comes to choosing foods before and during pregnancy. If women focus on a variety of minimally processed, wholesome foods, they can rest assured they're providing their babies with everything needed for healthy growth and development," says Maureen Murtaugh, Ph.D., R.D., an assistant professor in the Department of Foods and Nutrition at Rush-Presbyterian–St. Luke's Medical Center in Chicago.

Are You Ready for Pregnancy?

Even if you are a woman who pays close attention to her diet, there is room for improvement as you prepare for pregnancy. According to a Gallup poll conducted by Weight Watchers and the American Dietetic Association, 90 percent of women think their diets are pretty healthy. Most of them are delusional.

The latest national nutrition survey of Americans' eating habits found that only 1 percent of us meet even minimum standards of a balanced diet. According to a U.S. Department of Agriculture (USDA) study of women who rated their diets as excellent, only 18.7 percent actually ate reasonably well; women under the age of thirty-nine were the ones most likely to eat poorly. Consequently, many women enter pregnancy nutritionally challenged, with diets low in critical nutrients, such as iron, vitamin A, zinc, magnesium, folic acid, selenium, and vitamin D.

"Our eating styles are more like an hourglass than a pyramid," says Judith Putnam, an economist at USDA. We gobble lots of sugar and fat from the top of the food pyramid and platters of refined grains from the bottom tier, but we are sorely lacking in the vegetables, fruits, low-fat milk products, and other nutritious foods in the middle of the pyramid. "Fat, sugar, and refined grains are found together in the same processed foods, and women don't want to admit they eat much of these," says Putnam.

It's not that we don't know better. Nine out of ten women know it's important to limit sugary and fatty foods, yet we're gobbling up these foods in record amounts. Only a third of us meet the recommendations to keep fat at no more than 30 percent of calories, many of us unknowingly eat too much cholesterol, and we're whole-grain phobic. "Most Americans are missing out on whole grains, often consuming less than one serving a day, yet are eating record amounts of refined grains," says Putnam.

Of course there are also a few of us who are too hard on ourselves. "Many women think they are doing worse than they are," says Debra Waterhouse, M.P.H., a registered dietitian and author of *Outsmarting*

Female Fatigue (Hyperion, 2001). They think they are eating too much fat, sugar, and calories, when in fact they are doing just fine. "That's why I encourage women to 'eat write,' that is write down everything they eat so they have a clear picture of how they really are eating. Many find they are eating too much, but a surprising number of women find they are eating too little," says Waterhouse.

OK, so some of us are in serious diet denial. The good news is it takes only a few minor changes in what we're eating to produce big-time results now and during pregnancy. "If women focused on increasing their vegetables, fruits, and whole grains, and minimizing added fats, especially when eating out, they would be well on their way to eating better," says Amy Subar, Ph.D., R.D., research nutritionist at the National Cancer Institute in Bethesda, Maryland.

A nutritionally well-stocked woman is better prepared for the first few weeks of her baby's life—when cell division and growth are so rapid that all of the vital organs have been formed before a woman even knows she is pregnant—and for the nutritionally intense nine-month process of making a baby. Eating right also helps you recover quickly after the baby is born. The sooner you start the better; however, it is never too late to begin. (Take Quiz 1.1 at the end of this chapter to get an objective view of your present diet.)

Iron Blues

Iron is of particular concern for all women, but especially for a woman preparing for pregnancy. One out of every ten women is iron deficient, according to researchers at the Centers for Disease Control and Prevention in Atlanta, who found that approximately 11 percent of adolescent girls and women of childbearing age were low in iron. Those percentages equate to 7.8 million iron-deficient women in the United States, and another 3.3 million women who are anemic. Iron deficiency statistics vary from one study to another, with rates as high as 80 percent in certain populations, such as women athletes.

The developing baby and expanding blood volume will take a toll on a mother's iron reserves. If you enter pregnancy with these reserves already drained, it will be even more difficult to maintain optimal iron status and you are likely to suffer more complications during your pregnancy, including fatigue, vaginal bleeding, preterm delivery, an increased risk for delivering a low-birth-weight baby, delivering a baby who also is iron deficient, and prolonged fatigue after the baby is born. Because of the frequency of iron deficiency in women during the childbearing years and the consequences during pregnancy, researchers at the University of California, Davis, recommend that even women who have "reasonable iron stores" entering pregnancy should supplement with this mineral.

How Do You Know If You're Iron Deficient? Routine blood tests, such as hemoglobin and hematocrit, reflect final iron deficiency anemia, so ask for more sensitive tests, such as serum ferritin or total iron binding capacity (TIBC), which reflect tissue iron stores and identify iron deficiency before it has progressed to anemia. Most women of childbearing age who have complained to me about feeling tired and who have had a serum ferritin test done, found they were iron deficient. Be your own health advocate and ask for a copy of the lab report; don't settle for an "everything is normal" verbal report from your health-care provider. Serum ferritin levels less than 20 mcg/L or a TIBC greater than 450 mcg/L is a sign your tissue iron levels are depleted.

How Much Iron Do You Need? If a blood test verifies you are iron deficient, an aggressive supplement program should be undertaken several months prior to conception, since it takes three months or more to build iron reserves. Usually, physicians prescribe 60 mg to 120 mg of iron daily until blood values return to normal and 30 mg to 60 mg daily thereafter. If you experience digestive tract problems as a result of iron supplements, such as stomach upsets, diarrhea, or constipation, try taking a half dose and gradually increase to the full dose or divide the pill in two and take half twice a day. (See Table 1.1.)

Folic Acid: A Must before Pregnancy. Neural tube defects (NTD) are the second leading cause of death among infants who die from birth defects in this country (Down's syndrome is the leading cause). One nutrient known to prevent NTDs is folic acid. Numerous studies since the early 1990s have consistently found that folic acid supplementation in women around the time of conception and during pregnancy reduces the risk of NTD, especially spina bifida and anencephaly. Women who supplement with folic acid also deliver babies at low risk for urinary tract, cardiovascular, and limb defects. You also tend to improve your fertility, are less likely to miscarry, and should suffer less from nausea.

The problem is many women who enter pregnancy aren't getting enough folic acid. Researchers at the March of Dimes questioned women about whether they took supplements containing folic acid. Only 30 per-

TABLE 1.1

Iron Up

You should consume at least 18 mg of iron each day prior to pregnancy, more if you menstruate heavily or use the IUD as birth control. If a blood test shows you are iron deficient, your iron needs are even higher.

Food	Amount	Iron (mg)
Oysters, raw	1 cup	16.6
Tofu, firm	½ cup	13.2
Baked beans	1 cup	5.0
Refried beans, fat free	1 cup	4.5
Chard, cooked	1 cup	4.0
Black beans, cooked	1 cup	3.6
Wheat germ	½ cup	3.3
Spinach, cooked	1 cup	3.0
Beet greens, cooked	1 cup	2.7
Whole-wheat bread	2 slices	2.4
Sunflower seed kernels	¼ cup	2.4
Mango, fresh	1 cup sliced	2.1
Avocado	1 whole	2.0
Beef, extra lean, cooked	3 ounces	2.0
English muffin	1	1.7
Raisins	½ cup	1.5
Almonds	¼ cup	1.3

cent of all nonpregnant women said yes. Fewer than one in every five young women took supplements containing folic acid. Only 23 percent of the women who had been pregnant in the preceding two years said they had taken daily vitamins with folic acid before their pregnancies. In another study, from the University of Minnesota in Minneapolis, one in every eight women had folic acid levels low enough to place them at risk for having a baby with birth defects.

How Much Do You Need? Every woman during the childbearing years should take multiple vitamin and mineral supplements that contain folic acid, according to Andrew Czeizel, M.D., director of the Department of Human Genetics and Teratology at the National Institute of Hygiene in Budapest and an expert on folic acid. He recommends that "a woman should supplement a folic acid–rich diet with a 400 mcg supplement of folic acid or, in the event her diet is low in folic acid, supplement with at least 800 mcg of folic acid prior to and during her pregnancy." Women who already have given birth to babies with NTDs should supplement with 4 mg of folic acid prior to and after conception to reduce the risk of recurrence. Richard B. Johnston Jr., M.D., medical director of the March of Dimes, adds, "Since nearly half of all pregnancies in this country are unplanned and since folic acid is only effective in preventing birth defects when consumed before conception and during the first four weeks of pregnancy, all women capable of having a baby should be consuming folic acid every day."

Which Is Best, Supplements or Food? Supplements are better than food when it comes to raising blood levels of this B vitamin and reducing birth defects. Researchers at the University of Ulster in Northern Ireland assessed the effectiveness of 400 mcg of folic acid, given as a supplement, in fortified foods, or as dietary folate. Folic acid levels in the blood increased only in the women who supplemented or consumed fortified foods, while dietary intake of folic acid–rich foods produced no change in folate status. The researchers concluded that "compared with supplements and fortified foods, consumption of extra folate as natural food folate is relatively ineffective at increasing folate status . . . [and] advice to women to consume folate-rich foods as a means to optimize folate status is misleading." Your best bet is to include two or more servings of folic acid–rich foods in your daily diet AND take a supplement that includes at least 400 mcg of folic acid. (See Table 1.2.)

Other Nutrients and Birth Defects

Preventing birth defects goes beyond folic acid. Dr. Czeizel emphasizes that other nutrients affect NTD occurrence, including vitamin B_{12}, vitamin C, and zinc. In fact, women who take multiple vitamin and mineral supplements along with foods rich in these three nutrients prior to and during pregnancy are significantly less likely to give birth to babies with NTD as compared to women who do not supplement. The benefits are greatest when women take a multiple for at least three months prior to conception and during the first trimester of pregnancy; benefits are less pronounced if supplementation begins in the second trimester, and if started in the third trimester of pregnancy, there is little effect on preventing NTD.

TABLE 1.2

Fortifying Your Diet with Folic Acid

During the childbearing years, women should consume at least 400 mcg of folic acid daily from both food and supplements.

Food	Amount	Folic acid (mcg)
Lentils, cooked	1 cup	358
Brewer's yeast	1 tbsp.	313
Pinto beans, cooked	1 cup	294
Spinach, cooked	1 cup	262
Red kidney beans, cooked	1 cup	229
Wheat germ, toasted	½ cup	199
Chickpeas, cooked	1 cup	160
Lima beans, dried and cooked	1 cup	156
Asparagus, cooked	½ cup	132
Collards, cooked	1 cup	129
Split peas, cooked	1 cup	123
Spinach, fresh	1 cup	109
Orange juice, frozen	1 cup	109
Fortified breakfast cereal	½ to 1½ cups	100 to 400
Tomato juice	1 cup	48
Folic acid–fortified white bread	1 slice	38

Weight Issues and Birth Defects

Folic acid might be the main factor for preventing birth defects, but your weight also plays a role. The risk of having a baby with NTD escalates with increasing prepregnancy weight or body mass index (BMI) regardless of folic acid intake, according to researchers at Boston University School of Public Health. In their study, both elevated prepregnancy body weight (more than 176 pounds) and BMI (> 29) were linked with NTD risk, with the heaviest women having a threefold greater risk regardless of folic acid intake. In contrast, NTD risk was cut in half in lean women with high folic acid intakes.

Prepregnancy Reasons to Supplement

Anyone worth their weight in nutrition credentials will tell you to turn to food first for your nutritional needs during pregnancy. "We eat food, not nutrients, and foods are packages of vitamins, minerals, fiber, other nutrients, and the thousands of health-enhancing phytochemicals. Supplements won't compensate for poor food choices," says Dr. Murtaugh.

Granted, supplements don't make up for bad diets, but there is still reason to supplement a good diet. For one thing, several studies show that women who supplement prior to pregnancy, especially with folic acid and zinc, have a lower risk for birth defects and better pregnancy outcomes than women who don't supplement. "All women should be taking a moderate-dose multiple vitamin and mineral. Even if the only airtight proof that supplements are beneficial is with folic acid and its ability to prevent birth defects, that's reason enough to take the offensive," says Walter Willett, M.D., Dr.P.H., chairman of the nutrition department at Harvard School of Public Health. In addition, women who take a multiple vitamin and mineral supplement have a higher rate of conception and a shorter time to conception than do women who take only a trace mineral supplement, adds Dr. Czeizel.

The main reason to supplement, however, is that many women don't eat enough of the right foods prior to, during, and following pregnancy to guarantee optimal intake of all nutrients. Rather than an either/or issue, a woman's best bet is to combine an excellent diet with a well-balanced supplement program.

What Supplements Do You Need? The secret to supplementation is to do it sensibly. Choose a multiple vitamin and mineral that supplies at least 400 mcg of folic acid and approximately 100 to 200 percent of the Daily Value for all other nutrients. If you don't consume daily at least two calcium-rich foods, such as nonfat milk and fortified soy milk, and lots of magnesium-rich whole grains, wheat germ, and legumes, then consider supplementing your multiple with extra calcium (500 mg) and magnesium (250 mg) since no one-pill multiple contains enough of these two minerals. In addition, you will need additional iron if blood or tissue iron levels are low.

Can I Take Too Much? Some vitamins are best obtained from foods, rather than supplements. Vitamin A, for example, is a potent teratogen (a substance that causes birth defects) when consumed in excessive amounts during pregnancy. A study published in the *New England Journal of Medicine* found that women who consumed as little as 10,000 IU of vitamin A daily during pregnancy were at greater risk for birth defects. While subsequent studies found vitamin A safe at doses greater than 8,000 IU, it is wise to err on the side of caution and limit supplemental vitamin A to the Daily Value or 5,000 IU. (See Chapter 5 for guidelines on supplementation.)

Dispelling Myths and Debunking Misconceptions

People have been giving dietary advice to pregnant women since the dawn of civilization. Most of these beliefs about how food affects pregnancy are more fiction than fact, but some are worth heeding.

The first and foremost myth regarding diet and pregnancy is that you can rely on your physician for all your nutritional needs. Although your OB-GYN is your ally and the expert in all medical-related issues regarding your pregnancy, many physicians spend little time talking about diet. Many pregnant women, at best, receive a booklet on the four food groups. Few are asked even basic questions, such as whether they drink milk, take a supplement, smoke or drink alcohol, or eat dark green leafy vegetables daily. According to a survey conducted by New York Hospital and Cornell University Medical Center, more than half of the OB-GYNs interviewed admitted they rarely questioned their patients about their diets. Thus, gearing up for pregnancy means doing your own nutrition homework.

Thin Is Beautiful

Many women diet, and even those who don't often consume suboptimal amounts of calories, which implies that semi-fasting has become normal to many women. The average daily intake for women in the United States is approximately 1,600 calories, 600 calories short of the 2,200 calories recommended for most women. The "thin is beautiful" mystique that plagues American women prior to pregnancy could have lifelong damaging and irreversible effects on their developing babies and the outcome of their pregnancies, especially in light of the new research showing that restricting food prior to and during pregnancy might program your child for lifelong health problems.

Pregnancy is not the time to worry about your hips and thighs. All get-thin-quick fad diets are nutritional nightmares, including the latest high-protein, low-carbohydrate, food combining, and sugar-addict diets. When gearing up for pregnancy, focus on stockpiling the nutrient stores in your tissues and attaining or maintaining a desirable, healthy weight. Eating disorders, including anorexia, bulimia, and compulsive eating, can have serious and irreversible effects on the unborn child, so a woman should obviously resolve these problems prior to considering pregnancy.

How Thin Is Too Thin? Women who are below 10 percent of their desirable body weight prior to conception are at higher risk for complications during pregnancy that may affect the developing baby. A woman needs at least 18 percent body fat for ovulation to proceed. Even if an underweight woman does conceive, she is more likely to have a premature or low-birth-weight infant who has difficulty "catching up" in terms of growth and who shows delayed neurological development and reduced IQ later in life. Underweight women are also more likely to develop anemia and premature rupture of the amniotic membranes during their pregnancies than are normal-weight women.

How Heavy Is Too Heavy? Overweight women, that is, 20 percent or more above desirable weight, should not attempt to use pregnancy as a way to use up extra body fat, since stored body fat is not the stuff from which babies are made. The obese woman entering pregnancy is more likely to develop complications, such as hypertension and diabetes, and to have more trouble during labor and delivery. Overweight women also might have higher levels of some pesticide residues in their bodies than leaner women, according to a study from Duke University Medical Center in Chapel Hill, North Carolina. Losing weight before pregnancy would help lower the baby's exposure to these pesticides. Ideally, an overweight woman should lose excess body fat one to two months before she conceives, so that she enters pregnancy with well-stocked nutrient stores in her tissues and is within 10 to 20 percent of her desirable weight.

What Is the Best Way to Lose Weight? It is not only weight loss, but the method of weight loss that is important. "Women must de-emphasize weight loss and emphasize healthy behaviors. Anyone can lose weight doing a variety of tricks, many of which are not healthful. For the vast majority of people it's exercise and a healthful diet that will keep the weight off," recommends David Williamson, Ph.D., at the Division of Nutrition at the Centers for Disease Control and Prevention in Atlanta. Ironically, a side effect of adopting a healthy lifestyle and following the Baby-wise Diet is that women typically lose weight. "Once people adopt lifelong healthful behaviors, the weight takes care of itself," says Dr. Williamson.

Nutrition and exercise go hand in hand. Women who exercise are most likely to lose weight and keep it off. Yet, exercise is only effective when combined with a low-calorie diet. And the combination must be a lifelong commitment. "Even if people lose weight, they must continue to eat low-fat foods and exercise daily, or it's a sure thing they'll regain the weight and place themselves in a higher disease-risk category," says Steven Blair, Ph.D., director of epidemiology at the Cooper Institute for Aerobics Research in Dallas. In short, if you are 120 percent or more of your desirable weight, begin losing weight slowly prior to pregnancy so you have attained a more healthful weight by the time of conception. (See Worksheet 1.1 at the end of this chapter for developing a good weight-loss program.)

Fertility Foods

One in five married couples in the United States has fertility problems. Age may have something to do with this, since more couples are waiting to start a family, and infertility (that is, the inability to conceive after twelve months or more of unprotected intercourse) increases as you age, with up to 25 percent of couples in their mid to late thirties and as much as 50 percent of couples in their forties experiencing infertility problems. In addition, male fertility is suspected to be declining. A study in Denmark found a 50 percent decrease in sperm concentration in the past half century alone! While what you eat plays a part in fertility, it is important to sift the few facts from the wealth of fiction when it comes to how much food can do for your conception rate.

Fertile Fiction

Since the beginning of civilization, people have turned to food to enhance fertility and sexual prowess. In fact, eating and loving are so closely entwined that we often speak of "eating our hearts out," "feasting our eyes," or having "lusty appetites."

Before the turn of the century, people had little understanding of the chemical and nutritional content of foods, so much of the fertility-food links were based on hundreds of years of symbolism. Thus, plants shaped like human sexual organs, such as onions that resemble testicles or oysters and figs which resemble female anatomy, were thought to enhance sexual potency. The sexual organs and meat from animals known to reproduce easily, such as rabbits, have at one time or another been used to enhance fertility. These naive views were based entirely on superstition and hearsay.

Other diet myths about sexuality included a mistaken belief that if a spicy food raised blood pressure or pulse rate this was a sign of increased sexual potency. Rare or exotic foods, from hyena eyes in the distant past to ginseng and ginkgo biloba today, also were thought to supply a fertility or potency factor. Again, not a word of this advice was true.

Fertile Facts

While history is filled with food myths, there are a few foods that might boost your chances to conceive.

General Nutrition: There is strong evidence that reversing the effects of general malnutrition will improve conception rates. Anytime a woman follows a strict diet that severely limits calories or anytime she experiences severe weight loss (below 10 percent of desirable body weight), she is likely to experience a disruption in ovulation. Men undergoing strict dieting also are likely to show reduced sperm formation, possibly because of reduced blood flow to the sex organs. Usually, restoring a healthful eating pattern helps normalize reproductive function. This is especially true for people with serious eating disorders (such as bulimia and anorexia), women who engage in frequent strenuous exercise that has resulted in amenorrhea (cessation of the menstrual cycle), or even in women eating nutritionally unbalanced vegetarian diets. On the other hand, overnutrition, in the form of obesity, also affects the menstrual cycle and can interfere with ovulation and fertility, while gradual weight loss improves an overweight woman's chances of conception. In short, too few or too many calories or too much body fat interferes with a woman's ability to conceive.

Magnesium: Men who suffer from premature ejaculation might consider boosting their intake of magnesium. According to a study from Kuwait University in Safat, men who ejaculate prematurely also have lower seminal plasma magnesium levels compared to other men. The researchers speculate that marginal magnesium status results in constriction of the blood vessels in the penis and altered levels of hormone-like compounds called prostaglandins, which could lead to premature emission and ejaculation processes. Since magnesium also affects sperm transport, it is wise to tell your man to boost his intake of magnesium-rich whole grains, dark green leafy vegetables, beans, and nuts.

Zinc: The belief that oysters increase fertility might have some scientific basis. Oysters are the richest dietary source of zinc, supplying as much as 13 mg of zinc per oyster (the Recommended Dietary Allowance for adults is 12 mg to 15 mg). Even short-term inadequate intake of this trace mineral reduces fertility in men, including reduced semen volume, blood testosterone (the male sex hormone) levels, and zinc concentrations in semen. Zinc also plays a role in ovulation and fertilization in women. However, this research should be viewed in perspective. While attaining and maintaining normal zinc status by consuming 15 mg of zinc each day will help sustain a person's normal sexual function, consuming larger doses will not produce superhuman fertility rates or turn a jalopy-style reproductive system into a hot rod. (See Table 1.3.)

Vitamin D and Selenium: Other dietary and lifestyle habits also have been linked to fertility. Researchers at the University of Wisconsin at Madison investigated the effectiveness of vitamin D supplements on reversing male infertility caused by poor diet, and they found that the combined effect of increasing vitamin D and calcium intake (to 400 IU and 1,000 mg, respectively) might improve fertility rates. Both excessive and inadequate intakes of selenium are linked to reduced fertility rates, while consuming several selenium-rich foods, such as seafood, whole grains, and extra-lean meats, enhances conception.

TABLE 1.3

Galvanizing Your Reproductive System

You should consume approximately 15 mg of zinc each day. Here are a few ways to increase your zinc intake.

Food	Amount	Zinc (mg)
Oysters, raw	6 medium	76.70
Amaranth grain	1 cup	6.20
Wheat germ	½ cup	6.15
Ground beef, extra lean	3 ounces	4.44
Baked beans, vegetarian	1 cup	3.55
Cashews	½ cup	3.09
Lentils, cooked	1 cup	2.50
Chicken, dark meat	3 ounces	2.38
Bean burrito	1	2.37
Rice, wild, cooked	1 cup	2.20
Clams, canned	½ cup	2.18
Yogurt, low-fat	1 cup	2.02
Tofu, firm	½ cup	1.98
Spinach, cooked	1 cup	1.37

Vitamins C and E: Antioxidants also might be one of nature's natural fertility pills, at least for smokers, according to a study from the University of Buenos Aires in Argentina. Oxidative damage to DNA in sperm and seminal levels of antioxidants, such as vitamin E and vitamin C, were measured in male smokers and nonsmokers. DNA damage was 50 percent higher and vitamin E levels were 32 percent lower in smokers compared to nonsmokers. Vitamin C also appears to protect sperm from free radical damage, while men who supplement with vitamin E might improve the ability of their sperm to fertilize an egg. Note: Since both smoking and exposure to other people's smoke can decrease fertilization rates, your best bet is to stop smoking and avoid passive smoke before, during, and after pregnancy.

Other Habits: No evidence supports the use of any nutritional supplement to improve libido, sexual function, or fertility in women. Herbs, such as yohimbine, ginkgo biloba, ginseng, and damiana, have not proven effective for boosting sexual function in men. There are a few habits, however, that improve your chances of conceiving:

1. Cut out tobacco, alcohol, and caffeine, since women who limit or avoid caffeine and cigarettes are up to four times more likely to get pregnant than drinkers and smokers.
2. Don't douche, since douching alters the normal acidity of the vagina and can interfere with sperm survival, reducing your chances of conceiving by up to 30 percent.
3. Exercise moderately.
4. Include some daily relaxation (chronic stress interferes with ovulation and fertility).
5. Limit salty foods (men only).
6. Limit medications to only those prescribed by a physician.
7. Don't use street drugs. Even moderate use of street drugs can affect fertility and could have lifelong and serious consequences on the developing infant. For example, marijuana use lowers sperm count in men and may affect menstrual cycles and ovulation in women, which are reversed when the drug is discontinued.

These habits might not be as enticing as rhino horn, ginseng, or figs, but will go much further in helping you optimize your chances of conceiving a healthy baby. (See Box 1.2 on page 17 and Box 1.3 on page 23.)

BOX 1.2 HERBS AND PREGNANCY

Which herbs benefit fertility, conception, or pregnancy? Which herbs should you avoid? Good questions! The research is scanty at best, and in most cases completely lacking when it comes to both safety and effectiveness of herbs during pregnancy. In all cases, consider this area a buyer-beware market.

Black cohosh: This herb is supposed to stimulate normal functioning of the uterus and ovaries, help with labor, and reduce backaches during pregnancy but can cause headaches and blood vessel dilation. Avoid or use with caution during pregnancy.

Dandelion root: This root is a liver tonic and might increase bile flow, aid in digestion, and decrease water retention. Also useful in helping prevent anemia.

Ephedra, guarana, and kola nut: All of these are stimulants and should be avoided prior to and during pregnancy.

Ginger: Fresh ginger shows promise in helping to curb nausea in pregnant women.

Goldenseal, barberry, and celandine: These herbs have been used as antifertility agents and might have a mild stimulating effect on the uterus. They should be avoided during pregnancy.

Licorice: Contrary to popular belief, licorice does not cause a drop in the male hormone testosterone, nor does it decrease libido in men.

Pennyroyal: The oil of pennyroyal is toxic, but small doses of pennyroyal tea or tincture probably are not harmful.

Red raspberry leaf: Makes a tonic for the uterus, increasing tone in a lax uterus and relaxing a uterus that is taut and irritable.

Rose hips: A safe and excellent source of vitamin C.

Siberian ginseng: Some ginseng contains steroidlike compounds and should be avoided during pregnancy.

Spearmint and peppermint: Add flavor and aid in digestion.

Stinging nettle: The leaves and stems of this plant might be useful in the prevention of preeclampsia (see Chapter 6).

Saint-John's-wort: Extracts from this herb are said to enhance uterine tone in animals. Although research is limited on side effects, it is probably wise to avoid this herb during the first trimester or if you have a history of preterm labor, and to use whole plant extracts not standardized extracts.

Wild yam: Calms spasming muscles. Contrary to popular belief, this herb has no hormonal activity.

Just Say No to Caffeine, Tobacco, Alcohol, and Drugs

Gearing up for pregnancy is a great opportunity to "clean up your act" when it comes to health-damaging habits. Many medications, all street drugs, and even everyday substances, such as tobacco, alcohol, and caffeine in cola or coffee, could have far-reaching effects on your unborn baby.

Coffee, Tea, or Baby?

On average, American women guzzle more than thirty gallons of caffeinated beverages each year. While caffeine is found in tea, many soft drinks, cocoa, chocolate, some prescription and over-the-counter (OTC) drugs, and diuretics, the most concentrated source is coffee.

Starting in the late 1970s, concern was raised as to whether it was safe to consume coffee during pregnancy. Numerous studies on animals showed that even moderate amounts of caffeine caused birth defects, preterm delivery, reduced fertility, increased the risk for low-birth-weight offspring, and caused other reproductive problems. More recent studies show that caffeine has different effects on people.

How Much Can You Safely Drink? Caffeinated beverages don't appear to cause birth defects or preterm labor or delivery in people, but they might increase the risk for other pregnancy mishaps. Brenda Eskenazi, Ph.D., associate professor of Maternal and Child Health in the School of Public Health at the University of California, Berkeley, says, "The most consistent findings, if any, are with fetal growth retardation, miscarriage, and low birth weight. Women who consume more than 300 mg of caffeine daily are at highest risk." That's the equivalent of three five-ounce cups of coffee. It also appears that pregnant women who smoke and drink coffee have an even greater risk for giving birth to a baby with stunted growth; however, smoking is by far the greater sin.

Another concern is that although women avoid coffee while they are nauseated in their first trimester, they often switch to diet colas, which also are a source of caffeine, or return to coffee in the last trimester when infant growth is at its peak, says Dr. Eskenazi. Caffeine consumption (in amounts greater than 200 mg per day) in the later stages of pregnancy affects the unborn directly, including a disruption in normal sleep and activity patterns. Although a safe dose of caffeine has not been established, your best bet is to avoid all caffeinated beverages prior to and during the first trimester of pregnancy, and then, if you do drink caffeinated beverages in the second and third trimester, do so in moderation.

TABLE 1.4

Caffeine Counts

To be safe, you should avoid caffeine prior to and during the first trimester of pregnancy. Although no limit has been set, it is best to limit caffeine in the second six months of pregnancy to no more than 200 mg a day, from all sources.

Item	Caffeine (mg)
Coffee (5-oz. cup)*	
Brewed, drip method	60–180
Instant	30–120
Espresso	51–130
Irish cream coffee mix, 6 oz.	53
Cappuccino, latte, café mocha, 8 oz.	50–70
Decaffeinated	1–5
Tea (5-oz. cup—steeped 4 minutes)*	
Brewed	38–77
Instant	25–50
Iced (12-oz. glass)	67–76
Cocoa beverage (5-oz. cup)	2–20
Chocolate milk (8 oz.)	2–7
Dark chocolate, semisweet (1 oz.)	5–35
Baker's chocolate (1 oz.)	25
Milk chocolate, chocolate syrup (1 oz.)	4–6
Chocolate pudding (½ cup), mousse pie (⅛ pie)	2–6
Soft drinks, colas (12-oz. serving)	
Jolt	72
Java Johnny Water	70
Sugar-Free Mr. Pibb	59
Mountain Dew	54
Cola soft drinks	36–47
Nonprescription drugs	
Dexatrim/Dex-a-Diet Plus/Dietac	200
Vivarin	200
Prolamine	140
Aqua-Ban diuretic	100
NoDoz/Appedrine	100
Excedrin	65
Anacin, Midol, Vanquish, Dristan	30–33
Prescription drugs	
Cafergot (migraine headaches)	100
Norgesic Forte (muscle relaxant)	60
Fiorinal (tension headache)	40
Darvon or Soma compound/Synalgos-DC (pain relief)	30–32

*Caffeine content will vary depending on the strength of the brew.

Don't Smoke, Don't Spend Time with Smokers

Tobacco and pregnancy don't mix. Cigarette smoke contains thousands of chemicals, many of which are toxic, including nicotine, cadmium, carbon dioxide, aromatic hydrocarbons, and vinyl chloride. Many pollutants found in cigarette smoke migrate into seminal fluids, are carried by the sperm cells when they fertilize the ovum, and continue to bombard the developing baby when the mother smokes or is exposed to tobacco smoke.

Women who smoke have smaller babies who are more likely to die soon after birth compared to women who avoid tobacco. Prepregnancy smoking doubles your risk of having a growth-retarded infant, possibly because tobacco use results in calcification of the placenta, which would severely restrict blood and nutrient flow to the baby. The carbon monoxide in tobacco smoke also constricts blood vessels to the placenta and interferes with the oxygenation of the blood. Since the baby depends on the placenta to supply a constant supply of oxygen and nutrients, every time a woman puffs on a cigarette or inhales other people's smoke she is suffocating her baby.

Women who smoke are more likely than nonsmokers to experience complications, such as preeclampsia during pregnancy, preterm labor, premature rupture of membranes, and premature delivery. Even exposure to other people's smoke, called passive smoking, can increase your risk for having a low-birth-weight baby. Men who smoke have a considerably higher risk of having children with birth defects and childhood cancer, possibly as a result of smoking's effect on lowering vitamin C levels in seminal fluids and sperm. The best nutrition in the world can't make up for the damage done by smoking or passive smoking!

The damages to the growing baby persist into later life. Children born to mothers or fathers who smoked during the pregnancy are at increased risk for developing cancer. They are more susceptible to middle-ear infections, asthma, chronic bronchitis, and wheezing; score lower on intelligence tests later in life; and are more likely to develop hypertension, as well as neurological and behavioral problems such as attention deficit disorder compared to children born in a smoke-free environment.

Finally, women who smoke are twelve times more likely to die prematurely from lung cancer and three times more likely to die from strokes than are nonsmokers. Therefore, they are much less likely to live to see their children grow up or be there when their grandchildren are born.

Is There a Safe Dose for Tobacco? No. Don't smoke if you are trying to conceive and avoid all tobacco smoke prior to, during, and following pregnancy. For the future health of your child, keep your home smoke-free. Husbands, partners, and family members who can't quit should at least cut back to less than ten cigarettes a day, smoke outdoors where the air will help dilute the sidestream smoke, and avoid exposing children to smoke.

Don't Drink Alcohol

Alcohol and pregnancy don't mix. Alcohol freely crosses the placenta, directly exposing the developing baby to its toxic effects. The alcohol travels in the baby's bloodstream in the same concentration as that of the mother; if you drink enough to feel "tipsy," your baby is tipsy, too. However, the baby's immature nervous system, liver, and kidneys are not prepared to detoxify alcohol as quickly or efficiently as an adult body. Consequently, alcohol lingers in the unborn's body much longer than in the mother's body.

Alcohol can have a devastating and irreversible effect on your baby. Many babies born to women who drank alcohol during their pregnancy have a condition called "fetal alcohol syndrome" or FAS. They are shorter and lighter in weight than other babies, and they don't catch up even with special postnatal care. They have abnormally small heads, facial irregularities, joint and limb abnormalities, heart defects, and poor coordination. Many are mentally retarded and may develop behavior problems as they grow up, including hyperactivity, extreme nervousness, and poor attention spans. Some babies develop all of these physical and emotional problems, others develop varying degrees of some of these problems, still others show no signs until irreversible behavioral and learning disabilities surface when the child enters school.

Numerous marginal nutrient deficiencies that result from alcohol intake compound the risk for birth defects, including vitamin A, the B vitamins, vitamin C, vitamin D, vitamin E, calcium, magnesium, copper, iodine, manganese, and zinc. Alcohol consumption also increases your risk for miscarriage, stillbirth, and death in early infancy; heavy drinkers are two to four times more likely to have a miscarriage than are women who don't drink.

The strongest relationship between the mother's alcohol consumption and FAS seems to exist between the month prior to conception and the first missed menstrual period or pregnancy test, although alcohol can exert its effects anytime during pregnancy. The risk of birth defects increases with even two ounces of alcohol, or the equivalent of two drinks. You also can't "save up" by abstaining all week then downing six drinks on Saturday night; even a single high dose during one night or weekend of heavy drinking could be all it takes to change the course of your baby's life.

How Much Alcohol Is Safe? No one knows exactly how much alcohol it takes to damage your baby. Since alcohol causes permanent physical and mental birth defects and no safe amount has been found, your best bet is to abstain from all alcoholic beverages prior to and during pregnancy. Be aware of the alcohol content of foods and drugs you might not suspect; for example, Irish coffee, wine coolers, rum and fruit cakes, liquor-laced desserts, and cough medicines contain alcohol.

Drugs: Illicit, Prescription, and Over-the-Counter

Doctors used to think that the placenta formed an impenetrable barrier, protecting the developing baby from any harmful substances. Today, we know this is not true. Although the placenta is amazing, it is not flawless. Most drugs, chemicals, and other substances can cross it so that the baby is an unprotected recipient. While most people are well aware of the harm "hard" drugs, such as heroin, can have on maternal and infant health, some people are more lax when it comes to other street drugs, such as marijuana or cocaine, or commonly used over-the-counter or prescription medications.

Along with reduced fertility in women who use drugs, babies born to drug users are at higher risk for sudden infant death syndrome (SIDS), the third leading cause of infant mortality. Women who use drugs are more likely to deliver prematurely, and to give birth to a baby with a small head circumference, decreased birth weight, and reduced mental and motor development. Children who were born to mothers who used marijuana during pregnancy show learning deficits and short attention spans later in life.

The Bottom Line on Drugs: The recommendations for taking any type of street drug prior to and during pregnancy is as simple as "don't, not even a little."

Fortunately, most women have a healthy skepticism about taking over-the-counter (OTC) or prescription medications. On the other hand, people are accustomed to popping a pill at the first sign of an ache, pain,

---

BOX 1.3 MEDICATIONS AND YOUR BABY

Always consult your physician before taking any medication, even aspirin, while attempting to conceive. For example,

- The female hormones estrogen and progestin taken during the first few weeks of pregnancy can increase the risk for birth defects, including limb and heart defects, and increase the likelihood that a baby girl will develop cervical cancer later in life. Women who discontinue taking the birth control pill, which contains these hormones, should wait at least three months before attempting to conceive and should use another form of birth control in the meantime.
- Avoid drugs that interfere with folic acid—including trimethoprim, triamterene, phenytoin, phenobarbital, and primidone. These drugs increase the risk for neural tube defects, defects of the heart and urinary tract, and cleft palate.
- Tetracycline-like antibiotics taken during pregnancy cause permanent discoloration of the child's teeth, while erythromycin might cause liver damage and streptomycin can cause nerve deafness.
- Tranquilizers, such as Librium, Miltown, and Valium, taken by the mother during pregnancy might increase the risk that her baby will be born with a cleft lip or palate.
- Isotretinoin (Accutane), a vitamin A analog used to treat cystic acne, also causes birth defects, including mental retardation and facial deformities.
- Aspirin and many other pain relievers contain a compound called salicylate that might prolong pregnancy and labor and may cause excessive bleeding before and after delivery.

---

cold, or cough under the assumption that if it is readily available without a prescription, it must be safe to take during pregnancy. While some of these medications are safe, others aren't and almost all medications— OTC or prescription—come with risks as well as benefits. Even more important is that many of the potential physical defects to the unborn child caused by drugs occur within the first few weeks before you know you are pregnant.

A general rule of thumb: never self-medicate when you are planning to get pregnant or during your pregnancy. Medications that are safe when you are not pregnant can be toxic to your developing baby. On the other hand, many prescription and OTC medications are safe before, during, and following pregnancy. So always confer with your physician before taking any medication, even if it is something as simple as cough syrup or a painkiller.

Get Moving: Exercise and Your Prepregnancy Plan

In the past, pregnancy was the time when a woman was told to slow down and "take it easy." Not anymore, at least when it comes to moderate activity. The key is to start before you are pregnant so that you are physically fit and in shape ahead of time. Pregnancy is not the time to begin a rigorous exercise program, but most physicians agree that a pregnant woman can continue an exercise program begun prior to pregnancy, usually with some modification during the second and third trimesters.

Why Is Exercise Important during Pregnancy? Physical activity improves your sense of well-being. You also are likely to have fewer pregnancy complications, a more timely onset of labor, a shorter labor, less difficulty with labor pain, and fewer obstetric interventions. In addition, babies born to moms who burned 1,000 calories a week through exercise weigh 5 percent more than infants born to inactive women; moms who burn 2,000 calories a week birth babies who are 10 percent heavier than the norm. This increase in weight shouldn't be taken lightly, since researchers say that heavier babies are healthier and better able to fight infection than are smaller babies. Exercise also helps prevent abnormalities in blood sugar regulation that are more frequent during pregnancy, helps you sleep better at night, and assists in controlling excessive weight gain (the more active you are the more calories you can eat without gaining too much weight).

In general, the guidelines of the American College of Obstetricians and Gynecologists recommend against vigorous exercise during pregnancy for previously sedentary women or for women with prior adverse outcomes or symptoms in the current pregnancy, such as premature labor, a history of miscarriages, bleeding, or ruptured membranes. For women who started exercising prior to conception, the guidelines suggest limiting exercise in terms of activity type, intensity (less than or equal to 140 heartbeats/minute), and duration. A woman should exercise no fewer than three days a week, rather than sporadic or intermittent activity, and she always should warm up and cool down before and after exercise.

These recommendations are conservative and were developed to serve a diverse population, so they might not apply to a physically fit woman who is accustomed to daily intense exercise. (See Chapter 6 for a detailed description of exercise guidelines during pregnancy.) Most important, you should monitor your body temperature response to exercise during early pregnancy (that is, from conception through the first trimester), since limited evidence suggests that an increased body core temperature could adversely affect the developing baby.

As part of this temperature regulation, remember to drink ample amounts of fluids prior to and following exercise. In all cases, consult with your physician, preferably several months before you conceive, to develop a physical activity plan that is safe and will fit into your daily schedule.

The Prepregnancy Diet

Starting now, continuing through your pregnancy, and up until your baby's first birthday, you should follow the guidelines outlined in the Baby-wise Diet in Chapter 2. The guidelines differ from prepregnancy through the trimesters of pregnancy and during the recuperation year following pregnancy only in the minimum number of servings recommended from each of the following six food groupings:

1. Calcium-rich foods
2. Vegetables
3. Fruits
4. Extra-lean meats and legumes
5. Grains
6. Quenchers

Of course, the maximum number of calories, and therefore foods, you consume is based on your height and desirable body weight, your activity level, and your individual metabolism. In all cases, when you must cut back on servings to maintain your weight, cut fat and sugar before you reduce the number of servings of the more nutritious foods recommended. Here's the what, how much, and whys of your prepregnancy diet.

Calcium-Rich Foods

How Much? Two servings or more (1 serving = 1 cup nonfat milk, nonfat yogurt, or fortified soy milk; 1 ounce low-fat cheese; 2 cups nonfat cottage cheese).

Why? These foods provide:

- calcium and vitamin D (milk and fortified soy milk only) to build strong bones. Calcium prevents lead mobilization from bone tissue, thus reducing exposure to this toxic metal.
- vitamin B_{12} and vitamin B_6 to aid in nerve development.
- protein for the formation of muscles, hormones, enzymes, and nerve chemicals.
- no saturated fat. One study from Harvard Medical School in Boston found that women who consumed diets high in saturated fats from dairy foods and meat during the months before they conceived were more likely to suffer severe morning sickness during their pregnancies compared to women who ate lower-fat diets.

Fruits and Vegetables

How Much? At least 5, preferably 9, servings. At least two of these should be from the selections marked with an * in the "Fantastic Vegetables" list on page 34; these are folic acid–rich selections. Two selections should be from the selections marked with an * in the "Fabulous Fruits" list on pages 34–35; these are vitamin C–rich selections. Fried potatoes and iceberg lettuce don't count. (1 serving = 1 piece, ½ cup cooked or canned, 1 cup raw, 6 ounces juice.)

Why? These foods provide:

- the antioxidant nutrients, such as vitamin C and beta carotene, which protect your and your baby's tissues from damage from highly reactive oxygen fragments called free radicals; help form connective tissue, the most abundant tissue in the body and the "glue" that holds all other tissues together (vitamin C); aid in normal cell division and in the formation of skin and all the linings in the body, from the lungs and bladder to the blood vessels (beta carotene).
- folic acid, the B vitamin that prevents neural tube defects in the early stages of pregnancy and preterm deliveries in the last trimester.

Quiz 1.1 My Diet: What Needs Improvement?

Pondering pregnancy or already there? Here's a quick assessment of how you are doing. Any questions answered no are areas that need improvement.

_____ 1. I am within 10 percent of my desirable body weight.

_____ 2. I consume at least 2,000 calories a day of nutritious foods, and take a moderate-dose vitamin and mineral supplement that includes at least 400 mcg of folic acid and at least 18 mg of iron.

_____ 3. I consume at least eight servings daily of fresh fruits and vegetables. At least two servings are vitamin C–rich selections, such as citrus fruit, and two servings are dark green leafy vegetables.

_____ 4. I consume at least six servings daily of grains, and at least four are 100 percent whole grain breads and cereals.

_____ 5. I consume two servings daily of extra-lean meat (i.e., 7 percent fat calories or less by weight), poultry without the skin, seafood, or cooked dried beans and peas. At least one serving is beans or seafood. (If you are a vegetarian, you should consume daily at least four 1-cup servings of cooked dried beans and peas.)

_____ 6. I consume two or more servings each day of calcium-rich foods, such as low-fat or nonfat milk and milk products, fortified soy milk or orange juice, dark green leafy vegetables (i.e., kale, chard, spinach, or romaine lettuce), or other alternative sources of calcium.

_____ 7. I am fat conscious and usually bake, steam, broil, poach, or grill food, rather than fry, saute, or use sauces and gravies that contain fat; avoid ordering fatty foods in restaurants; and purchase mostly low-fat foods.

_____ 8. I include fish or another source of omega-3 fatty acids in my weekly diet.

_____ 9. I drink at least five glasses of water and other nutritious fluids each day.

_____10. I limit intake of salty foods and avoid using salt in food preparation or at the table.

_____11. I limit my intake of processed foods and sweets.

_____12. I avoid alcoholic beverages.

_____13. I limit coffee, caffeinated soft drinks, and other caffeine-containing beverages to 1 serving or less a day, and I do not take caffeine-containing medications.

_____14. I've had my iron levels checked and am taking extra iron when my serum ferritin levels are below 20 mcg/L.

_____15. I exercise at least three days a week for a half hour or more.

_____16. I don't smoke and I avoid breathing other people's smoke.

_____17. I have a strong, supportive group of friends and/or family members.

_____18. I take time every week to relax and enjoy life.

_____19. I've checked with my physician on the safety during pregnancy of all my medications, including over-the-counter ones.

Extra-Lean Meats and Legumes

How Much? Two servings from "Extra-Lean Meats and Legumes" on page 35. At least one serving of fish or legumes. (1 serving = 1 cup beans, 8 ounces tofu, 3 ounces chicken, fish, meat.)

Why? These foods provide:

- protein for the formation of hormones, enzymes, and nerve chemicals.
- vitamin B_6, a nutrient essential in the development of your baby's nervous system, formation of all tissues, and protein metabolism.
- vitamin B_{12} for red blood cell formation (beans and tofu are not good sources of this vitamin).
- iron for red blood cell formation.

Grains

How Much? Six servings or more. At least four of these should be whole grains from the selections marked with an * in the "Great Grains" list on pages 35–36; these are trace mineral–rich selections. (1 serving = 1 slice of bread; ½ cup cooked pasta, rice, or cereal; 1 ounce ready-to-eat cereal.)

Why? These foods provide:

- fiber to keep you regular.
- carbohydrates to fuel the billions of daily cell divisions and metabolic processes that will make a baby.
- B vitamins, which help convert calories into energy and promote normal growth and development.
- magnesium, which is essential for relaxation of the uterine muscular lining, building bones, and regulating nerves.
- trace minerals, such as copper, help prevent birth defects, aid in the formation of connective tissue, and are essential for the development and maintenance of a baby's heart, arteries, and blood vessels; the skeletal system; and the nervous system.

Quenchers

How Much? Five servings or more from the Quenchers (beverages) group on page 36.

Why? "Getting enough nourishing fluids, like water, fruit juices, or milk, is so important throughout pregnancy to provide for the expanding blood volume that carries oxygen and nutrients to both the mother's tissues and to the developing baby," says Dr. Murtaugh. You lose two to three quarts of water every day, through perspiration and urination. To restock this loss, place a water bottle at your desk and fill it up several times during the day. When home, fill eight glasses with water and place them in sight so you know when you've met your goal.

To make your own diet checklist, see Worksheet 1.2, on page 31.

Worksheet 1.1   Gearing Up for Pregnancy: A Sensible Weight-Loss Plan

Unless advised and monitored by a physician, you should lose no more than two pounds a week, with a long-term goal of achieving between 90 and 120 percent of your desirable weight prior to conception. To determine how long it will take you to reach this goal:

1. Identify your target weight and subtract that weight from your current weight to achieve the total pounds to be lost.
2. Divide this figure by 2 pounds per week.
3. Starting with this week, count off on the calendar the number of weeks it will take to reach your goal.
4. Use the following worksheet to track your success.

Current weight: _____   Target weight: _____
Pounds to lose: _____   Weeks needed (@2 pounds/week): _____

Once a week, fill in your weight in the lefthand column of the chart, beginning with your starting weight. Mark the appropriate box to the right and connect the marks to create a graph. (Each square represents two pounds.) See the filled-in chart on the next page for an example.

WEIGHT	PRE-PROGRAM	WEEK 1	WEEK 2	WEEK 3	WEEK 4	WEEK 5	WEEK 6	WEEK 7	WEEK 8	WEEK 9	WEEK 10	WEEK 11	WEEK 12
STARTING WEIGHT													

WEIGHT	PRE-PROGRAM	WEEK 1	WEEK 2	WEEK 3	WEEK 4	WEEK 5	WEEK 6	WEEK 7	WEEK 8	WEEK 9	WEEK 10	WEEK 11	WEEK 12
165													
163													
161													
159													
157													
155													
153													
151													
149													
147													

STARTING WEIGHT (161)

Worksheet 1.2   My Prepregnancy Daily Checklist

Copy this master sheet to complete daily.

Food Groups	Minimum Servings	Actual Intake
Calcium-rich foods	2	_____
Vegetables (at least 2 folic acid–rich choices)	5	_____
Fruits (at least 2 vitamin C–rich choices)	3	_____
Extra-lean meats and legumes	2	_____
Grains (at least 4 whole-grain choices)	6	_____
Quenchers	5	_____

Did I reach my goals? _____

What needs improvement? _____

What will I do differently next week? _____

Chapter 2

❧

The Baby-wise Diet

This chapter spells out exactly how you should be eating before, during, and following pregnancy. If you do nothing else but follow the guidelines for the Baby-wise Diet in this chapter, you will be well on your way to giving your baby the best start toward a long, happy, and healthy life.

"The general public has been educated on the need to cut the fat and increase high-quality complex carbohydrates, whole grains, legumes, fruits, and vegetables, but the same guidelines are not being emphasized for pregnant women, even though they are just as important," says Janet King, Ph.D., R.D., professor in the Department of Nutritional Sciences at the University of California, Berkeley. "Those simple guidelines alone would improve the mother's overall health during pregnancy and could increase the nutrient supply to the developing baby."

The guidelines are simple and easy to follow. In a nutshell, plan your meals and snacks around fresh fruits and vegetables, grains, and legumes, with ample amounts of calcium-rich and protein-rich foods. The Baby-wise Diet is based on six food groupings:

1. Calcium-rich foods
2. Vegetables
3. Fruits
4. Extra-lean meats and legumes
5. Grains
6. Quenchers

These food groups are outlined in the lists below. On page 36 you'll find additional high-value foods that can be consumed in moderation, and page 38 lists foods to be avoided.

The number of servings from each group varies somewhat depending on your stage of pregnancy—from preparing for pregnancy, through the three trimesters, to restocking your body's nutrient stores after the baby is born. Later chapters in this book provide specific guidelines on how to apply the Baby-wise Diet to each of these specific stages of pregnancy.

You still can eat your favorite foods, enjoy your favorite recipes, and go to your favorite restaurants. You even can eat foods out of a bag or box. Just make sure you first eat the number of nutritious foods in the Baby-wise Diet. When, where, and how much you eat is flexible, and often is governed by necessity. You might choose little meals and snacks throughout the day and a large evening meal during the first trimester if you suffer from morning sickness, but select a larger breakfast and a light evening meal in the last trimester when heartburn is more of a problem.

Calcium-Rich Foods

A cup of milk provides approximately 300 mg of calcium. The following foods supply a similar amount of calcium. A woman should consume 1,000 mg calcium (at least 3 servings of the following calcium-rich foods, plus calcium from other sources), before, during, and after pregnancy. If you are eighteen years old or younger and pregnant, you should consume at least 1,300 mg daily (3 to 4 servings). With so many new calcium-fortified foods and beverages on the market, it's easy to reach your daily quota!

Food	Amount
Milk, nonfat or 1 percent fat	1 cup
Milk, skim evaporated	½ cup
Black-eyed peas, cooked	1½ cups
Bok choy, cooked	2 cups
Broccoli, cooked	3 cups
Low-fat cheese	1½ to 2 ounces
Collard greens, cooked	2 cups
Cottage cheese, low-fat	2 cups
Dandelion greens, cooked	2 cups
Figs, dried	1 cup
Mustard greens, cooked	1½ cups

Orange juice, fortified	1 cup
PowerBar, all flavors	1
Rice Dream Original Enriched drink	1 cup
Soy milk, fortified	1 cup
Spinach, cooked	1¼ cups
Tofu, firm	¾ cup
Turnip greens, cooked	1½ cups
Waffles, Kellogg's Eggo Homestyle frozen	2 waffles
Whole-grain Total cereal	1 cup
Yogurt, low-fat	¾ cup

Fantastic Vegetables

In general, one portion is equal to one cup raw, one whole piece (such as one carrot), or ½ cup cooked. Vegetables marked with an * are also high in folic acid. If you are gearing up for pregnancy or in your first trimester, include at least five portions daily of these foods. During the second two trimesters of pregnancy and during breast-feeding, consume at least six servings daily.

*Asparagus	*Chard	*Peas, green
Bean sprouts	*Collards	*Romaine lettuce
Beans, green	*Dandelion	*Spinach
Beets	greens	Squash, winter
*Broccoli	Eggplant	Succotash
Brussels sprouts	*Kale	Sweet potato
Cabbage	*Mustard greens	Tomato
Carrots	Okra	*Turnip greens
Cauliflower	Pea pods	Zucchini

Fabulous Fruits

In general, one portion is equal to one piece (as in an apple or an orange), ½ cup cubed or sauced, or 1 cup whole (as in strawberries or cherries). The fruits marked with an * are especially high in vitamin C. If you are gearing up for pregnancy or in your first trimester, include at least three portions daily of these foods. During the second two trimesters of pregnancy and during breast-feeding, consume at least four servings daily.

Apple	Berries:	*Cantaloupe
Applesauce	Blackberries	Casaba melon
Apricots	Blueberries	Cherries
Banana	*Strawberries	Fruit cocktail

*Grapefruit	*Mango	Pineapple
Grapes	Nectarine	Plum
*Kiwi	*Orange	Prunes
*Honeydew melon	*Papaya	*Tangerine
*Mandarin	Peach	Watermelon
oranges	Pear	

Extra-Lean Meats and Legumes
In general, a portion is three ounces of cooked extra-lean meat, skinless poultry, fish, or one cup cooked dried beans and peas.

Cooked dried beans and peas, such as kidney, black, garbanzo, great northern white, or lima beans; lentils; split or chickpeas; soybeans or tofu
Beef, such as chipped beef, flank steak, London broil, round steak, stew meat, or ground round marked as 7 percent fat by weight
Pork, such as boiled ham, Canadian bacon (high in salt), and tenderloin
Poultry, preferably breast meat, which is lowest in saturated fat
Seafood (see page 42 for best selections)
Veal, such as chop, steak, or roast
Luncheon meat (95 percent fat-free)
Egg (limit to no more than 5 per week)
Egg substitute

Great Grains
In general, one portion is equal to one slice of bread; ½ bagel, English muffin, or pita bread; ½ cup cooked pasta, rice, or cereal; or 1 ounce of ready-to-eat cereal. Foods marked with an * are especially high in trace minerals. If you are gearing up for pregnancy or in your first trimester, include at least six portions daily of these foods, with at least four servings being whole grains. During the second two trimesters of pregnancy and during breast-feeding, consume at least seven servings daily, with at least five of those being whole grain.

*Bagel, whole wheat	Bread, white, French, or sourdough
Bagel, egg, raisin, or plain	*Cereal, cooked, i.e., oatmeal,
*Bread, whole wheat	barley, farina

Corn bread
Crackers, i.e., Ry-Krisp, SnackWell's,
    low-salt whole-wheat saltines
English muffin, whole grain
Hamburger bun, made with
    whole wheat
Hot dog bun, made with whole
    wheat
*Noodles or pasta, whole wheat or
    regular
Pancake, made from low-fat
    mix or homemade

*Pita bread, whole wheat
Popcorn, plain, air-popped
Pretzels
*Rice, brown
Rice, white
Rice cakes
Tortilla, corn, whole wheat, or
    low-fat flour
Waffle, made with whole
    wheat
*Wheat germ

Quenchers

In general, a portion is one 8-ounce glass. Drinks marked with an * are especially high in vitamin C; drinks marked with a † are especially high in beta carotene. Gearing up for pregnancy and during the first trimester, you should include at least five glasses daily of these fluids; more if you exercise. Fruit or vegetable juices can double as servings of fruits or vegetables. During the second two trimesters of pregnancy, drink at least six glasses and during breast-feeding, drink no less than eight glasses of fluid daily.

Water
Sparkling water
Juices:
Apple cider
Apple juice
†Apricot nectar
†Carrot juice
*Grapefruit
Grape
*Orange

*Papaya nectar
†Passion fruit
    juice
Peach nectar
Pear nectar
Pineapple juice
Prune
Tomato juice
V8 juice

Nutritious Additions

The following foods are high in fat or sugar, but also supply a hefty dose of vitamins and minerals. They are OK in moderation.

Avocado
Cake, angel food
Cookies, i.e., vanilla wafers or
    animal crackers

Dried fruit, i.e., dates, figs, and
    raisins
Ice cream, preferably low-fat
    or fat-free varieties

| Nuts, i.e., almonds, cashews, peanuts, pecans, pistachios, or walnuts
 Peanut butter | Pudding
 Seeds, i.e., pumpkin, sesame, or sunflower seeds |

How Often Should I Eat?

How you mix and match these selections is up to you. Keep in mind that vitamins and minerals are best absorbed and a desirable body weight is best maintained when food is divided into little meals and snacks evenly distributed (i.e., every three to five hours during waking hours) throughout the day. Ideally, you should aim for an eating plan that includes three meals and two to three snacks, each snack including at least one fruit or vegetable and one serving from the other food groups, such as grains or calcium-rich foods. The menus in the Appendix are based on this eating style.

However, you are most likely to stick with an eating plan if it fits into your schedule. So, if three square meals is your eating style, then plan them accordingly. As your pregnancy progresses, everything from morning sickness in the first trimester to a bulging tummy in the third trimester may dictate when and how much you eat at any one sitting.

Start the Day Off Right

One rule in the Baby-wise Diet is that you must eat breakfast. At no other time in life is breakfast more important than during pregnancy. Breakfast will help you maintain a more desirable weight and will help prevent fatigue. Women who skip breakfast in an effort to cut calories often do more snacking later in the day and overeat at evening meals. In addition, a woman who skips breakfast might initially feel energized in the morning, but waning blood-sugar levels eventually lead to fatigue. Even if you try to catch up by eating a well-balanced lunch, you never will regain the energy you would have had if you had taken ten minutes to eat a nutritious breakfast. Finally, allowing too much time to lapse between meals can be stressful to your baby during pregnancy, since a constant supply of nutrients and calories is needed for the minute-by-minute growth that is taking place.

Even if you are not particularly hungry, eat at least a small snack in the morning, preferably one that includes some protein and some carbohydrates. Even a toasted whole-grain English muffin with a slice of low-fat cheese and a glass of orange juice, or a small bowl of ready-to-eat whole-grain cereal with fruit and nonfat milk will suffice.

What about Foods Not on the Lists?

The basic foods in the Baby-wise Diet are low in fat, salt, and sugar. If you follow this meal plan, you automatically will consume about 2,000 calories with 25 to 30 percent of those calories coming from fat and very little or none coming from refined sugars. This meal plan also provides about 25 to 35 grams of fiber. If you exercise daily and/or can maintain a desirable weight on more calories, then feel free to include other foods, such as foods listed as "Nutritious Additions" on pages 36–37.

There is nothing wrong with a few high-fat or high-sugar foods as long as they don't replace more nutritious foods. Problems arise when potato chips, greasy fast foods, fried foods, cookies, salad dressings, cakes, pies, and other sweet-and-creamy foods are chosen instead of fruits, vegetables, and whole grains. If you're drinking soda pop instead of milk, you and your baby might suffer during and following pregnancy for lack of calcium. If you snack on ice cream instead of blueberries, you might gain more weight than you bargained for. If you munch on potato chips instead of baby carrots, you're likely to pack in too many calories and too much fat and salt. (Salt will be discussed in more detail in Chapter 6.) Vegetable oils used in food preparation or in salad dressings, convenience snack foods such as chips or granola bars, or desserts can be included in your meal plan, but ideally only after you have met the recommended number of servings from each of the six food groups in the Baby-wise Diet.

Now I Can Eat All I Want, Right?

Not quite. It takes about 55,000 extra calories to make a healthy baby. That might seem like a lot, but it's only 300 extra calories a day (the equivalent of a glass of low-fat milk, a slice of bread, and an apple), and that's only in the last two trimesters. Calorie needs don't budge an inch in the first trimester when your baby grows no longer than a green bean. However, your vitamin and mineral needs skyrocket. You need more than twice as much vitamin A, folic acid, and iron; up to 50 percent more vitamin B_1 and calcium; and lots more of most other nutrients. That means:

BOX 2.1   THE NO-NO LIST FOR PREGNANCY

The following foods supply few nutrients; are very high in fat, sugar, or salt; or contain harmful substances. They should be avoided or consumed in very small amounts.

Alcohol, including hard liquor, wine, and beer
Caffeinated beverages, such as coffee, colas, or tea
Candy
Candied fruit, including maraschino cherries
Cereals sweetened with sugar
Cookies, cakes, pies, brownies, or commercial sweetened pie fillings
Doughnuts
Fruit drinks made with sugar, concentrated pear, or high-fructose corn syrup (HFCS)
Luncheon meats that are less than 95 percent fat-free
Nondairy creamers
Olives
Potato chips, corn chips, and other commercial snack foods high in fat and salt
Relishes and pickles
Soda pop
Soups, commercial dry or canned varieties that are not "low sodium"
Sour cream (unless it is fat-free)
Sugar, corn syrup, honey, or fructose
Sundae toppings
Whipping cream or commercial whipped toppings

1. a lot more fruits, vegetables, whole grains, legumes, and nonfat milk, and
2. little room for extra chocolate cake, Ding Dongs, Cheez Whiz, and chips.

Your best bet is to consume foods that are as close to their natural, wholesome forms as possible. That is, choose minimally processed whole grains, such as whole wheat or brown rice, more often than highly refined grains, such as white bread or rice. Opt for low-fat or nonfat milk instead of ice cream, and fresh fruit instead of fruits canned in heavy syrup. Choose oatmeal over granola bars, steamed broccoli over broccoli with cheese sauce, blueberries over blueberry muffins. . . . You get the picture. Just as you wouldn't dream of feeding your newborn a diet of hot dogs, cola, and French fries, remember to give your unborn the same consideration.

That doesn't mean you can't enjoy your favorite foods, just make sure nutritious foods far outnumber fatty, sugary, or salty items. You still can eat pizza on occasion; just say no to the fatty salami and sausage and complement it with a large spinach salad and a glass of nonfat milk. (For a list of foods to avoid, see "The No-No List for Pregnancy" on page 39.)

Unconscious Eating

Unplanned eating is likely to get you into trouble. You find yourself nibbling from the refrigerator when you return home from work, grab a candy bar at a vending machine or a cinnamon roll while shopping, or order your turkey sandwich without specifying you want it on whole-wheat bread. While these eating habits have only minor effects on your overall health at other times of life, they are indiscretions you can't afford to tolerate before, during, and following pregnancy. So, think before you eat and make every bite count. Plan ahead so you won't be caught hungry with only the vending machine to curb your appetite.

Think before you DON'T eat, too. Your nutrient needs are at an all-time high and your baby will need a constant supply of calories, fluids, and nutrients. You can't afford to skip meals now. Eat regularly, or approximately every four hours.

Protein: A Little More Is More Than Enough

Once you're pregnant, you'll need more protein than at any other time in your life. The extra servings of nonfat or low-fat milk and extra-lean protein-rich foods recommended in the Baby-wise Diet will more than accommodate any increases in protein needs. There is no reason to use protein powders or tablets. Women following a strict vegetarian diet that includes no foods of animal origin must be particularly careful to include ample amounts of protein-rich legumes, nuts, and soy products.

Carbs Count More Than Ever

Starches and other complex carbohydrates remain the mainstay of the diet, just as they did prior to pregnancy, especially if they are high-quality whole grains and starchy vegetables. Now they also serve an added bonus by helping to fend off morning sickness. In addition, carbohydrate loading, the same dietary practice used by athletes prior to a marathon, might increase tissue glycogen stores and help supply extra energy for labor and delivery.

Fat: Not Too Much

Fat adds calories without much nutritional clout and should be limited in the pregnant woman's diet to no more than 25 to 30 percent of total calories. The main culprit here is saturated fats in meat and dairy foods, while some fats in vegetable oils and fish are healthy additions to the pregnancy menu. If you use oil in cooking or in salad dressing, choose safflower oil, preferably the cold-pressed versions, which contain more vitamin E than the bleached and other highly processed oils, or choose canola or olive oils, which contain heart-healthy monounsaturated fats. Also, include at least two to three servings of fish during the week.

What about Fish?

Fish is a healthful alternative to red meat and supplies hefty amounts of the type of oils needed for the development of vision and the nervous system. However, some seafood is safer than others.

The biggest concerns about eating fish during pregnancy are bacterial food poisoning and chemical contaminants in fish that come from polluted waters. Although purchasing fresh fish and proper handling and cooking will reduce or kill bacteria, you have less control over chemical contaminants. Some environmental residues, such as PCBs and PBBs, have leached into the water supply and accumulate in some freshwater fish. PCBs and related contaminants have been associated with a reduced birth weight, neonatal behavioral problems, and poorer recognition and memory in infants. The toxic metal mercury also accumulates in some fish and is known to cause nerve damage.

According to a *Consumer Reports* study, up to 30 percent of sampled fish is of poor quality; half the fish analyzed was contaminated by bacteria, and some samples were contaminated with PCBs and mercury. Although the sample size in this study was small and might not be representative of the total supply of edible fish, it does provide food for thought and sheds doubt on the safety of some fish for pregnant women.

What Can You Do? A general guideline is to choose low-fat fish, since most contaminants are stored in fatty tissue. The fish most likely to be contaminated with harmful pesticides or metals are those from freshwater sources. Marine fish—with the exception of tuna, shark, mackerel, tilefish, and swordfish, and inshore species such as bluefish and striped bass—are relatively safe. However, a recent report from the Environmental Working Group warned the FDA that other fish should be avoided during pregnancy because of mercury contamination, including Gulf Coast oysters, sea bass, halibut, marlin, pike, and white croaker. Your safest bets in order of safety from least likely to most likely to be contaminated, are:

Freshwater:	*Near shore:*	*Offshore:*
Yellow perch	Pink salmon	Cod
White perch	Chum salmon	Haddock
Brook trout	Sockeye salmon	Pollack
Rainbow trout		

Vitamins and Minerals: How Much of What and Why?

It takes a wide variety of unprocessed foods consumed daily to ensure optimal intake of all the vitamins, minerals, fiber, phytochemicals, protein, and more needed to build a perfect baby.

- The fruits and vegetables in the Baby-wise Diet supply beta carotene, vitamin C, and folic acid. Some also provide iron, calcium, and other minerals. All fruits and vegetables are excellent sources of health-enhancing phytochemicals. All of these nutrients are essential for your baby and your pregnancy, although folic acid has received particular attention because of its ability to help prevent birth defects. (See Chapters 1 and 3 for more on folic acid.)
- The whole-grain breads and cereals in the Baby-wise Diet contribute trace minerals, such as chromium, iron, and selenium, and B vitamins. They also provide fiber to help prevent constipation, hemorrhoids, and other inconveniences of pregnancy.
- The nonfat and low-fat milk products supply protein, calcium, vitamin B_{12}, vitamin B_2, and magnesium, nutrients essential for normal bone, muscle, and nerve development and function. Milk also is an excellent source of vitamin D.
- The two to three servings of extra-lean meat and legumes provide protein, iron, magnesium, zinc, vitamin B_6, vitamin B_{12}, and other B vitamins.

Avoiding any of these foods could result in nutrient deficiencies that would have far-reaching effects on the developing infant and your pregnancy. For example, low calcium intake increases the risk for elevated blood pressure in both the mother and the newborn, while calcium intake of 1,000 mg or more each day lowers blood pressure and reduces the risk of eclampsia in pregnant women. A vitamin B_6 deficiency is linked to reduced Apgar scores, increased irritability, and reduced mother-infant bonding. (The Apgar score reflects a baby's condition sixty minutes after delivery, based on heart rate, respiratory effort, muscle tone, reflexes, and color.) Marginal zinc intake increases the risk for pregnancy complications and premature delivery.

TABLE 2.1

Super Foods for Pregnancy

While any natural food is a healthy inclusion in your diet, some offer an extra nutritional punch. Here are ten of Mother Nature's finest foods.

1. *Spinach:* One cup of cooked spinach supplies only 41 calories, yet boosts your zinc intake by almost 2 mg. It also comes packaged with a hefty dose of calcium, magnesium, iron, and folic acid.
2. *Kidney beans:* One cup, sprinkled onto a salad, added to vegetable soup, mixed with couscous to make a meal, or rolled into a tortilla with cheese and salsa supplies almost one-third of a pregnant woman's daily need for iron, and lots of protein, potassium, folic acid, and vitamin B_1, all for only 219 calories and no fat!
3. *Strawberries:* A woman gearing up for pregnancy or in her first trimester who consumes only 2,000 to 2,200 calories each day must get approximately 1 mg of iron for every 100 calories to ensure optimal iron intake. Strawberries are one fruit that exceeds this limit, supplying 1.23 mg per 100-calorie serving (about 2 cups of fresh strawberries), along with lots of fiber and vitamin C.
4. *Tofu:* This bean curd made from soybeans may be the closest thing to the perfect food. A ½-cup serving of firm tofu supplies more than 13 mg of iron! It also is a low-fat, low-sodium, low-cost source of protein, B vitamins, calcium, magnesium, and zinc.
5. *Wheat germ:* A ½-cup serving of toasted wheat germ supplies more than half of your daily magnesium needs, as well as husky amounts of vitamins (including 100 percent of your daily need for folic acid and 50 percent of your vitamin E requirement), iron (2.58 mg), zinc (more than 4 mg), and other trace minerals.
6. *Broccoli:* This cruciferous vegetable is high in folic acid, vitamin C, beta carotene, iron, magnesium, calcium, vitamin B_2, and just about every other vitamin and mineral. It also comes with a phytochemical mixture that lowers your risk for cancer, heart disease, and other diseases.

TABLE 2.1 continued

7. *Papaya:* This tropical fruit supplies more than twice your day's need for vitamin C, more than your daily allotment for vitamin A (as beta carotene, the nontoxic form of this vitamin), and hefty amounts of magnesium, calcium, and potassium, all for only 117 calories!
8. *Salmon:* One of the best dietary sources of the omega-3 fats that aid in normal development of vision and brain function in your developing baby.
9. *Nonfat milk:* You'll be hard-pressed to meet your calcium and vitamin D needs without this super food.
10. *Water:* The most important food of all. You need at least five to eight glasses daily during pregnancy, even more if you breast-feed.

Since marginal vitamin and mineral intakes are common in women and can have far-reaching effects on the health of your baby even before you know you're pregnant, it is wise to consider taking a moderate-dose vitamin and mineral supplement that contains at least 400 mcg of folic acid and 18 mg of iron. (See Chapters 1, 3, and 5 for more on vitamin and mineral supplements.)

How Do I Change My Eating Habits?

You'll have the most success at eating better and well during pregnancy if you slowly make changes in your diet during the months prior to conception. Make the Baby-wise Diet your goal and slowly work toward that goal. Become a fat, sugar, and salt sleuth by learning what foods are high in these substances. Then, slowly reduce them in your diet, while emphasizing vegetables, fruits, and whole grains.

In most cases, only minor changes in fat, sugar, or salt intake make dramatic differences in the nutritional quality of a day's menu. Reducing your butter serving from 1 tablespoon to 2 teaspoons (a difference of only 1 teaspoon) could drop the fat calories from 39 to 31 percent in a breakfast. Sprinkling a quarter, rather than a half, teaspoon of salt on a potato can cut the day's sodium intake by 25 percent or more. Switch from fruited yogurt to plain yogurt with fresh fruit and reduce your sugar intake by several teaspoons.

While fat, salt, and sugar should be reduced, they shouldn't be eliminated. Fat is needed to help absorb the fat-soluble vitamins (A, D, E, and K), supply the essential fat called linoleic acid, and add variety to the diet. Your body needs some salt (i.e, sodium) during pregnancy to regulate muscle and nerve function and maintain its natural fluid balance. Sugar adds taste and pleasure to a meal or snack. So, set your sights on reducing, but not eliminating, these ingredients.

Finally, "don't sweat the small stuff." Minor fluctuations in fat, salt, or sugar have little or no impact on the total day's food intake. Sodium may fluctuate 100 mg or more, fat intake may vary a few percentage points, a teaspoon of sugar one way or the other is not important. Your goal is not a food-by-food or even a meal-by-meal inventory, but rather an overall daily and weekly reduction in fat, sugar, and salt.

The Vegetarian Diet and Pregnancy

Avoiding meat is no longer fringy business. With meat linked to everything from heart disease to cancer, many women have taken the plunge and gone vegetarian. But are vegetarian diets the best, or even safe, during pregnancy and nursing? Can you meet all of your increased nutrient needs without a meat-and-potatoes diet? Must you resort to bizarre foods and eating habits to ensure optimal nutrition for you and your baby? You might be surprised at the answers to those and other important questions.

Meat consumption, with its high amount of saturated fat and cholesterol, is positively correlated with heart disease in both men and women. Women who daily eat meat have a 50 percent higher risk of developing heart disease compared to vegetarian women. Disease risk increases as both the length of time and frequency of meat consumption increases. Consequently, people who adopt a vegetarian diet early in life have a lower risk of disease than do people who wait until after age fifty to switch from meat to beans.

In all fairness to meat, it might not be the harmful effects of a T-bone steak per se, but the protective effects of other foods in the vegetarian diet that is the real issue. Studies on Seventh-Day Adventists, a group with a high percentage of vegetarians and a lower cancer rate than that found in the general public, concluded that meat was not a significant factor in the development of certain types of cancer. However, people who ate lots of whole grains, legumes, and vegetables were at much lower risk for certain cancers, probably because they simply didn't have as much room in their diets for other fattier foods.

Whether it's an issue of a lower meat intake, a higher intake of fruits, vegetables, and legumes, or both, vegetarian diets can be a safe and healthful alternative to typical Western diets when you're pregnant. "The vegetarian diet is a good thing [for your health]," recommends Bonnie

Worthington-Roberts, Ph.D., former professor of nutritional sciences at the University of Washington in Seattle. "But, even with a good thing, you must do it right." With careful planning, both a lactovegetarian (who eats milk products) and a lacto-ovovegetarian (who eats milk products and eggs) can obtain all the necessary vitamins, minerals, protein, and other nutrients essential to health.

"The research on Seventh-Day Adventists shows there are good reproductive outcomes with vegetarian diets," says Johanna Dwyer, D.Sc., R.D., professor at Tufts University School of Medicine and the director of the Nutrition Center at the New England Medical Center in Boston. In fact, most women who eliminate meat from their diets actually consume more nutrient-rich diets than meat eaters, probably because they include more fruits and vegetables and fewer fatty animal products.

Lacto-ovovegetarians: Women on lactovegetarian or lacto-ovovegetarian diets should consume basically the same diet plans when gearing up for pregnancy, minus the meat and with extra servings of cooked dried beans and peas. A moderate-dose vitamin/mineral supplement that includes iron, zinc, and folic acid should fill in the gaps and help the vegetarian woman prepare for pregnancy.

Strict Vegetarians or Vegans: Women on strict vegetarian diets (who consume only whole grains, fruits, vegetables, cooked dried beans and peas, and nuts and seeds) have greater nutritional challenges. These women must consume adequate calories to ensure optimal weight and to spare protein from being used for energy. They also must choose several servings of high-quality protein by combining grains and legumes.

Without milk, these women must look for other sources of vitamin D, vitamin B_2, vitamin B_{12}, and calcium. Increased amounts of iron, zinc, and other trace minerals must be consumed to compensate for the lack of meat and the added phytates (in unleavened whole grains), oxalates (in spinach and other dark green vegetables), and fiber in these diets, which interfere with mineral absorption.

The strict vegetarian diet should include at least the following:

- 7 servings of vegetables
- 3 servings of fruits
- 6 to 11 servings of whole grains
- 4 servings of cooked dried beans and peas, nuts, and seeds
- 4 servings of calcium-rich foods
- a source of vitamin B_{12}

Fermented soy products such as miso and tempeh that contain vitamin B_{12}, brewer's yeast, fortified soy milk, and wheat germ are nutrient-rich sources in the strict vegetarian's diet. In general, most strict vegetarians getting ready for pregnancy would benefit from a multiple vitamin and mineral supplement that contains 2 mcg of vitamin B_{12} and 400 IU of vitamin D.

Nutrition: 1, 2, 3

Eating well is essential for the health of your baby—from conception throughout life. It does not mean resorting to odd eating habits or having to eat bizarre foods. Eating well does mean planning your meals and snacks around foods of plant origin plus two to three servings daily of both protein-rich and calcium-rich foods. Three rules of thumb are:

1. Two-thirds to three-quarters of your plate should be heaped with a variety of whole grains, vegetables, and fruits, with the rest coming from extra-lean protein-rich and low-fat calcium-rich items. Another way to say this is that for every one protein-rich or calcium-rich food you consume, choose at least three servings of fruits and vegetables, and two servings of whole grains.
2. Include at least one whole grain and two fruits and/or vegetables at every meal and one fruit or vegetable at every snack. Vary your choices.
3. Before you eat something, always ask yourself "Is this good for me and my baby?" If you answer yes, then go ahead and eat it. If you answer no, try to find something that will satisfy the same taste and hunger needs, but will be a healthier choice.

This eating plan is a family affair that includes you, your unborn baby, and your partner. The father-to-be will need his stamina just as much as Mom. He also plays an important role in supporting your nourishing efforts during pregnancy and will be a major role model for your child in the coming years. So, choose foods that look good, taste good, and are good for you and your family.

Stocking the Kitchen

Eating well begins with taking stock of your kitchen and learning a few shopping tips to survive the supermarket experience. Take a quick trip through your cupboards and refrigerator. What takes up the most room?

- Are your shelves jammed with canned beans, fruit canned in their own juice, and bags of whole-wheat noodles? Or, do you see dried soup mixes, bags of potato chips, and gravy mixes?
- Is your freezer filled with frozen plain vegetables, frozen blueberries, and concentrated orange juice, or ice cream and bags of frozen French fries?
- Is your refrigerator bulging with nonfat milk, yogurt, and fresh fruits and vegetables, or bottles of soda pop, luncheon meats, and margarine? Is what you see what you want to feed your developing baby?

TABLE 2.2

Healthy Snacks for Pregnancy

- A small slice of angel food cake topped with 1 cup fresh or thawed berries.
- Whole-wheat pita bread dunked in hummus and topped with sliced red peppers.
- Tomato soup made with nonfat milk and topped with cilantro.
- Chicken noodle soup with added green peas.
- Whole-wheat toast topped with almond butter and pineapple chunks.
- Asparagus spears lightly sauteed in chicken broth and garlic, then cooled for a crunchy snack.
- A sweet potato, sliced into strips and baked until crispy.
- Pitted lemon-flavored dried plums with an almond stuffed into each.
- Cantaloupe cubes drizzled with lime juice.
- A glass of chocolate-flavored fortified soy milk with graham crackers.
- A handful of chocolate morsels, dried cranberries, and almonds.

Toss It Out: Not-so-nutritious foods can be tempting. So, your first step is to discard anything in the kitchen that will interfere with your eating plans. Basically, you want to keep the wholesome foods and limit the highly processed ones. Granted, the old standby, "out of sight, out of mind," isn't foolproof, but it will help you stay on track. Remember, the father-to-be is part of this team effort. One way he can help is by not bringing home the pizza, chips, beer, and other foods that tempt you to revert back to less nutritious eating patterns.

The Snack Center: Think of your kitchen as the quick-fix snack center.

Stop buying the potato chips, cookies, soda pop, and ice cream and start stocking the kitchen with low-fat, low-sugar items.

- Fill apothecary jars on the kitchen counter with nuts, dried fruit, fat-free crackers, low-fat fruit bars, dried vegetable snacks, low-salt pretzels, and other healthy snacks.
- Keep nutritious snacks at arm's reach in the freezer and fridge: non-fat yogurt, baby carrots, cut-up fruit, celery sticks filled with peanut butter and raisins, string cheese, frozen blueberries and grapes, frozen fresh-fruit pops, frozen yogurt (top with fresh fruit).
- Keep the cupboards stocked with nutritious munchies: soft microwave pretzels, raisin bread to dunk in apple-spice yogurt, whole-wheat pita bread to fill with fat-free cream cheese and peaches, microwave fat-free popcorn, canned tomato soup to be made with nonfat milk.
- Bring foods with you. Fill your purse, glove compartment, or brief-case with baby carrots, yogurt, whole-wheat crackers, and bags of air-popped popcorn.
- Place a bowl of cut-up fruit in the refrigerator or on the table after a meal. You'll chow down on vitamin-packed fruit, not fat-packed chips.

Your next step is to assemble a list of healthful foods that you enjoy and that complement your favorite recipes. The "Sample Shopping List" (Table 2.3) provides a workable model that you can revise to fit your needs. Make sure to avoid impulse buying, always shop from a list, and never shop when hungry. In addition, planning the week's menus in advance allows you to shop only once a week, which can save precious time.

At the Store

Shop primarily around the periphery of the grocery store. Choose a wide variety of fresh fruits and vegetables from the produce department; a mix of whole grains from the bakery section; nonfat or low-fat milk or soy milk products from the dairy case; and extra-lean meats, poultry, and fish from the meat department. Venture into the aisles to purchase low-fat cereals and crackers, dried beans and peas, and low-fat convenience foods. Selecting nutritious foods is as easy as one-two-three.

TABLE 2.3

A Sample Shopping List

The following shopping list is a sample of the types of foods recommended in the Baby-wise Diet.

What	*How Much*
At the Produce Department: Fresh fruits and vegetables	Purchase enough for 8–10 servings daily per person.
At the Bakery: Whole-wheat bread, bagels, bread sticks, corn tortillas	Purchase enough for 6–8 servings daily per person.
At the Dairy Case: Nonfat or low-fat milk or yogurt, low-fat cheeses, calcium-fortified soy milk, eggs or egg substitutes	Purchase enough for 2–4 servings daily per person.
At the Meat Department: Extra-lean cuts of beef, chicken, pork, turkey, or veal	Purchase enough for 1–2 three-ounce servings daily per person.
At the Seafood Counter: Fresh fish and shellfish	Purchase enough for at least 1–2 three-ounce servings weekly per person.
Along the Canned and Dry Goods Aisles: Dried beans and peas; rice, pasta, flour, and other grains; canned fruit; nonfat evaporated milk, low-fat soups, fat-free tomato sauce	Purchase enough for at least 1 serving daily per person. Keep the kitchen shelves well stocked, preferably with whole-grain varieties; select fruit canned in its own juice; keep 1–2 cans each of soups and sauces in the cupboard.
Along the Cereal Aisle: To cook: oatmeal, barley, farina Ready-to-eat: low-fat, whole grain, such as Grape-Nuts, Shredded Wheat, NutriGrain Wheat germ	Keep a supply on hand.
At the Frozen Foods Department: Concentrated fruit juice, low-fat frozen entrees, whole-wheat waffles	Keep a supply on hand.

Nutritious Additions:
Dried fruit, nuts and seeds,   As needed.
popcorn, low-salt pretzels,
oven-baked chips, angel food
cake, vanilla wafers

Herbs, Oils, and Condiments:
All-fruit jam, herbs and spices,   As needed.
ketchup, lemon juice, mustard,
nonfat salad dressings, safflower
oil, low-fat mayonnaise, salsa,
vanilla

---

1. *Read labels:* Learn to identify which foods contain fat. A rule of thumb is to select foods that contain no more than 3 grams of fat for every 100 calories (i.e., if a food supplies 300 calories per serving, it should contain no more than 9 grams of fat per serving). Ignore the "Calories from Fat" and the "% Daily Value" on the label; these numbers provide little practical information for planning menus.

   Unfortunately, labels lump together all sugars, both natural and refined. Consequently, a food low in refined sugar, such as plain yogurt or fruit canned in its own juice, may appear high only because the food contains natural sugars, such as lactose or fructose. The only way to identify sugar-laden foods is to eyeball the ingredients list. If sugar (as sucrose, corn syrup, high-fructose corn syrup, or other added sugars) appears in the first three items, it is a good bet the food is high in refined sugar.

2. *Focus on real food:* The more refined and processed a food, the higher the fat, sugar, salt, and calorie content is likely to be and the lower the vitamin, mineral, and fiber content. For example, a potato is a fat-free source of vitamins, minerals, and fiber. Frozen scalloped potatoes contain 1 teaspoon of fat per serving and a bag of potato chips contains several teaspoons of fat, while the vitamin, mineral, and fiber content is dramatically reduced.

3. *Be wary of label claims and promises:* Although foods labeled "low-calorie" must contain no more than 40 calories per serving, check the serving size to make sure it is not unrealistically small! Low-fat milk contains 2 percent fat *by weight*, but 35 percent of the calories come

from fat! When in doubt, return to the 3-grams-of-fat-per-100-calories rule and read the ingredients list for sources of sugar and fat.

Menu Planning

When you sit down to plan your menus, plan for the whole week. This saves time, helps prevent last-minute food choices, and allows you to plan a more varied and appealing eating plan. A seven-day plan also makes it easier to do your grocery shopping; clean and store enough raw vegetables for several days; cook enough of some foods to use for more than one meal; and plan for social engagements. Of course, you probably will modify the plans throughout the week, but you are more likely to follow the dietary guidelines outlined in the Baby-wise Diet when you have stocked your kitchen with the necessary supplies. If you can plan for only three or four days at a time, then schedule more planning time midweek. Remember, *failure to plan is planning to fail.* (See the four weeks of menus at the back of this book.)

Plan meals and snacks with vegetables, fruits, and whole grains in mind. Since nine out of every ten women do not consume even five servings daily of fresh fruits and vegetables, it probably will take an "attitude shift" to make sure you get enough of these nutrient-packed foods. In general, include vegetables in everything you prepare. Rather than six ounces of beef and an iceberg lettuce salad, be creative and add vegetables to the following:

- Spaghetti and pizza sauce: add grated carrots, onions, mushrooms, green or red peppers.
- Lasagna: substitute a layer of broccoli or spinach in place of all or part of the meat and cheese.
- Casseroles: stir in green peas, corn, green beans, carrots, celery, onion, green/red/yellow peppers, squashes, sweet potatoes.
- Baked beans, chili, meat loaf: grated carrots, extra tomato sauce, canned tomatoes, green beans.
- Potato salad: add carrots, peas, peppers, red onions.
- Canned soups: add extra vegetables such as potatoes, corn, beans, peas, carrots, squash.
- Baked potato: stuff with spinach and low-fat yogurt; broccoli, mushrooms, and part-skim ricotta cheese; or nonfat cottage cheese and salsa.
- Corn bread and muffins: grated carrots, zucchini, corn, green chilies.

- Shish kebab: at least twice as many vegetables, such as mushrooms, carrots, eggplant, cherry tomatoes, zucchini, onion, or potato, as extra-lean meat, chicken, or shellfish.
- Tortillas: filled with ricotta or cottage cheese and spinach sprinkled with nutmeg; black beans, plain nonfat yogurt, and salsa; grated carrot and zucchini, low-fat cheese, and green chili peppers; no-fat refried beans, cilantro, tomato, and grated carrot.
- Salads: carrot-raisin; Waldorf (apples, celery, green pepper, nuts); spinach and orange slices; or marinated vegetables such as carrots, celery, tomatoes, broccoli, cauliflower, beans, yellow squash, mushroom combined with a low-fat or nonfat vinaigrette dressing.

Recipe Makeover

Gradually converting your eating style to one that will nourish your growing baby does not mean you throw out all of your favorite recipes. Most recipes just need a low-fat face-lift. Those that include a mixture of ingredients, such as most soups, stir-fries, bean dishes, or tomato sauces, adapt well, as will recipes that feature vegetables, grains, and small amounts of extra-lean meat and dairy products. Quick breads, muffins, and other desserts also can be easily revised. Try reducing the fat and sugar by half in a recipe and continue to cut back as you reeducate your palate. Even packaged grain dishes, such as rice or noodle side dishes, can be fat-modified by eliminating the suggested added fats and using nonfat or 1 percent low-fat milk instead of whole milk or cream. Eating aspartame-sweetened desserts or reducing the serving size of packaged desserts are two ways to cut back on sugar. Many of the commercial no-fat desserts, such as cakes and cookies, have increased the sugar content to make up for the lack of fat, so never assume that a low-fat food is a low-calorie food; always read the label. Table 2.4, "Healthy Sweet Treats," offers several guiltless desserts loaded with taste and nutrition.

The Working Mother: Quick Meals and Snacks on the Job

Pregnant women get hungry at the oddest times. At the library, on the bus, at the makeup counter of a department store, at the playground, or waiting in rush-hour traffic. More likely than not, you'll be hungry someplace other than your kitchen. So plan ahead. Stock your purse, briefcase, glove compartment, and/or office desk drawer with healthful snacks, such as fat-free whole-grain crackers, bread sticks, fresh fruit, crunchy vegetables, or dried fruit. Take a thermos of nonfat milk, fruit juice, or vegetable juice or a mini-brown-bag lunch wherever you go.

TABLE 2.4

Healthy Sweet Treats

Watch out for "low-fat" desserts. They are just as high in calories and even higher in sugar than their original versions. Instead, let the sweet tooth work to your nutritional favor. For example,

- *Whipped Cream Mountain:* Layer fresh fruit in a parfait glass and top with a dollop of low-fat whipped cream.
- *Peanut Butter Candy:* Blend peanut butter, honey, and wheat germ and spread on whole-wheat bread.
- *Superman Oatmeal:* Cook oatmeal in nonfat milk and add wheat germ and brown sugar.
- *Milk Shaker:* Add a teaspoon of chocolate syrup to nonfat or 1 percent low-fat milk. Blend with ice.
- *Sweet Fruits:* Switch from fruit canned in heavy syrup to fruit canned in juice.
- *Spiced Apples:* Sprinkle apple slices with cinnamon sugar for a sweet taste.
- *Popsicle Power:* Blend fresh fruit, pour mixture into a paper cup, insert a Popsicle stick in the middle, and freeze for an all-fruit dessert.
- *I Can't Believe It's Fruit:* Make fruit smoothies with nonfat milk, a banana, and a handful of strawberries whipped in a blender.
- *Tropical Snack:* Serve pineapple chunks dipped in strawberry yogurt.
- *Fruit-Yogurt Parfait:* Mix low-fat kiwi-strawberry yogurt with 1 chopped fresh kiwifruit.
- *Strawberries and Chocolate:* Dunk two cups fresh strawberries in ¼ cup dark chocolate syrup.
- *Chocolate Chews:* 5 chocolate-dipped dried apricots.
- *Pudding Parfait:* Add a dollop of light whipped cream to lemon-flavored custard-style yogurt.
- *Sorbet-ish:* 2 cups frozen blueberries.
- *Ginger Oranges:* Mix ½ cup canned mandarin oranges with 1 teaspoon crystalized ginger.
- *Late-Night Comfort Food:* Two fig bars and a cup of nonfat milk warmed and flavored with almond flavoring.
- *Glacéed Grapes:* Roll rinsed grapes lightly in sugar.
- *Nut Bread Spread:* Top a thin slice of date-nut bread with fat-free cream cheese and diced dates.

Brown-bag lunches and snacks are a must for any expectant mother. First, invest in an insulated lunch box with a dry ice unit that can be refrozen at night. Second, pack your lunch the night before to save time in the morning. Table 2.5, "Brown-Bag Lunchables," provides additional lunch ideas.

TABLE 2.5

Brown-Bag Lunchables

- Include leftovers from the previous night's dinner, such as soup, pizza, spaghetti, or chicken breast and rice casserole. (You can pack your lunch as you clean up after dinner.)
- Pack sandwich fillings and bread separately to avoid soggy sandwiches.
- Prepare an assortment of raw vegetables, whole-grain crackers, and a filling dip made from well-seasoned thick bean soup.
- Stuff whole-wheat pita pocket bread with meat loaf (made from extra-lean meat) and salad greens, or chicken salad and sprouts.
- Make a rolled sandwich from a warmed whole-wheat tortilla, mashed beans, and crumbled feta cheese. Pack a cup of salsa to dip the rolled sandwich.
- Pack a tortilla, a container of leftover vegetables, and some grated cheese. Combine the ingredients just before warming.
- Stuff a baked potato with part-skim ricotta cheese and reheated steamed vegetables.
- Bring Southwest Tuscany Soup* in a thermos and a fruit salad.
- Pack two muffins with two slices of low-fat cheese, an orange, and a bag of baby carrots.
- Top a portion of fat-free cottage cheese or low-fat yogurt with a mixture of cut-up fresh fruit and a topping of low-fat granola or wheat nugget cereal.
- If you have a microwave at work, bring leftover Spinach-Cheese Manicotti* along with a tossed salad.
- Always pack cut-up vegetables to eat with lunch or as emergency snacks.

* Recipes appear in the Appendix.

The vending machine might be your only option at work if you forget to bring a snack or lunch. For the most part, office vending machines should be viewed as reminders of the importance of planning ahead. They typically are filled with high-sugar, high-fat items, not the stuff on which babies are made. If you are in need of a snack with only a vending machine as a cure, quickly scan for the best options, including fruit, fruit juice, whole-grain crackers, fig cookies, or low-fat or nonfat milk. If all else fails, choose starch over candy, preferably pretzels, but potato chips or corn chips are last-resort options. The latter are high in fat, but have less sugar than candy.

Will It Cost More to Eat Well?

As a nutritionist, I've promised people for more than two decades that it won't cost any more to eat well—or take any more time—than it does to eat poorly. Most people don't believe me. "Come on, how can it cost less to eat California plums and imported olive oil?" is a typical response. OK, fresh raspberries out of season are pricey and grilled salmon and a spinach salad cost more than a Happy Meal, but my promise holds true: If you make smart choices, shop carefully, and adopt some cheap-shopping tricks, you can boost your health and shave enough off your food bill to afford a part-time housekeeper.

A study at the Research Institute at Bassett Health Care in Cooperstown, New York, found that a person following a heart-healthy diet reduced the shopping bill by up to $8 a week. For a family of four, that could mean about $1,664 in annual savings. Dietitians at the 5-A-Day program also made a few healthful changes in a typical menu and saved almost $1.00 a day. Why the discrepancy in the findings? "It's a difficult subject to study, since people can eat poorly on a tight or loose budget, just as they can eat well for more or less," says Susan Krebs-Smith, Ph.D., research nutritionist for the National Cancer Institute in Bethesda.

Even if humongous Big Gulps and football-sized hamburgers and doughnuts provide the most calories for the least cost—known in the trade as the "cal-a-buck ratio"—there are hidden costs of eating poorly. "Supersized portions of cheap food appear to be a great deal, but when you factor in the added costs of wardrobes, weight-management programs, health-care costs, and lost days of work due to complications of being overweight, it's not such a bargain," says Barbara Rolls, Ph.D., at Pennsylvania State University in University Park and author of *Volumetrics* (HarperCollins, 2000). More than one in every two of us is eating too much, with the extra pounds costing a person more than $5,000 in added health-care bills, plus the more than $33 billion spent annually in this country on weight-loss products and services. Obviously, getting the most calories for your buck—i.e., a good cal-a-buck ratio—isn't cost effective, while getting the most nutrients for your buck is.

You don't need to spend freely to eat well. The first place to start is with meat, which accounts for a third of our food bills. You can save money by redefining this one item as a complement, not the main attraction. For example, instead of steak, serve beef stew made with extra-lean meat, carrots, potatoes, celery, mushrooms, and onions, and cut your dinner bill by up to one-half. Not only that, but while the steak gets 66 percent of its calories from fat, the stew was only 29 percent.

In general, the less processed a food, the more nutritious and less costly it is. For example, a serving of frozen hash browns costs 70 percent more than an equal serving of potato. Or cut the cost of breakfast in half by switching from cinnamon-flavored oatmeal to plain instant oatmeal. Frozen plain vegetables also tend to be cheaper than canned.

Snack on fruits and vegetables. Highly processed snack items aren't as cheap as they look. Price a bag of potato chips by the pound and you'll find it costs more than steak! Switch to the same pounds of oranges and you'll save more than $32 alone on snacks! Check out other ways to cut your food costs in Table 2.6, "Cheap Tricks."

TABLE 2.6

Cheap Tricks

Want to get the biggest nutritional bang for your buck? Follow these tried-and-true cost-saving tips and you might just shave enough money off your yearly food bill to afford a regular day's pampering at a local spa!

1. Buy less expensive produce. Apples, oranges, bananas, carrots, cabbage, and onions are usually less expensive year-round. Use the expensive mangos, arugula, or papaya to garnish an occasional dish.
2. Look for specials/use coupons. Buy these discounted foods in quantity and store or freeze. For example, purchase bananas when they go on sale for 33 cents a pound. Peel and freeze to use in smoothies later.
3. Buy in bulk. Oatmeal, rice, nuts, tea, dried fruit, seasonings, sugar, and many other dry goods are now available in bulk bins at supermarkets, health-food stores, discount groceries, and food co-ops. You can buy the exact amount you need *and* cut costs.
4. Shop at warehouse clubs. Granted, you buy in larger quantities at these stores, but comparison shopping can save you big bucks. No place to store the box of apples or case of water-packed tuna? Shop with friends and split the food.
5. Buy in season. Raspberries might cost $10 a basket in March, but be patient and enjoy them for a fraction of that cost in July.

TABLE 2.6   continued

6. Bean it up. Americans average more than 8 ounces of meat per person per day, accounting for a third of our food dollars. Switch to beans a couple of times a week and you'll save hundreds of dollars over the course of the year! One bag of kidney beans costs less than a dollar and provides 12 servings, not to mention the fiber, B vitamins, minerals, and protein! Even canned beans are well under a dollar a pound!

7. Think quantity. Make extra servings of that stir-fry, stew, soup, or grilled chicken and freeze them in individual containers for future quick-fix instant dinners. Freeze batches of basic sauces, such as tomato-based sauce or low-fat creamed sauces that can be thawed and seasoned (add Italian spices or clams for pasta dishes, peppers and cumin for enchiladas, tuna or shrimp for a creamed dish over rice) for instant meals.

8. Grow your own. If you have the space and the time, there is nothing fresher and more rewarding than lettuce, carrots, corn, or other vegetables straight out of your garden. You're also likely to eat more produce when you grow your own. If your family eats a lot of whole-grain bread, consider investing in a bread-making machine, make weekly batches, and save a dollar or more on every loaf.

9. Visit farmer's markets. Locally grown produce often is less expensive and fresher than store bought.

10. Bring food with you. Stuff your purse, briefcase, glove compartment, diaper bag, or desk drawer with low-fat cheese, peanut butter, whole-wheat breads, oranges, apples, carrot sticks, and other nutritious, low-cost foods so you're less tempted to put a dollar in the vending machine for a candy bar or pull up to a drive-up window for a cheeseburger.

11. Beware of impulse buying. That sushi from the deli looked good, but you never got around to eating it. How many bags of lettuce were tossed after sitting in the fridge for a week? Eat before you shop and bring a list to cut back on these wasted food dollars.

12. What will you really eat? Take a hard look at your food wastes. If you buy fresh pineapple or peaches, but throw out more than you eat, then purchase canned fruit (in its own juice), which can sit on the shelf longer. Bottled lemon juice might be more cost-efficient than the real thing if you usually end up throwing out the moldy lemon.

13. Compare prices. Sure, the whole chicken appears cheaper than the boned and skinned chicken thighs, but when you factor in the amount that is thrown away—up to a third to a half the weight is skin, bones, and unusable parts—you might find that the more expensive cut is actually cheaper. When purchasing produce, consider which fruits and vegetables give you the most edible food for your buck.

14. Eat in more. We're spending 47.5 percent of our food dollars in restaurants these days, where food choices are higher in calories, fat, saturated fat, cholesterol, and cost than homemade food. Limit dining out and you'll be

healthier *and* have pocket money for that white-water rafting trip or spa vacation.

15. **Store it right.** Store vegetables, such as peppers, broccoli, carrots, cauliflower, green onions, and lettuce, in the crisper bin. Artichokes, asparagus, brussels sprouts, corn, and mushrooms should be stored in the refrigerator, but not the crisper. Keep in mind that even the freshest produce stored under perfect temperature and humidity conditions maintains best quality for only a few days.

16. **Buy generic.** Store brands of frozen vegetables, canned fruit, milk, and other items usually cost less than brand names. Quality can vary, so pick and choose which brands are worth the extra cost.

The Five-Minute Meal

If you have time to pull up to a drive-up window at a fast-food restaurant or grab a box of buttered popcorn at the movies, then you also have time to eat right to feel your best. The tricks to preparing quick, low-calorie meals and snacks are advanced planning, a basic inventory of ingredients, and the right time-saving equipment.

A well-stocked pantry and freezer will provide your basic ingredients. Time-saving cooking equipment includes a microwave oven for reheating foods and cooking vegetables and fish and a slow-cooker for meals that can be started in the morning and are ready when you get home in the evening. (You also can slow-cook brown rice on high for two to three hours in a slow-cooker.) A wok or a large, nonstick skillet is handy for stir-frying vegetables. A blender is great for whipping up a fruit and milk "smoothie" at breakfast.

Some foods are quicker to prepare than others. For example, fish is the fastest-cooking animal protein. A fresh fish fillet or fish steak can be cooked in the microwave in less than ten minutes. A frozen fish fillet can be oven-baked in less than thirty minutes. Soup and salad is a fast and satisfying quick fix for lunch or dinner. You can start with a low-fat, low-sodium canned soup from your pantry and tailor it to your taste by adding fresh or frozen vegetables, canned kidney beans, or extra noodles. Or, you can reheat a homemade soup from a previous meal and add fresh vegetables, herbs, or a fast-cooking grain like quick-cooking rice or bulgur wheat. Another five-minute meal is to toss a salad from your already-prepared stash of vegetables and toast a piece of whole-grain bread while the soup is heating.

Hey, who said you even had to cook to eat well? Serve raw vegetables and fruits or foods that come straight from the refrigerator and cupboard. For example, serve cold chicken or tofu salads on a bed of fresh greens, surrounded by marinated vegetables and whole-grain crackers. Even a few slices of low-fat turkey, a hunk of low-fat cheese, a handful of whole-wheat crackers, and a bag of baby carrots can be a nutritious quick meal. Or, you can choose from the wide variety of frozen entrees that are low-fat and low-sugar, and supplement them with a salad, frozen vegetables, orange juice, and/or milk. Other ideas include:

- Breakfast foods for dinner: scramble a low-fat egg substitute with a small amount of low-fat bacon and serve with whole-grain toast and fresh fruits. Or make pancakes with pureed fruit toppings and non-fat yogurt.
- Chef's salad: layer salad greens, chopped vegetables, beans, sliced chicken or turkey, grated low-fat cheese, sweet potato strips, and/or pretzel bits. Serve with a nonfat dressing, whole-grain roll, and fresh fruit.
- Baked sweet potatoes: top with fat-free sour cream, yogurt, or cottage cheese. Serve with steamed broccoli sprinkled with nutmeg and cinnamon.
- Grilled sandwiches: use whole-grain bread, low-fat cheese, deli-sliced lean meat, grated carrots, canned chilies, and a nonstick pan. Serve with fat-free baked tortilla chips and fruit slices.

There is no excuse for not eating a nutritious breakfast. To speed the process on hectic mornings and reduce your chances of skipping the day's most important meal, try the following:

1. Set out bowls, plates, silverware, and cups the night before.
2. Assemble dry ingredients for hot cereal in a bowl the night before. In the morning, add the liquid and microwave the cereal.
3. For a breakfast burrito, chop an onion and low-fat turkey bacon and store in the refrigerator the night before. In the morning, saute the onion and bacon until tender in a nonstick skillet coated with vegetable spray. Add prepared fat-free egg substitute and scramble until done. Roll up in a whole-wheat tortilla.

4. Split a whole-grain bagel and sprinkle low-fat or fat-free grated cheese on each half. Wrap in plastic and store in refrigerator. In the morning, add slices of fresh tomato or apple and microwave.
5. Peel, wrap, and freeze chunks of bananas or other fruits in advance. In the morning toss frozen fruit chunks in the blender with nonfat yogurt and orange juice. Toast a bagel while your shake blends until smooth.

Snack Right

Snacks play an important role in the Baby-wise Diet. Snacks provide up to 25 percent of a woman's calorie intake and, if properly selected, can be a prime source of nutrients. As a further benefit, women who eat more frequently throughout the day have an easier time maintaining desirable weight gain during pregnancy than women who stick to the "three square meals" plan.

Before you race to the vending machine with a license to snack, keep in mind that nibbling can make or break the nutritional quality of your diet, your stamina, and your baby's development, depending on what you choose.

Keep It Simple: A nutritious snack must be convenient, i.e., it must be readily available, take little time to prepare, and taste great.

Consider Snacks Part of Your Total Diet: Snacks are a perfect way to meet your daily quota for nutrient-packed, low-fat, and low-sugar foods. Include at least two of the following groups at any one snack and make one choice either fruits and vegetables or whole grains.

1. nonfat or low-fat milk products, such as yogurt or cheese
2. fresh vegetables and fruits
3. extra-lean meats
4. cooked dried beans and peas
5. whole-grain breads and cereals
6. nuts and seeds

Focus on Minimally Processed Foods: Most commercial cookies, chips, flavored popcorn, and candy are high in fat, salt, or sugar. Choose fruit, unsalted pretzels, apple-cinnamon rice cakes, bagels, crunchy carrots, and other nutritious snacks instead.

Snack Only When Hungry: Listen to your body and your mood and snack only when you're hungry. See Table 2.2, "Healthy Snacks for Pregnancy," on page 48, for more snack ideas.

Eating Out

Even the most conscientious person can find eating away from home a challenge. Social and situational pressures and disruption of daily habits can undermine the best intentions. Sometimes the stress of travel can foster emotional eating, sleep disturbances, or other moods that, in turn, cause you to throw dietary caution to the wind.

At the Restaurant: Occasional social events or restaurant meals probably will have little impact on your overall plan, even if you "just wing it," that is, as long as you don't allow a minor slip to progress to a major relapse. However, unless you exercise regularly, you probably are on a tight nutritional budget during pregnancy and need to make every bite count. The good news is that most restaurants are willing to accommodate special requests, especially from a pregnant woman!

The same rules apply to eating out as they do for eating at home:

- Choose low-fat fare, fill your plate with vegetables and grains, and complement the meal with moderate amounts of low-fat protein-rich and calcium-rich foods.
- Never assume anything; always ask how a food is prepared ("grilled" could mean grilled in butter) and request lower-fat preparation methods where needed.
- Order off the menu. For example, ask the server if you could get grilled salmon with a huge side of steamed vegetables.
- Also, state specifically what you *don't* want. When ordering scrambled eggs with a side of sliced tomatoes, whole-wheat toast no butter, and a glass of orange juice, also specify that you don't want the hash browns, sausage, or butter on the side.
- Split entrees with your partner and fill in with a side salad or bowl of vegetable soup.

At the Party: Parties and social engagements at other people's homes are another chance to test your assertiveness skills. If you know the person well, you can discuss your food preferences openly and can offer to bring something to add to the meal. For example, you might want to bring sparkling water if only alcoholic beverages or soda pop will be served. If you do not know your hosts well, you must decide whether you want to risk eating a high-fat and/or high-sugar meal, avoid the high-fat or high-sugar foods that are served and risk having less to eat, or discuss your eating plan with the hosts and offer to bring something to add to the meal. In all cases, making specific plans ahead of time will help you avoid spur-of-the-moment decision making.

Take Charge

Now is the best time to make changes in what and how you eat. You probably want the very best for your baby, so you'll be more motivated to spend the extra time it takes to develop new eating habits. Once established, these habits will be yours and your baby's for life. Getting by is no longer good enough. Now you should be striving for optimal.

So,

- Take charge of your kitchen (by stocking only nutritious foods),
- Shop well (by reading labels and not being swayed by advertising gimmicks), and
- Focus on healthy meal preparation (by revising recipes), and always be prepared (by carrying nutritious snacks wherever you go).

Chapter 3

❧

The Nutrition Primer for Pregnancy

We all know that eating well before, during, and after pregnancy is essential, but research is accumulating to show it's even more important than we realize. According to a recent review from Emory University, increased intake of foods rich in zinc, calcium, and magnesium improves birth weight, reduces the risk for premature birth, and lowers the risk for pregnancy-induced hypertension. Folic acid prevents birth defects, while adequate intake of iodine protects against miscarriage, mental retardation, and cretinism. Vitamin A–rich foods reduce the risk for low-birth-weight babies, and vitamin C–rich fruits and vegetables might protect against premature birth. The B vitamins, copper, and selenium also are important in protecting the mother and baby. And that's just the beginning!

Unfortunately, we do not instinctively choose a good diet. If we did, sales for soda pop and fast food would not have skyrocketed in the past three decades, while consumption of dark green leafy vegetables went from too little to even less. The first step in guaranteeing the very best diet for you and your baby is to understand what you need, why you need it, and what foods are the best sources. Here is a quick course on the nutrients most important as you plan for and experience your pregnancy, as well as the nutrients you will need to recover after the baby is born. Table 3.1, "Pregnancy Nutrients at a Glance," gives a summary of which nutrients you need, how much, and what foods are the best sources.

TABLE 3.1

Pregnancy Nutrients at a Glance

Protein

Requirement: 60 grams
Needed for: Helps build baby's tissues, placenta, and red blood cells in mother.
Sources: Extra-lean meat, chicken, fish, low-fat milk products, cooked dried beans and peas, soy products.

Vitamin A/Beta Carotene

Requirement: 800 mcg (4,000 IU)
Needed for: Aids reproduction. Helps maintain immune system, vision, cell, and tissue growth.
Sources: Vitamin A: Liver, eggs. Beta carotene: Dark green or orange vegetables, cantaloupe, peaches.

Vitamin D

Requirement: 5 mcg (200 IU)
Needed for: Helps build strong bones in baby and maintain bones in mother.
Sources: Fortified milk (not milk products), salmon, sardines, fortified cereals, egg yolk.

Vitamin E

Requirement: 10 mg (22 IU)
Needed for: Helps protect tissues in baby and mother from free-radical damage. Might help prevent vision damage in premature infants.
Sources: Wheat germ, safflower oil, nuts, spinach.

Vitamin K

Requirement: 65 mcg
Needed for: Aids in blood clotting and bone formation.
Sources: Dark green leafy vegetables.

Vitamin B_1

Requirement: 1.4 mg
Needed for: Energy metabolism. Aids in digestion. Essential for formation of nervous system and normal growth of body and brain.
Sources: Whole grains, wheat germ, peanuts, green peas, dark green leafy vegetables, lean pork, cooked dried beans and peas.

TABLE 3.1   continued

Vitamin B₂

Requirement: 1.4 mg
Needed for: Energy metabolism. Necessary for growth and building of all tissues.
Sources: Milk products, avocado, dark green leafy vegetables, salmon, asparagus, whole grains, cooked dried beans and peas.

Niacin

Requirement: 18 mg
Needed for: Energy metabolism. Necessary for growth and building of all tissues; promotes development of healthy skin, nerves, and digestive tract.
Sources: Chicken, fish, peanut butter, green peas, wheat germ, whole grains, cooked dried beans and peas, low-fat milk products.

Vitamin B₆

Requirement: 1.9 mg
Needed for: Energy metabolism. Helps build proteins, such as hormones, enzymes, red blood cells, and nerve chemicals. Essential in development of baby's brain and nerve tissue.
Sources: Chicken, fish, extra-lean meat, avocado, potatoes, bananas, whole grains, wheat germ, cooked dried beans and peas, nuts and seeds.

Folic Acid

Requirement: 400 mcg of folic acid from supplements or 600 mcg from a mixture of food and supplements (4 mg for women with a history of neural tube defects)
Needed for: Normal cell division and the prevention of birth defects. Red blood cell formation. Normal growth and optimal birth weight.
Sources: Dark green leafy vegetables, asparagus, broccoli, orange juice, wheat germ, cooked dried beans and peas, fortified grains.

Vitamin B₁₂

Requirement: 2.6 mg
Needed for: Normal formation of proteins. Essential for normal cell and tissue growth, especially brain, nerve, and red blood cells. Helps prevent anemia.
Sources: Extra-lean meat, chicken, fish, eggs, milk, tempeh, miso.

Biotin

Requirement: 30 to 100 mcg
Needed for: Prevents dry skin, hair loss, nerve problems. Pregnant women often show marginal biotin status.
Sources: Oatmeal, soybeans, clams, eggs, peanut butter, salmon, milk.

Pantothenic Acid

Requirement: 4 to 7 mg
Needed for: Energy metabolism. Helps make fats, cholesterol, bile, some hormones, red blood cells, and vitamin D.
Sources: Fish, chicken, cheese, whole grains, avocados, vegetables, and legumes.

Vitamin C

Requirement: 70 mg
Needed for: Normal function of all cells. Formation of connective tissue, bones, teeth, and blood vessels. Aids in formation of some nerve chemicals.
Sources: Citrus fruits, brussels sprouts, strawberries, green and red peppers, dark green leafy vegetables.

Calcium

Requirement: 1,000 mg for pregnant women over nineteen years old; 1,300 mg for pregnant women eighteen years old and younger
Needed for: Helps build baby's bones and maintains mother's bones. Possibly helps prevent pregnancy-induced high blood pressure. Inhibits lead mobilization from bones. (See page 220 for more information.)
Sources: Low-fat milk products, sardines, canned salmon with bones, tofu, dark green leafy vegetables, dried beans and peas.

Chromium

Requirement: 50 to 200 mg
Needed for: Helps regulate blood sugar. Builds proteins in baby's developing tissues. Might aid baby's growth and reduce pregnancy-induced diabetes (gestational diabetes).
Sources: Whole grains, wheat germ, orange juice.

Copper

Requirement: 1.5 to 3.0 mg
Needed for: Essential for normal pregnancy outcome, energy metabolism, connective tissue and red blood cell formation. Aids in development and maintenance of a baby's heart, arteries, and blood vessels, skeletal system, and nervous system.
Sources: Chicken, fish, extra-lean meat, organ meats, whole grains, nuts and seeds, soybeans, dark green leafy vegetables.

Fluoride

Requirements: 3.0 mg
Needed for: Strengthens bones and teeth, reducing risk for cavities in mother and baby.
Sources: Fluoridated water.

TABLE 3.1   continued

Iodine

Requirements: 175 mcg
Needed for: An essential component of the thyroid gland.
Sources: Iodized salt, seafood.

Iron

Requirement: 30 mg
Needed for: Prevents anemia. Helps baby develop and gain weight. Prevents premature delivery.
Sources: Extra-lean meat, fish, poultry, cooked dried beans and peas, dried apricots, dark green leafy vegetables, raisins, whole grains.

Magnesium

Requirement: 350 mg for pregnant women over age nineteen; 400 mg for pregnant women eighteen years old and younger.
Needed for: Energy metabolism. Blood sugar regulation. Helps develop normal muscle contraction and nerve transmission. Maintains uterine relaxation during pregnancy and aids in contraction during labor.
Sources: Low-fat milk, peanuts, bananas, wheat germ, whole grains, cooked dried beans and peas, dark green leafy vegetables, oysters.

Manganese

Requirement: 2.0 to 5.0 mg
Needed for: Component of several enzymes.
Sources: Whole grains, fruits, vegetables, tea.

Molybdenum

Requirement: 75 to 250 mcg
Needed for: A component of several enzymes.
Sources: Whole grains, beans, milk.

Selenium

Requirement: 65 mcg
Needed for: Essential to growth. Protects tissues in baby and mother from free-radical damage.
Sources: Whole grains, seafood, lean meat, low-fat milk products.

Zinc

Requirement: 15 mg
Needed for: Essential for conception. Reduces risk for spontaneous abortions and premature delivery. Helps prevent birth defects. Aids normal growth. Helps in development of bones, vision, and taste.
Sources: Extra-lean meat, turkey, cooked dried beans and peas, wheat germ, whole grains.

The Calorie-Containing Nutrients

Protein, carbohydrate, and fat are the calorie-containing nutrients. They supply the energy you and your baby need to produce the miracle of life. Protein and carbohydrates (including both sugar and starch) supply four calories per gram, while fat supplies nine calories. Except for sugar (which is pure carbohydrate) and oils, butter, and other fats (which are pure fat), most foods are a combination of two or more of these nutrients. For example, a bowl of oatmeal is primarily carbohydrate, but supplies a little protein and a trace of fat. A protein-rich chicken breast also contains some fat, while peanut butter is high in fat, but also contains protein and carbohydrate.

Protein

Protein is the essential building block for muscle, organs, skin, and all tissues. It also is essential for making antibodies, hormones, nerve chemicals, and red blood cells. More than a quarter of the protein you eat goes directly to the placenta and uterus.

Protein is essential, yet your protein needs prior to and during the first trimester of pregnancy are the same as during any other time in your adult life. It is during the second and third trimesters of pregnancy that you will need a little more protein, about 10 grams more (the amount of protein in a glass of milk). The extra servings of nonfat milk and low-fat protein-rich foods, such as cooked dried beans and peas, chicken without the skin, and fish, recommended in the Baby-wise Diet, will more than accommodate this increased requirement. In fact, protein is the least likely nutrient to be low in your diet, since most of us already consume more than twice our protein needs. You won't need extra protein in the form of powders or tablets.

Vegetarian Diets: One exception is women following strict vegetarian diets (no animal products). These women must be very careful to plan adequate amounts of protein into their daily menus, since poor protein intake can reduce placental growth and function, limit the growth of the baby, impair normal brain development, and jeopardize survival rates. Several servings daily of cooked dried beans and peas combined with whole grains and pasta, as well as tofu, soy milk, and nuts will help ensure adequate protein intake for strict vegetarians (also called vegans). See Chapter 2, pages 45 to 47, for more on vegetarian diets.

Carbohydrates

Starches and other complex carbohydrates remain the mainstay of the diet. Carbohydrate comes in two packages—the complex starches in breads, pasta, rice, grains, potatoes, legumes, and vegetables, and the simple sugars naturally found in milk (lactose) and fruit (fructose) or the refined or concentrated sugars in table sugar, honey, brown sugar, corn syrup, and "raw" sugar.

The starches in whole grains and naturally occurring sugars in fruit come packaged with vitamins, minerals, fiber, phytochemicals, and other essential nutrients. Wholesome, minimally processed, low-fat versions of these foods are essential to building a healthy baby and are the mainstay of the Baby-wise Diet. On the other hand, prior to and during pregnancy you should minimize foods high in refined starches and sugars, including desserts, sweet snack foods, sweetened fruit drinks, processed noodles and bread, sugary cereals, and most convenience foods, since there is little room in your diet for these nutrient-poor selections. Inevitably, they either replace more nutritious foods and jeopardize your health and your baby's welfare or are eaten in addition to all the other nutritious foods you need, thus causing excessive weight gain.

Fat

Fat adds calories quickly, so you need to be judicious in what type of fats you use. Limit total fat intake to 25 to 30 percent of total calories by cutting back on saturated fats in fatty meats and dairy products, and other fats in processed foods.

The Good Fats: The best fats for you and your baby are those in olive or canola oils, nuts, seeds, avocados, and fish. You need some of these healthy fats to build brain tissue and aid in the development of vision, so don't get carried away and cut fat too low. Fish oils also might help prevent or treat some pregnancy-related disorders, such as preeclampsia and high blood pressure. In the case of diabetes or heart disease where pregnancy raises blood cholesterol levels as much as 40 percent, reducing fat intake to less than 25 percent of total calories might be warranted, but should be recommended and monitored by a physician and dietitian. (See Chapter 6 for more information on gestational diabetes, fish oils, and pregnancy-related disorders and Chapter 9 for more information on fish oils and infant formulas).

Trans Fatty Acids: Processed foods often contain altered fats that you also want to limit. Hydrogenated fats are liquid vegetable oils made creamy when manufacturers convert some of the unsaturated fats into saturated ones through a process called hydrogenation. This process also rearranges some of the remaining unsaturated fats so their natural "cis" shape is transformed into an abnormal "trans" shape. These fats are known as trans fatty acids or TFAs.

While TFAs are found naturally only in minute amounts, they constitute up to 60 percent of the fat in processed foods that contain hydrogenated fats, such as cookies, potato chips, and other snack foods. Margarine and vegetable shortening are two prime sources of these fats. TFAs are polyunsaturated fats but they act more like saturated fats by raising LDL levels (the "bad" cholesterol) and increasing heart disease risk by as much as 27 percent. In addition, they might accumulate in the baby's tissues and have been associated with lower birth weights. Researchers at the University of Munich in Germany who studied the effects of TFAs during pregnancy caution that their findings shed doubt on the safety of these processed fats during pregnancy and the months preceding and following birth. See Table 3.2, "Reading between the Lines: Trans Sleuthing."

You can't eat butter because its high saturated fat content increases the risk for heart disease, and now margarine is a no-no. Is this a nutritional catch-22? No. The bottom line is eat less fat. Limit your intake of any processed product that contains "hydrogenated vegetable oil" in the ingredient list. Use diet or whipped margarine in moderate amounts, since they contain less TFAs than tub or stick margarine, or make your own spread by whipping a stick of butter with a half cup of canola oil. This blend is lower in saturated fat than butter and is TFA-free.

Vitamins, Minerals, and Phytochemicals

The best place for the mother-to-be to obtain all the essential vitamins, minerals, fiber, phytochemicals, and other nutrients is from food. The trick is getting enough. As long as you follow the Baby-wise Diet, your diet will supply everything you need. A moderate-dose multiple that contains extra iron and folic acid will fill in any nutritional gaps on the days when you don't eat perfectly.

TABLE 3.2

Reading between the Lines: Trans Sleuthing

Food labels do not require that trans fatty acid (TFA) content be listed directly on the label. However, they also do not allow any unsaturated fat that has been converted to a trans fatty acid to appear as part of the total fat content. So when it comes to TFAs, what you don't see is what you get. For example, a label on a bag of potato chips might read:

Total fat: 15 grams
    Polyunsaturated fat: 5 grams
    Saturated fat: 2 grams
    Monounsaturated fat: 1 gram

The remaining 7 grams of fat (15 grams − 8 grams = 7 grams) probably are trans fatty acids.

The following has been organized by food groups that, in general, are the best sources of the listed vitamins and minerals. Keep in mind, however, that all wholesome, minimally processed foods supply varied combinations of nutrients, so that while vegetables are generally a good source of vitamin C, beta carotene, and/or folic acid, some vegetables are also excellent sources of vitamin B_2 and calcium (nutrients typically high in milk products), while other vegetables are better sources of vitamin E or copper. Most milk products are excellent sources of calcium, but some also supply ample amounts of zinc.

Fruits and Vegetables: Vitamins A and C, Folic Acid, Phytochemicals
The fruits and vegetables in the Baby-wise Diet supply a wealth of nutrients, including beta carotene, vitamin C, folic acid, and phytochemicals. All of these nutrients are essential for your baby.

Vitamin A: Beta carotene is converted to vitamin A in the body, a fat-soluble vitamin essential in reproduction, the immune system, vision, and cellular differentiation. The latter function is particularly critical during periods of rapid growth and tissue development, as in pregnancy, infancy, and early childhood. Too little vitamin A during pregnancy also might damage the baby's developing nervous system and suppress the immune system, increasing your baby's risk during the first few months of life for diarrhea, measles, respiratory infections, and other illnesses. During pregnancy and especially during the first trimester, the supply must be closely regulated to ensure that the developing baby is exposed to neither too little nor too much vitamin A, since both conditions can cause birth defects. Deep orange or dark green fruits and vegetables are the best place to get your vitamin A, since it is virtually impossible to consume a toxic dose of beta carotene from dietary sources.

Vitamin C: This vitamin is essential in the formation and maintenance of collagen, a protein that forms the basis for the most abundant tissue in the body—connective tissue. The shape and function of all tissues depend on collagen, which acts as a cementing substance between cells. Collagen is found in the bones and teeth, tendons, skin, the cornea of the eye, and blood vessel walls. It maintains the shape of the disks of the backbone, allows the joints to move, and binds muscles together. Limited evidence suggests that consuming adequate vitamin C during pregnancy might help lower a woman's risk for premature rupture of the membranes surrounding the baby during pregnancy by maintaining optimal collagen formation.

Vitamin C also helps maintain the immune system and a person's resistance to infection and disease. This vitamin promotes the healing of tissues and helps prevent the development of numerous diseases, from cancer and cataracts to heart disease. Vitamin C is in most fruits and vegetables, with some of the best sources being citrus fruits, kiwi, papaya, broccoli, and strawberries.

Folic Acid: As discussed in detail in Chapter 1, this B vitamin is essential in the first few weeks surrounding conception for the formation of normal nerve tissue and in the prevention of neural tube defects. Low intake of folic acid throughout pregnancy also increases the risk of spontaneous abortion, pregnancy complications such as placental abruption and preeclampsia, preterm delivery, low birth weight, and slowed growth. Your best sources of this B vitamin are dark green leafy vegetables, asparagus, broccoli, and orange juice. Other sources include wheat germ, legumes, and fortified grains.

Phytochemicals: Fruits and vegetables are jam-packed with vitamins, minerals, and fiber, all of which are essential for a healthy pregnancy. But there are thousands of other compounds in foods (12,000 to be a bit more exact) that are not strictly nutrients, yet pack an extra health-enhancing punch.

These naturally occurring compounds, called "phytochemicals" or plant nutrients, evolved because they provide plants with a natural protection against disease, insects, and sun damage. But, by the benevolent hand of Mother Nature, these compounds also are beneficial to people. Every spinach leaf, every slice of tomato, every spear of broccoli is literally a bumper crop of health-enhancing compounds. For example,

- A clove of garlic supplies next to nothing when it comes to vitamins and minerals, but it is a gold mine for other health-enhancing compounds, including the sulfur-containing compounds allicin, alliin, and ajoene that lower heart-disease risk and boost immunity.
- Beta carotene is an antioxidant that lowers cancer risk. It is one of more than 600 related compounds, called carotenoids, found in dark green leafy vegetables, tomatoes, broccoli, carrots, and more, that have health-enhancing capabilities.
- Tomatoes top the list as a source of a carotene-like substance called lycopene, which is one of the most potent antioxidants in preventing damage to cells and tissues. Tomatoes also contain p-coumaric acid and chloragenic acid, which prevent the formation of carcinogens.
- Ellagic acid in strawberries and grapes neutralizes carcinogens that otherwise attack the cell's DNA and initiate abnormal cell growth.
- Cabbage is loaded with phenethyl isothiocyanate (PEITC), which inhibits the growth of lung cancer.
- The bioflavonoids, including rutin; the flavonones—hesperidins, eriocitrin, naringen, and naringenin; the flavones; and the flavonols, packed into citrus fruits and vegetables, reduce blood clots associated with stroke and inhibit the oxidation of LDL that turns harmless cholesterol in the blood into the sticky glue that clogs artery walls. They also stimulate the immune system, have antioxidant capabilities, and might strengthen blood vessel walls.
- Spinach and other greens (such as collards, mustard, and turnip) are the best dietary sources of lutein, another carotene-like compound that has antioxidant capabilities. Lutein also helps prevent normal cells from converting to abnormal cells by improving cell-to-cell communication.
- Broccoli contains sulforaphane, an antioxidant that bolsters the body's natural defense mechanisms. This plant nutrient also might boost the production of detoxifying enzymes that usher harmful substances out of cells before they can cause problems.
- Oranges and other citrus fruits contain an antioxidant called limonene that might enhance the activity of enzymes that help dispose of harmful substances before they jeopardize health.

The list is endless and is growing daily as researchers uncover more about these plant nutrients. Granted, researchers haven't investigated how phytochemicals enhance pregnancy, but it's a sure bet that a healthy pregnant mom stacks the deck in favor of having a healthy, robust baby.

Whole Grains: Trace Minerals, B Vitamins, Fiber

The whole-grain breads and cereals in the Baby-wise Diet contribute trace minerals, such as chromium, iron (see Chapters 1 and 6), and selenium, and some of the B vitamins. They also provide fiber to help prevent constipation, hemorrhoids, and other inconveniences during pregnancy.

Chromium: This trace mineral is essential for the normal regulation of blood sugar and, in concert with insulin (the hormone secreted from the pancreas that regulates blood sugar levels), stimulates the synthesis of protein in the unborn's developing tissues. Consequently, poor chromium intake is associated with pregnancy-induced diabetes, also called gestational diabetes (see Chapter 6), and possibly poor fetal development.

Limited evidence shows that pregnancy might be associated with low chromium levels, either because of poor dietary intake or increased requirements. This is not surprising, since nine out of ten adults consume suboptimal amounts of this mineral. It is essential that several servings daily of chromium-rich foods, including whole grains, wheat germ, and orange juice, be included in the diet. (Refined and "enriched" breads, rice, and noodles are poor sources for this essential nutrient.)

Selenium: Selenium is an antioxidant mineral that is important for your body's defense against disease. As a component of the antioxidant enzyme called glutathione peroxidase, selenium protects red blood cells and cell membranes from damage by highly reactive oxygen fragments called free radicals. Selenium also is important for maintaining a strong immune system in both you and your baby.

While no studies have been conducted on humans, there is evidence that blood levels of selenium and its enzyme decrease during pregnancy, suggesting that unless you eat well, you might not get enough of this mineral to maintain normal body stores. Switching from refined to whole grains improves your chance of having a healthy full-term baby. Whole grains are excellent sources of selenium, supplying approximately 12 mcg per serving; six servings daily will supply 72 mcg or more than the Recommended Dietary Allowance for pregnant women.

B Vitamins: Whole grains are also excellent sources of several of the B vitamins, including vitamin B_1, vitamin B_2, niacin, and pantothenic acid.

These B vitamins function primarily in the release of energy from the calorie-containing nutrient—fat, carbohydrate, and protein—and their need increases in proportion to the increase in calories during the second and third trimesters. Optimal intake ensures a readily available supply of energy to fuel the processes of developing a baby and building the support tissues of pregnancy, such as the placenta.

The Baby-wise Diet emphasizes whole grains. Don't waste your carbohydrate quota on too many "enriched" processed grain products, such as white bread, white rice, or egg noodles. While vitamin B_1, vitamin B_2, niacin, and folic acid have been added to these refined "enriched" grains, they are poor nutritional alternatives when it comes to other B vitamins, such as vitamin B_6 and pantothenic acid. They also contain as little as 4 percent of the original amount of vitamin E, fiber, magnesium, zinc, chromium, copper, and manganese.

Fiber: You'll be hard-pressed to make it through pregnancy without a daily dose of fiber-rich foods. Whole grains—along with vegetables, legumes, and fruits—supply insoluble fibers that absorb water in the digestive tract, increase stool bulk, speed the movement of waste products through the digestive tract, and help prevent colon cancer, constipation, diverticulosis, irritable bowel syndrome, and hemorrhoids. The soluble fibers, such as the vegetable gums and pectin, are found in oat bran (fruits and cooked dried beans and peas, too). These fibers assist in curbing erratic swings in blood sugar levels and lower blood cholesterol, thus helping prevent or treat diabetes and cardiovascular disease. They also aid in filling you up without adding unnecessary calories, so you'll be more likely to gain just enough, but not too much weight.

Low-Fat Milk and Soy Milk Products: Calcium, Magnesium, Vitamin D

Low-fat milk products, including nonfat and low-fat milk, yogurt, and cheese, and some fortified soy milk, supply protein, calcium, vitamin B_{12}, vitamin B_2, and magnesium, nutrients essential for normal bone, muscle, and nerve development and function. Fortified milk and fortified soy milk are the only reliable dietary sources of vitamin D (all other milk products, from yogurt to cottage cheese, contain little or no vitamin D).

Calcium: This mineral builds bones. Approximately 200 mg of calcium per day is deposited into the baby's skeleton during the last trimester of pregnancy. A similar amount is secreted daily in breast milk, although this varies depending on how much breast milk is produced and how much

BOX 3.1   IODINE AND FLUORIDE

Iodine and fluoride are two minerals essential to your baby's health that do not have reliable dietary sources, so they must be added to the diet by fortifying salt (in the case of iodine) or water (in the case of fluoride).

Iodine is a component of the hormone thyroxine that regulates your body's metabolism, including when, where, and how much energy is used for any given task. Inadequate intake of iodine causes thyroxine levels to drop. The thyroid gland tries to compensate by working harder and a condition called goiter results. During pregnancy, an iodine deficiency can cause permanent malformations and mental retardation, a condition called cretinism, primarily because the nervous system requires adequate thyroid hormone exposure for normal development. Goiter and cretinism are rare because of the addition of iodine to salt. Using iodized salt sparingly during pregnancy plus consuming other sources of iodine, such as milk, brewer's yeast, and eggs will help meet your needs for this mineral.

Fluoridation of water (at a level of one part per million, the equivalent of a few drops in a swimming pool) is the most efficient and economical way to reduce dental caries. Fluoride helps bond calcium and phosphorus in bones and teeth, making them strong and resistant to decay. Your baby's teeth begin to form about the tenth week of pregnancy; permanent molars and incisors begin developing in the second and third trimesters. A study from the Children's Dental Research Society in Florida found that 2 mg a day of fluoride throughout pregnancy and then fluoride either in water or in a weighted dose (0.25 mg/day until two years old, 0.5 mg/day from two to three years old, etc.) after the baby is born help prevent tooth decay later in life.

calcium a woman consumes while pregnant, with some women secreting more than 300 mg daily. The total calcium cost of pregnancy for a woman who has had two babies and has breast-fed them both for three months is approximately 100,000 mg, the equivalent of more than 333 extra glasses of nonfat milk!

The bones are the storage shed for 99 percent of the body's calcium. If a woman does not consume enough of this essential mineral to ensure optimal growth of the baby's skeleton, either the baby's growth is affected or calcium is drained from her bones. Optimal calcium intake might decrease risk for pregnancy-induced high blood pressure in the mother, lowered blood pressure in the infant (see Chapter 6), and reduced risk for nerve damage from toxic metals such as lead.

Your body performs a miracle in the way it handles calcium while you're pregnant and nursing. During gestation, it helps compensate for higher calcium needs by increasing the average amount absorbed into your bones from food—from about 20 to 25 percent prior to pregnancy to as much as 50 percent during pregnancy. While nursing, your body compensates for the loss in breast milk by reducing calcium losses in the urine. But, miracles must be matched with personal responsibility. Regardless of absorption, you need to make sure you get enough of this mineral prior to, during, and after pregnancy. Calcium intake should remain optimal throughout the childbearing years, since one in every two pregnancies is unplanned.

More than half of all women drink less than one glass of milk a day; only 18 percent consume the recommended three daily servings. Three out of every four women entering pregnancy are marginally nourished in calcium, averaging only 600 mg when they should be getting twice that much. Pregnancy and nursing increase daily requirements even higher and you might need up to 2,000 mg daily if you are at high risk for preeclampsia.

Milk and fortified soy milk are the best sources of calcium. In fact, people in Western countries are hard-pressed to meet their nutrient needs without it, since milk supplies up to 75 percent of an adult's calcium intake. "It is very difficult to get enough calcium from diets that exclude milk because there are so few foods as rich in calcium that people are willing to eat frequently," states Bess Dawson-Hughes, chief of the Calcium and Bone Metabolism Laboratory at USDA Human Nutrition Research Center at Tufts University in Boston. Janet King, Ph.D., R.D., a professor in the Department of Nutritional Sciences at the University of California, Berkeley, agrees and adds, "A woman must keep in mind that milk also supplies other essential nutrients, such as vitamin D and vitamin B_2, that are difficult to get anywhere else." Luckily, many calcium-fortified foods are now available, including breads, orange juice, and rice mixes. Only fortified soy milk, however, contains all the nutrients found in milk, including calcium, vitamin D, and vitamins B_2 and B_{12}.

Of course, you can take several calcium pills each day instead of drinking milk, but this goes against all dietary recommendations to turn first to food and only to supplements as a last resort. "There is no evidence that calcium supplements are superior to milk [in preventing osteoporosis] and food always should be a person's first choice when it comes to obtaining optimal nutrition," says Dr. Dawson-Hughes.

For those women who cannot meet the two-to-three servings goal for low-fat milk, fortified soy milk or orange juice, and other calcium-rich foods, supplements are a must. "It's prudent to take a 1,000 mg supplement of calcium, since most women average only 600 mg of calcium from their diets," says Robert Heaney, M.D., a calcium expert at Creighton University in Omaha, Nebraska. Avoid the "natural source" calcium pills, such as oyster shell and bone meal, since they might contain the toxic metal lead.

Magnesium: This mineral doesn't get a lot of attention, but magnesium is an important nutrient during pregnancy and for the prevention of numerous health problems, from heart disease and high blood pressure to diabetes.

Magnesium functions in more than 300 processes essential to the development of a healthy baby, including the metabolism of carbohydrate, protein, and fat. It is one of the most abundant minerals in muscle, liver, heart, and other soft tissues, and is essential in the regulation of insulin and blood sugar regulation, nerve transmission, the manufacture of proteins that synthesize the cells' genetic material, and in the removal of toxic waste products from the body. Magnesium also aids in muscle (including the uterus) contraction and relaxation. In fact, optimal blood levels of magnesium during pregnancy might help maintain uterine relaxation up until the thirty-fifth week, while dropping levels thereafter might favor the onset of labor. Optimal magnesium intake during pregnancy also might lower the risk for cerebral palsy and retardation in newborns.

Magnesium and calcium work as a team. For example, excess intake of magnesium inhibits bone formation, while consuming too much calcium interferes with magnesium metabolism. The balance between these two minerals is reflected in their role in muscle contraction; calcium stimulates muscles to contract, while magnesium relaxes muscles. Milk is one food that supplies both calcium and magnesium.

When it comes to magnesium, Americans often don't get enough. The Recommended Dietary Allowance (RDA) is 320 mg for a pregnant woman, but a typical diet in the United States provides 120 mg of magnesium for every 1,000 calories; consequently, a woman consuming less than 2,000 calories might consume suboptimal amounts of magnesium. In addition, many researchers suspect the RDAs are inadequate to help prevent heart disease, high blood pressure, and diabetes. The RDAs for magnesium are based on 2.1 mg to 2.3 mg for every one pound of body weight. How-ever, studies show some people require up to 2.7 mg or more per pound of body weight, the equivalent of 368 mg for a 135-pound woman.

You will obtain optimal amounts of magnesium if you follow the Baby-wise Diet, which contains ample amounts of magnesium-rich foods, including nonfat or low-fat milk, nuts, cooked dried beans and peas, whole-grain breads and cereals, fortified soy milk, and seafood. Excep-tions to this rule are women who have lost extra magnesium because of chronic diarrhea or repeated vomiting. In these cases, additional magnesium-rich foods should be consumed or a moderate-dose supple-ment that contains approximately 400 mg per day should be considered. (See Table 3.3, "What Foods Supply Magnesium?")

Vitamin D: This fat-soluble vitamin is essential for making sure cal-cium is absorbed and then deposited into bones. Our bodies can manufac-ture this vitamin when skin is exposed to sunlight. But in the winter months or if you always use sunscreen (which you should!), this source of vitamin D is unpredictable, so dietary sources become more important. Only milk and fortified soy milk are reliable sources of vitamin D in the diet. You must drink at least two glasses or one pint of nonfat milk or soy milk to meet your minimum requirement for this vitamin, or make sure you are out in the sun on a regular basis without a hat or sunscreen.

Low intake of vitamin D during pregnancy can adversely affect growth, bone mineralization, tooth enamel formation, and even normal calcium balance in you and your unborn child. Dr. Dawson-Hughes's research shows that increasing vitamin D intake, even without extra calcium, can help reduce bone fractures and slow the progression of osteoporosis. Poor intake also might increase the risk for giving birth to a low-birth-weight baby. Congenital rickets, a condition in the newborn characterized by malformed bones, knocked knees or bowlegs, skull malformations, and deformed rib cage, is the most common result of poor dietary intake of vi-tamin D. Low intake of vitamin D when breast-feeding reduces amounts of the vitamin in the milk, so a baby is even more dependent on sunlight to get enough of this bone-building nutrient.

Getting enough vitamin D is essential, but getting too much can be dangerous. Vitamin D is a fat-soluble vitamin and can accumulate in the body to potentially toxic levels with excessive intake. Make sure your total day's intake from fortified foods, milk, soy milk, and supplements does not exceed 100 to 200 percent of the RDA for vitamin D, or a total of 200 IU to 400 IU. Don't worry about getting too much vitamin D from sun exposure; your body will regulate how much vitamin D is made based on need, not exposure.

TABLE 3.3

What Foods Supply Magnesium?

Food	Amount	How Much? (mg)
Wheat germ	¼ cup	112
Peanuts	¼ cup	63
Banana	1 medium	58
Avocado	½	56
Cashews	9 medium	52
Milk, low-fat	1 cup	40
Brewer's yeast	2 tbsp.	36
Mustard greens	1 cup	31
Bread,		
whole wheat	1 slice	19
white	1 slice	5

Extra-Lean Meats and Legumes: B Vitamins, Trace Minerals

Most people equate this group with protein, but meat and legumes also are the best sources of iron, magnesium, zinc, vitamin B_6, and other B vitamins. Dried beans and peas and lentils are excellent sources of fiber and, except for soybeans, are essentially fat-free. Extra-lean meat, chicken, and fish also supply vitamin B_{12}.

Vitamin B_6: Vitamin B_6 is essential in the buildup and breakdown of carbohydrates, proteins, and fats; however, its main function is building proteins. That means vitamin B_6 is essential in the formation of all tissues, from the brain and nervous system to the muscles. Hormones, enzymes, red blood cells, and neurotransmitters (the chemicals that relay messages from one nerve to the next) are all proteins dependent on vitamin B_6.

It is not surprising that low dietary intake of this B vitamin could have far-reaching effects on the physical, mental, and emotional development of your baby. Mothers who consume suboptimal amounts of vitamin B_6 during pregnancy are more likely than other mothers to give birth to babies who are irritable and not easily soothed. A deficiency is linked to reduced Apgar scores. Mothers and babies who have low blood vitamin B_6 levels also have trouble bonding after delivery.

The recommend daily intake for vitamin B_6 is 1.9 mg during pregnancy, a 0.6 mg increase over the prepregnancy allowance. Many women consume much less than this, averaging as little as 54 percent of their needs. In one study, only 6 percent of 400 pregnant and breast-feeding women met or exceeded their requirements for vitamin B_6. In addition, the adequacy of these standards has been questioned. Blood vitamin B_6 levels drop during pregnancy when women consume recommended levels, but are maintained with intakes two or more times higher than this, thus raising the suspicion that current recommended levels might not be enough to maintain optimal nutritional status. On the other hand, a pregnant woman should not consume huge amounts of vitamin B_6 without her physician's consent and monitoring, since this B vitamin can cause nerve damage at high doses.

Vitamin B_{12}: This B vitamin is important in the normal processing of energy from carbohydrates, protein, and fats; in the formation and maintenance of the nervous system; in the correct replication of the genetic code within each cell; and in the formation of all body tissues. Consequently, vitamin B_{12} has been indicated, along with folic acid, in the prevention of birth defects.

The most common symptom of vitamin B_{12} deficiency is a special type of anemia called macrocytic anemia (or pernicious anemia when the deficiency is caused by a lack of a digestive factor necessary for normal absorption of vitamin B_{12}). In addition, the nerves do not form or function correctly as a result of B_{12} deficiency, causing disorientation, numbness and tingling in the extremities, moodiness, irritability, and agitation, dimmed vision, and dizziness. Digestive tract disorders develop as a result of poor cell formation in these tissues. Fatigue and memory loss occur from the breakdown of the nervous system. Increased susceptibility to colds and infections result from faulty formation of white blood cells and other immune system cells and tissues. Poor cell production in the skin causes dermatitis and changes in the lips and tongue. While pregnancy does not dramatically increase vitamin B_{12} needs (from 2.4 mcg to 2.6 mcg), consuming enough to ensure optimal health and development of the baby is essential.

This vitamin differs from other B vitamins in that it is only found in foods of animal origin, such as meat, milk, and eggs. If a plant contains this B vitamin, it is because of bacterial fermentation, as is true in the case of fermented soybean products such as miso. Strict vegetarians who avoid all animal products must be especially careful to consume either vitamin B_{12}-fortified soy milk, supplements, or hefty amounts of other B_{12} sources, since there are reports of vitamin B_{12}–deficient infants born to vegetarian mothers.

Iron: A woman's biggest nutritional challenge is iron. As many as 80 percent of active women and 20 percent of women in general are iron deficient. Compared to men, women have almost twice the daily requirement for iron, but consume half as much in food. Pregnancy more than doubles your iron requirement, but has a minimal effect on your food allowance; consequently, the iron dilemma intensifies prior to, during, and following pregnancy. It's no wonder that one in every two women either enters pregnancy iron deficient or becomes anemic while pregnant.

According to Fergus Clydesdale, Ph.D., professor and head of the Department of Food Science at the University of Massachusetts in Amherst, a well-balanced diet supplies approximately 6 mg of iron for every 1,000 calories. Based on this ratio, you must consume at least 2,500 to 3,000 calories to meet your prepregnancy requirement of 15 mg to 18 mg (prepregnancy iron requirements are even higher if you menstruate heavily or have used the IUD for birth control). But women average well under 2,000 calories daily and consume as little as 8 mg of iron; consequently many women enter pregnancy already iron-depleted.

Iron deficiency can have serious consequences for you and your baby. As a component of hemoglobin in the blood and myoglobin within the cells, iron is the key oxygen carrier in the body. Poor iron intake means fewer red blood cells to carry oxygen to the tissues and your baby. Consequently, you are tired, have trouble concentrating, recover slowly after exercise, and feel weak. Poor regulation of body temperature and suppressed immunity increases susceptibility to infections and disease. An anemic woman also is more likely to miscarry. Blood loss during delivery can stress an already depleted system; the blood loss from a cesarean birth further depletes iron levels. Recovery after the baby is born takes longer, leaving you with less physical and emotional energy to adjust to the new baby and the hectic first three months before your baby is sleeping through the night. Your baby also is starved for oxygen. An anemic mother is three times more likely to deliver a low-birth-weight infant and twice as likely to deliver a premature infant than is a nonanemic woman. (See Chapter 6 for more on iron and fatigue.)

Iron deficiency is common in pregnancy, but should be differentiated from normal changes in blood iron levels. The expanding blood volume during pregnancy dilutes the concentration of iron-containing substances, such as the hemoglobin in red blood cells that carries oxygen to the tissues. Consequently, it is normal for hemoglobin and hematocrit values (typical tests for iron-deficiency anemia) to fall. However, these tests measure the final stages of iron deficiency, so a drop well below normal nonpregnant values in these scores indicates that a woman has been iron deficient for some time.

Serum ferritin is a much more sensitive indicator of tissue iron stores and the early stages of iron deficiency anemia. In one study, 112 out of 120 pregnant women (93 percent) had depleted their tissue iron stores to levels less than 20 mcg/L, even though all of these women had hemoglobin and hematocrit values within the normal range and were not anemic. (To get a rough idea of your iron needs, see quiz 3.1, "What Is Your Risk for Iron Deficiency?" at the end of this chapter.)

The iron costs of pregnancy are high. More than 246 mg of iron is stockpiled in the baby's tissues prior to delivery, another 134 mg is taken up by the placenta, and about 290 mg is used to expand the volume of the mother's blood. That equates to about 2.4 mg a day during pregnancy just to cover the iron costs of pregnancy. In addition, 1.0 mg or more is needed to maintain the mother's normal body processes. Since you absorb only about 10 percent of dietary intake (although iron absorption increases to as much as 50 percent during pregnancy in some women), you must consume about 30 to 60 mg or more of iron daily to ensure optimal iron status.

The iron in meat, called "heme" iron, is better absorbed than the iron in plants. While legumes, dark green leafy vegetables, and prunes are good sources of iron, as little as 5 percent of this iron is absorbed, while up to 30 percent of the iron in meat is absorbed. You don't need to guzzle sixteen-ounce steaks! Adding a small amount of meat to a dish with iron-rich plants increases the absorption of the plant iron. For example, adding extra-lean ground sirloin to spaghetti sauce or bits of lean meat to chili beans boosts the iron from both the pasta and the beans. (See Table 3.4, "The Balancing Act," for additional ways to boost iron absorption.)

The Baby-wise Diet provides about 18 mg of iron daily, so you will need to consider a supplement. Even with a good diet and supplementation, it may take up to two years to restock iron stores after pregnancy and return serum ferritin levels to optimal levels. (See Chapter 1 for more information on iron and the prepregnancy diet and Chapter 10 for more information on iron and preparing for the next pregnancy.)

Copper: This trace mineral is found in all tissues, but is especially high in the brain, heart, kidney, and liver. It is essential for the development and maintenance of your baby's heart, arteries, and blood vessels; the skeletal

---

TABLE 3.4

The Balancing Act

Iron intake involves a balance between iron promoters and iron inhibitors, and entails more than just eating iron-rich foods. Here are a few ways to maximize your promoters to guarantee you get the most from your diet:

1. Always consume a vitamin C–rich food with every meal, such as orange juice, a tossed salad, broccoli, or most fruits. Vitamin C improves the absorption of iron and counteracts some of the inhibitors in foods, such as phytates in whole grains and tannins in tea and coffee.
2. Consuming small amounts of red meat, such as extra-lean beef, with large amounts of iron-rich plants, such as split pea and ham soup, increases the absorption of the plant iron.
3. Cook in cast-iron skillets. The iron leaches out of the pot into the food, raising the iron content of the meal. Try this trick with Chunky Spaghetti Sauce in the recipe section.
4. Select iron-fortified foods.
5. Drink tea and coffee between meals. Tannins in these beverages (even if they are decaffeinated) reduce iron absorption by up to 80 percent if consumed with the food.
6. Take iron supplements on an empty stomach to improve absorption.

---

system; and the nervous system. Copper also is important in the development and maintenance of red blood cells, normal hair, and skin color.

Studies on animals show that a copper deficiency during pregnancy increases the risk for birth defects and spontaneous abortions, while increasing copper intake improves survival rates and reduces nerve damage and spontaneous abortions. Researchers at the University of California, Davis, state that copper deficiency during pregnancy results in numerous gross structural and biochemical abnormalities that affect free-radical defenses, connective tissue metabolism, and energy production in the developing baby's tissues. Even marginal copper deficiency might contribute to the more than 50 percent of human conceptions that fail to implant, the 30 percent that implant but fail to reach term, and the 3 percent of births with serious congenital malformations.

The only reported risk for copper deficiency in humans is when pregnant women take the drug penicillamine, which depletes copper from the tissues. However, the diets of many pregnant women might be marginal, since blood levels often are low and optimal copper status often is achieved only when women take multiple vitamin and mineral supplements that contain copper. The Baby-wise Diet supplies at least the recommended intake of 1.5 mg to 3.0 mg, so a supplement should not be necessary if you are eating according to this plan. Besides meat, legumes, and seafood, other good sources of copper include whole grains, nuts, seeds, and baked potatoes.

Beware of cooking acidic food such as spaghetti sauce or tomato-based soups in copper cookware. Cooking in copper pots destroys vitamin C, vitamin E, and folic acid and can increase the copper content of food to potentially toxic levels. While copper-bottomed stainless steel cookware is safe, avoid using copper pans that are not well lined.

Zinc: This trace mineral plays center stage from conception through delivery. Zinc is essential for the formation of sperm and the ovum, ovulation, and fertilization. During pregnancy, even a marginal zinc deficiency increases a woman's chance of having a spontaneous abortion and other complications, pregnancy-related toxemia, an extended pregnancy or premature delivery, and prolonged labor.

The baby also suffers. In studies on animals, pups born to mothers who are marginally nourished in zinc have an increased likelihood of malformation (including cleft palate and lip, brain and eye malformations, and numerous abnormalities of the heart, lung, and urogenital system), retarded growth, poor bone development, reduced taste acuity, visual impairment, and low birth weight.

Similar problems have been noted in humans. For example, malformations, preterm deliveries, and spontaneous abortions are more common in women with low blood zinc levels than in women with optimal zinc status. Zinc status is so important for pregnancy outcome, that researchers at the University of Alabama recommend checking the mother's blood zinc concentration during early pregnancy as a screening technique for preventing low-birth-weight infants.

Zinc also has lifelong effects on the well-being of your baby. Low zinc intake might contribute to the development of neural tube defects. Zinc-deficient babies also are less likely to survive, have compromised immune systems so are more susceptible to infections, show developmental and behavioral problems, and have a delayed onset of puberty later in life.

Why is zinc so critical to health? Zinc is needed every minute of pregnancy for all phases of growth and tissue maintenance. It stabilizes the genetic code in every cell and, therefore, maintains normal tissue growth and development during pregnancy. Zinc also plays an active role as a component of insulin, the hormone that regulates blood sugar—the primary energy source that fuels the baby-making process. In addition, zinc helps maintain the normal acid-base balance in the body, helps produce hormonelike compounds called prostaglandins that regulate numerous body processes, and aids in the functioning of the oil glands of the skin.

Pregnant women's diets are sometimes low in zinc. The requirement during pregnancy is 15 mg. Yet, many women consume only 9 mg to 10 mg daily. Fortunately, your body boosts absorption of this mineral when you breast-feed, possibly in response to the increased demand for zinc to manufacture milk. Your zinc needs will be met if you follow the Baby-wise Diet, especially if you regularly consume zinc-rich foods, such as seafood, extra-lean meats, whole grains, and legumes. However, if you are a vegetarian or cannot always eat well, a moderate-dose multiple vitamin and mineral supplement that contains 15 mg to 20 mg of zinc provides safe nutritional insurance.

Food or Supplements?

Eating well is a must during pregnancy. In every case, wholesome, minimally processed foods are your best source of vitamins, minerals, fiber, and other nutrients, and your only source of phytochemicals. For one thing, food supplies these nutrients in the proper ratio and balance, so your chances of consuming too little or too much or of creating a secondary deficiency by consuming excessive amounts of one at the expense of other nutrients is not likely.

In addition, a nutrient never works alone; vitamins and minerals always work as a team in any and all body processes. Calcium builds strong bones, but only with the help of magnesium, vitamin D, zinc, and other nutrients. Iron builds oxygen-rich blood, but only if the diet also supplies ample amounts of vitamin B_{12}, folic acid, vitamin C, vitamin B_6, and other vitamins and minerals. Science only understands a small part of this teamwork and until more is known, it is safe to say Mother Nature probably knows best how to mix and match nutrients for your and your baby's well-being.

Science knows even less about phytochemicals. Although we know that chemicals called indoles in cabbage reduce your risk for cancer and saponins in beans might lower your cholesterol, how these, and other as yet unidentified, compounds work together or with the nutrients is still to be explored, so a good diet is essential, with supplements as a backup for nutritional insurance.

It's obvious that women must take this nutrition more seriously, because adequate isn't good enough when it comes to building a better baby. Small changes are worthwhile, but don't stop there. You know how to push the limits when it comes to everything, from exercise to work deadlines. Now it's time to stretch a little to reach your nutritional potential for the health of your baby and the ease of your pregnancy. Making changes might seem time consuming at first, but the extra time up front is worth it when those goals become habit and you know you have given your baby the best possible start in life.

Quiz 3.1　What Is Your Risk for Iron Deficiency?

Answer the following questions yes or no.

_____ 1. When not pregnant, do you have heavy menstrual bleeding?
_____ 2. Do you eat less than 3 ounces of red meat every day?
_____ 3. Do you often skip a vitamin C–rich fruit, such as an orange or a dish of strawberries, with your meals or snacks?
_____ 4. Do you consume less than 2,500 calories daily of wholesome, minimally processed foods?
_____ 5. Do you exercise regularly?
_____ 6. Do you regularly take aspirin?
_____ 7. Have you donated blood in the past year?
_____ 8. Are you currently pregnant?
_____ 9. Have you been pregnant with another baby in the past two years?
_____10. Do you take iron supplements sporadically or not at all?

Although there is no set number of yes answers that will guarantee you are iron deficient, the more times you answered yes to the above questions, the more likely you are to be marginally nourished in this essential mineral. The best way to check is to request a serum ferritin test from your physician and ask to see the results. A score less than 20 mcg/L is a clear sign you are iron deficient.

❧

Chapter 4

Your Changing Body:
What to Expect

Before and throughout your pregnancy be sure to take care of:

1. **Nutrition:** Follow the Baby-wise Diet.
2. **Exercise:** Exercise daily.
3. **Safety:** Refrain from smoking, drinking alcohol, or taking any drugs or medications without your physician's approval. Wear your seat belt. Avoid hot tubs or saunas, especially during the first trimester when the risk for birth defects is highest. Notify health-care providers that you are pregnant before having any X rays. Read all labels for warnings and directions before you use cleaners, bug sprays, paint, and other chemicals.
4. **Medical/Dental Visits:** Keep all of your physician appointments. If you miss one, call and reschedule rather than wait until the next month. Brush and floss your teeth daily and see your dentist at least every six months.

Whether you are in touch with your body or you race through life barely aware of your body's subtle ups and downs, the next nine months of pregnancy (as well as the first few months after the baby is born) are likely to bring some surprises—physically, emotionally, and mentally.

Whereas a slight slump in your afternoon energy level prior to pregnancy was a minor inconvenience, the same symptom during pregnancy can escalate rapidly to exhaustion with no warning. The shrimp salad that sounded so good when you ordered it, now triggers an overwhelming surge of nausea when set in front of you. You are in a great mood one minute and sobbing the next. Even women who take pride in their self-control say they often had no idea how they would be feeling from one minute to the next during their pregnancies. While the first pregnancy usually brings the most surprises, subsequent pregnancies are seldom carbon copies of the first and usually come packaged in their own set of unique experiences.

Pregnancy can be one of life's little lessons, reminding us that we are only partly in control. On the other hand, at no other time in life is a woman more aware of her connection to a greater purpose. Many of the ups and downs of pregnancy are natural rhythms resulting from dramatic physical changes that must take place to build a new person. You can't stop Mother Nature—she's doing what she does best—but you do have some say over how you react to these changes.

Learning about your body's changes during pregnancy can help you understand why you are exhausted one minute and elated the next, why you crave foods you never would have eaten before pregnancy, or why at nine months it takes you longer to get off the couch than it used to take to run a mile! Your body will be experiencing some very dramatic changes and it knows how to do it all with no help from you. Knowing how that new life is forming inside you can help you be patient with the process and develop a deep appreciation for the miracle of life; this positive attitude will help foster an easier pregnancy and a healthy baby.

Your Pregnant Body from Head to Toe

Every part of your body, from the top of your head to the tip of your toes, is affected by the baby-making process. Long before your tummy begins to protrude or the scale shows a gain in weight, you'll feel the changes.

Throughout pregnancy, the most obvious changes are in your uterus, blood, breasts, and fat stores. Your pulse rate also increases, the heart enlarges, skin temperature rises, appetite fluctuates from nil to famished, nutrient absorption increases in the intestines, and your ligaments soften. Your body will secrete more than thirty different hormones, many of which are only present during pregnancy, while others such as estrogen are normally present, but now their levels are altered by the pregnant state. (See Table 4.1, "Hormones during Pregnancy: The Short List.")

Your uterus, which is usually a solid, pear-shaped organ, will expand and increase hundreds of times in volume. The walls will thicken to protect your fragile developing baby, and later will thin to accommodate changes in your growing baby's size and position. The lower end of the uterus, called the cervix, softens during pregnancy and forms a mucus plug that protects the uterus from bacterial infection.

TABLE 4.1

Hormones during Pregnancy: The Short List

Hormone	Primary Source	What Does It Do?
Estrogen	Placenta	Influences mood, alters thyroid function, controls growth and function of uterus, increases flexibility of connective tissues which facilitates delivery, causes fluid retention and puffiness or swelling, alters taste and smell
Progesterone	Placenta	Slows stomach emptying, stimulates fat accumulation in mother, increases urinary loss of salt, influences mood, relaxes uterus to allow growth, relaxes other muscles in digestive tract that allows increased nutrient absorption and constipation, increases respiration
Human placental lactogen (HPL)	Placenta	Increases availability of blood sugar
Human growth hormone (HGH)	Pituitary (brain)	Increases blood sugar, stimulates bone growth
Human chorionic thyrotropin (HCT)	Placenta	Stimulates thyroid function
Thyroxine	Thyroid gland	Regulates metabolism
Parathyroid hormone (PTH)	Parathyroid gland	Increases calcium absorption
Insulin	Pancreas	Reduces blood sugar levels, promotes energy production, aids in fat storage
Glucagon	Pancreas	Increases blood sugar
Calcitonin	Thyroid gland	Inhibits calcium loss from bone

TABLE 4.1   continued

Aldosterone	Adrenal glands	Maintains salt balance
Cortisone	Adrenal glands	Helps regulate glucose and protein metabolism
Renin-angiotensin	Kidneys	Regulates salt and water retention, increases thirst

If you are healthy, gain sufficient weight, and eat well, your blood volume will increase by about 50 percent. This increase is an indicator of your pregnancy outcome, since women who have a small increase in blood volume compared to women with a normal increase are more likely to have stillbirths, spontaneous abortions, and low-birth-weight infants. Another example is your skin. Both "pregnancy glow" and the dark blotches on the face, upper lips, cheeks, or forehead (a condition called chloasma or pregnancy mask) could result from changes in hormones.

Since the physical changes of pregnancy are too complicated to describe in detail, the following is a summary of how the changes in your body correspond to the growth of your baby.

The First Trimester (Weeks 1 through 13)

During the first three months of pregnancy, your body must adapt to very dramatic changes. The female hormones—estrogen and progesterone—are elevated, while another hormone called human chorionic gonadotropin (HCG) enters the bloodstream and maintains the growth of the uterine lining, called the endometrium, by keeping levels of estrogen and progesterone high. (HCG eventually will give you a positive reading on your pregnancy test.)

Settling In: The first signs of pregnancy are subtle: a missed period, tender breasts (probably as a result of increased estrogen levels), frequent urination (caused by the expanding uterus pushing against your bladder), or a sleepy haze that comes over you late in the afternoon (possibly caused by the elevated progesterone levels). These are just the tip of the iceberg, however, in terms of what is going on inside.

The fertilized egg divides rapidly as it moves down the fallopian tubes toward the uterus, which will be its home for the next nine months. By the time it implants in the uterus, about six to eleven days later, it already is a hollow ball made up of at least one hundred individual cells. Some of these cells create a bubble that fills with fluid; this will eventually become the amniotic fluid where the baby develops, lives, and is cushioned and nourished. Out of this bundle of cells, which is increasing in number every minute, the inner cells differentiate and go about becoming a baby, while the outer cells will form the placenta and other membranes. (See Box 4.1, "The Placenta: The Nutrient Highway.")

By the second week, some of the new cells form a type of barrier surrounding the embryo, which now contains three layers of immature tissues that will continue to differentiate into the entire body. The outer layer, or the ectoderm, will develop into the brain, nervous system, hair, and skin. The middle layer, or the mesoderm, develops into the muscles, bones, and cardiovascular and excretory systems The inner layer of cells, the endoderm, will develop into the digestive tract, lungs, and glands. This marks the end of the first phase of pregnancy called the blastogenesis stage. At this point, if your menstrual periods are regular, you will notice you have missed a period and might suspect you are pregnant. Most of the nutrients your baby has needed so far have come from those stored within the surrounding tissues and fluids.

Weeks 3 through 8: The second phase of pregnancy is called the embryonic stage, which begins about the third week and lasts through the second month. Your baby now is one-tenth of an inch long and has developed a rudimentary brain with two lobes and the beginnings of a spinal column. By the fourth week, the placenta has grown deeper in the endometrium and now is passing nutrients to your baby and carrying away waste.

On about the twenty-fifth day, the heart is beating, blood is flowing, and arm "buds" appear, followed two days later by leg "buds." By the fourth week, other organs, such as the liver, kidneys, and thyroid gland, are visible. The embryo is now about the size of a grain of rice (10,000 times larger than the original fertilized egg!), has a primitive vascular system, but no face.

It is about this time that you will experience more pronounced physical changes. Nausea, vomiting, food aversions, or food cravings might begin. You might be overcome with fatigue as your body adapts to the radical changes. Changes in blood pressure might make you feel dizzy or faint when you stand up too quickly, so avoid sudden movements. The increased levels of estrogen and progesterone also might be the cause of bleeding, inflamed, or tender gums, called pregnancy gingivitis. (See Table 4.2, "Red Flags of Concern," on page 95.)

BOX 4.1   THE PLACENTA: THE NUTRIENT HIGHWAY

The placenta is the nutrition highway between you and your baby. In addition to its role in producing several of the hormones responsible for the regulation of your baby's growth and development, it is the vital pipeline for nutrients to and waste products from the baby and it forms a somewhat permeable barrier against some harmful substances.

The placenta is a network of blood vessels and tissues attached to the uterine lining and to the baby via the umbilical cord. The umbilical cord contains one blood vessel that carries oxygen and nutrient-rich blood to the baby and two different blood vessels that return waste products and carbon dioxide to the placenta. These umbilical blood vessels branch out into the placenta in fingerlike projections called villi. Blood vessels from the mother also project into the placenta and blood pools around the fetal villi. It is here that nutrients, oxygen, and waste products are exchanged.

One of the unique capabilities of the placenta is that it contains two separate blood supplies—the mother's and the baby's—that communicate, but never touch. Consequently, when the mother eats and digests food, the nutrients dump into her blood system and make their way to the blood vessels in the placenta. Here the fetal blood vessels pick up the needed nutrients, fluids, oxygen, and other substances and release waste materials that are excreted by the mother via the kidneys.

The placenta is not a true barrier and cannot protect the baby from harmful substances. Size and chemical structure, not potential toxicity, determine what crosses from the mother's blood into the baby's environment. Many drugs, chemicals, and medications can pass into the baby's bloodstream and influence development. Other substances, such as alcohol or vitamins A and D, can accumulate to toxic levels in the developing baby if they remain high in the mother's blood.

A well-nourished woman builds a better placenta. Research shows that the growth of the placenta is directly related to the mother's food intake. Even a marginal nutrient deficiency can have significant effects on the size and functioning of the placenta, which in turn affects the nutrient supply to the developing baby.

TABLE 4.2

Red Flags of Concern

While most of the changes, discomforts, and symptoms a woman experiences during pregnancy are normal, there are a few warning signs that should be immediately checked by a physician.

Symptom	The Concern
Bleeding or cramping	Could be a sign of miscarriage (often accompanied by the absence of pregnancy symptoms; that is, you no longer feel tired, nauseous, or your breasts are no longer tender). An ectopic pregnancy (where the fertilized egg implants outside the uterus) also might cause bleeding and is life-threatening to the mother. Bleeding late in pregnancy could indicate problems with the placenta.
Pain	Continuous pain could signal nonpregnancy problems, such as appendicitis, or could be a sign that something unusual is happening with the pregnancy. Abruption—premature separation of the placenta from the uterine wall—also causes pain.
High blood pressure	Usually identified by your physician during your routine checkup. Also called pregnancy-induced hypertension or PIH, preeclampsia, and/or eclampsia, it will cause no symptoms, but often is accompanied by sudden weight gain of more than two pounds in a week and swelling of the face and hands. Headaches, pain, or blurred vision (seeing spots) also are signs of PIH. Left untreated, PIH can progress and cause seizures in the mother and a stillborn baby.

Emotional changes also crop up probably as a result of hormone storms. You might feel more irritable, weepy, depressed, or anxious. On the other hand, you might experience a newfound joy, elation, and excitement about life, which could spill over into an increased sex drive. Many normal emotions are amplified during the first months of pregnancy. If this is an unwanted pregnancy, you may be angry or in denial. If this is a wanted pregnancy, you may be fearful of a miscarriage (in reality, about 10 percent of women experience an early miscarriage, while ectopic or tubal pregnancies affect only one in every one hundred women).

By the fourth week, your baby's eyelids begin to appear and will be formed and closed around the developing eyes within another week. By the thirty-seventh day, the nose has formed, while the ears take shape around the fifth or sixth week and rudimentary hearing begins during the second month. During the second month, the kidneys begin to function, the stomach produces some digestive juices, and blood is forming in the liver. Muscles also are developing and lengthening.

Even though your baby is only slightly larger than a coffee bean by the sixth week, the skeleton already has formed. The early skeleton is composed of cartilage; cartilage makes way for calcium-containing bone around the forty-eighth day. The fingers you will eventually count and the toes you will kiss also have taken shape.

By the end of the second month, the embryo is now called a fetus and is about the size of your big toe, with arms and legs thinner than spaghetti and skin as thin as waxed paper. You barely know you are pregnant, but your baby has weathered its most critical time. Developing properly during these first two months greatly increases the baby's chances for survival.

As early as the first month or two you will notice changes in your breasts. Your milk glands and ducts enlarge and fatty tissues form to prepare for breast-feeding. You might even experience tingling in your breast tissue during this time. Increased blood supply to the breast might cause blue veins to become temporarily noticeable, while the areola around the nipples might darken. Raised white areas, called Montgomery's glands, begin to secrete oil to keep the nipples lubricated.

The Third Month: While your uterus grows to the size of a grapefruit and your waistline thickens, your baby is developing a rudimentary personality. The first ridges of the fingerprints appear, a lifelong mark of individuality. As internal organs and the nervous system mature enough to communicate back and forth, the brain can now send signals to the body. The fluttering (called quickening) feeling in your abdomen as if you swallowed a butterfly (or a feeling like someone is blowing a fine stream of bubbles inside your belly) is your four-inch-long baby letting out a kick with her fragile legs and newly formed muscles. Most women feel these tumbles by weeks sixteen to twenty.

Babies at this stage also can bend their wrists and elbows or form a fist. Your baby's face looks more human now and can make facial expressions, such as a frown or a squint. The vocal cords also begin to develop around the tenth week. The ribs and vertebrae begin to calcify, bones form in the hands, the nail beds start to form, and tooth formation has begun.

The two bony plates that make up the palate are combining at this stage. By the twelfth week, your baby develops sexual organs. In fact, by the end of the first trimester, the baby has developed all of the major systems and is giving clues as to whether he or she will be rambunctious or quiet.

Your blood volume has increased 30 to 40 percent. You also might be thirsty or perspire more as a result of increased fluid requirements and metabolic rate.

Fortunately for many women, by the end of the first trimester, much of the hormonal upheaval that caused the fatigue, nausea, mood swings, and other annoying symptoms has subsided and the body is in full-pregnancy swing. Even though a frequent need to urinate might disrupt sleep patterns, many women report feeling better by the end of the first trimester and some say the nausea and fatigue seem to vanish overnight, leaving them feeling calmer, more accepting, and more energetic. For other women, symptoms lessen, but they still set aside time for a quick nap in the afternoon or continue to experience nausea. A few women battle serious nausea, fatigue, or other discomforts well into the second trimester, and some are relieved from nausea only when the baby is born.

The Second Trimester (Weeks 14 through 27)

Many women consider the second trimester the easy part. Most women no longer have the fatigue, nausea, and mood swings of the first trimester, while the awkwardness that comes in the final weeks of pregnancy is far away. The size of your baby rapidly increases in the second trimester. In the fourth month, your baby could fit into a teacup; by twenty weeks it is half the birth length; by the end of the second trimester your baby will be twelve inches or longer and will weigh about one and a half pounds.

The bones continue to develop, which causes the fetus to straighten from its curled position. The tiny heart is pumping quarts of blood through its body, the facial features are becoming more distinct, hair is beginning to grow, and the air passageways are developed even though the baby isn't able to breathe. The muscles are more developed, so the gentle flutters you felt before now turn to tumbles, rolling waves, kicks, pokes, and even hiccups as your small baby still has plenty of room inside the uterus to test his or her new abilities.

Sounds can penetrate the uterus. Although the mother's voice reaches the womb more readily than other voices, men's voices carry better than higher-pitched women's voices. Your baby now can hear you and most of the outside racket, and may startle at a sudden noise.

Even though the organs are well developed, your baby could not survive outside the womb at four or five months, because the lungs, digestive organs, and skin are not completely developed. Your baby also develops a downy coat (called lanugo), which disappears before birth, and a waxy protective covering (called vernix caseosa) to protect the delicate skin from the mineralized amniotic fluid in which he or she is bathed.

Your weight gain begins to pick up during the second trimester and should average about one-half to one pound a week. In contrast to the first trimester, during which your baby's growth was primarily focused on developing organs, tissues, and cells, the second trimester is a time of rapid overall growth in body weight. Your weight gain also reflects changes in your body. Your blood volume increases to accommodate the increased nutrient demands of the baby and also might contribute to nosebleeds, bleeding gums, and headaches.

Your breast tissue increases as it prepares for breast-feeding. Your nipples might start secreting small amounts of colostrum, a yellowish fluid that will nourish your baby in the first few days of breast-feeding before mature milk is produced. (Nursing pads placed in your maternity bra will catch any leaks.) The placenta continues to grow, and your body is building fat stores to ensure there is enough fuel for making milk after the baby is born.

Increasing body weight and an expanding tummy might change your posture as your center of gravity shifts toward your back to compensate for the baby's weight in front. The increased pressure on your lower back can cause backaches, which are best treated by sleeping on a firm mattress, wearing comfortable flat shoes, and bending from the knees, not the waist, when lifting. Leg cramps also might develop and are probably caused by the enlarged uterus pressing against the major vein, called the vena cava, that returns blood from the lower body to the heart. This squeezing effect causes the pressure in the veins of the legs to increase, which might result in leg cramps, varicose veins, hemorrhoids, and edema in the legs and ankles. The elevated pressure returns to normal when a pregnant woman lies on her side and also immediately after delivery.

In addition, the hormone relaxin is now released to help soften your ligaments around the pelvis and hips so they will stretch more easily during labor. This effect, however, also might make rising from a chair or any sudden movement more difficult.

The Third Trimester (Weeks 28 through 40)

Now you're in the homestretch of pregnancy. Your baby's main job for the next three months is to gain weight at a rate of about one-half to three-quarters of a pound a week! By the end of the eighth month, your baby will weigh four to six pounds. During the ninth month, weight gain averages two ounces a day! As your baby gets bigger, there is less room available in the uterus for tumbling, so the energetic quick kicks and pokes you felt during the second trimester might gradually be replaced by slow, strong turns; you might even notice a foot, elbow, or fist when the baby bumps up against the wall of the abdomen. Your baby also spends increasingly more time in the fetal position.

Your baby's brain also is growing and developing, which allows the genetic blueprint for personality to express itself. For example, some babies are in constant motion as if they can hardly wait to get out and get going; others are content to sleep and snuggle peacefully in the womb. One baby will be a "night person" and want to tumble until dawn; another might be more active in the morning. One baby will be irritated by hiccups and start kicking and thumping within minutes of a hiccup attack; another baby might seem unaware of the experience.

The wrinkly, reddened skin at five months now begins to smooth out as the layer of "baby fat" just under the skin begins to accumulate. This fat pad will help regulate body temperature and provide energy stores after birth. Fingernails grow beyond the tips of the fingers and toenails reach the ends of the toes. The eyes are slate blue, with their true color developing within a few months after birth.

Your expanding tummy and the pressure of the large baby, who is three times heavier at delivery than at twenty-eight weeks, might aggravate backaches; press against your diaphragm, making breathing more difficult; limit your stomach's capacity, making big meals an impossibility; and press on the pelvic veins, possibly causing some edema in the legs and feet, as mentioned above.

Sleep becomes a bittersweet experience. You might be more uncomfortable now and have to urinate more frequently, both of which interfere with a good night's sleep. Lack of sleep and the extra energy required to move might cause some fatigue and possibly some moodiness or irritability. Naps, elevating your feet, avoiding standing for long periods of time, daily exercise to keep the blood circulating, and general self-nurturing are essential now. You also might feel flushes of warmth probably because your baby's body heat is passing through the placenta and your metabolism is working overtime during this trimester.

Although active and growing, a baby at seven months usually can survive outside the womb only with specialized care in a neonatal nursery. (Some infants survive at earlier ages with intensive neonatal care.) By eight months, however, a baby has a good chance of survival outside the womb, even though some functions, such as the lungs and digestive tract, and the immune system, still might be undeveloped. During the ninth month, these tissues and systems mature and antibodies from your blood are transferred to the baby to provide protection against disease and infection. This passive protection continues if you choose to breast-feed.

By the ninth month, you and your baby are ready for delivery. About one to two weeks before delivery, the placenta begins to change in shape and function, becoming less fibrous and more tough, and its blood vessels begin to deteriorate. This signals the baby that it is time to make an entry into the world. You might experience Braxton Hicks' contractions, which are mild, irregular uterine cramps sometimes mistaken for labor. You will note that your baby has "dropped" or "engaged"—that is, settled into a head-down position—and moved lower into your abdomen (a process called "lightening" that happens as the baby positions itself correctly for birth). This might ease some of the pressure against your stomach and lungs and make breathing and eating a little easier.

A rise in estrogen levels boosts a last growth surge in the baby, but also causes the mother to retain more fluids. This results in some puffiness and swelling in the face, legs, ankles, and feet, a harmless condition that shouldn't be mistaken for the more serious edema of pregnancy-induced hypertension or PHI (see Chapter 6). The swelling is aggravated by gravity and the pressure of the growing baby and uterus on your blood vessels. Exercise will help circulation, while elevating your feet regularly and avoiding tight shoes or stockings (if you can even reach your feet anymore!) will help reduce the pressure on your veins and lessen the fluid accumulation in your ankles and feet.

Your cervix also becomes softer and begins to thin (efface). This action might expel the mucus plug that protected your uterus or even cause your water (the amniotic fluid that has bathed your baby for the past nine months) to break before you are in actual labor. On the other hand, you might not expel the mucus plug or have your water break until you are in labor. Labor begins when you start experiencing mild, rhythmic contractions that gain in intensity, causing your cervix to experience pro-gressive changes that ultimately lead to birth. Keep in mind that leakage of the amniotic fluid, with or without labor, is an indicator that you should see your physician.

How Diet Impacts on You and Your Baby

At every moment along the assembly line, your baby depends on you to provide the right mix of fuel, the optimal amount of the forty-plus nutri-ents, and regular feedings. From conception to birth, your baby's body weight increases from a fraction of a gram (less than the weight of an ant) to eight and a half pounds or more. From the eighth week of pregnancy to birth, your baby's weight increases more than four-hundred-fold! (See Graph 4.1, "What Makes Up Weight Gain during Pregnancy?") Your new-born's weight doubles from birth to four months and triples by the first birthday. That miracle demands optimal nutrition.

The diversity and rate of growth are greater during the first nine months prior to birth than at any other time of life. The first two years of life are the second fastest and most demanding growth period. Many growth processes that occur during these two critical periods happen at no other time in life; therefore, anything that interferes with this rapidly growing body could have lifelong consequences. While most of the changes in your body and your growing baby that occur during pregnancy proceed with no conscious help from you, your diet is one aspect over which you have complete control.

Weight Gain: Eating the best foods and gaining the right amount of weight affects your baby at every stage of pregnancy. In the first trimester, numerous factors including low prepregnancy weight or low weight gain can slow the baby's growth, including head circumference. As a result, a mother is more likely to give birth to a small for gestational age or SGA infant whose growth continues to lag behind the norm even into the first year of life. Slowed infant growth during the second trimester—caused by excessive exercise or fatigue, poor maternal weight gain, iron deficiency, and more—can contribute to a baby's risk for insulin insensitivity and a higher risk for diabetes, heart disease, and hypertension later in life. Poor infant growth in the third trimester impairs the growth of the baby's thymus, which is important in regulating the immune response later in life and preventing asthma. Interestingly, although a baby with poor growth in the last trimester might be of normal birth weight with shorter than average length, he is more prone to obesity later in life. Poor nutrition during pregnancy also affects your unborn baby's future fertility, intelligence, and risk for a variety of problems from polycystic ovaries to acne.

Optimal Nutrition: The development and growth of each organ, from the kidneys to the liver, and each tissue, from the muscles to the nerves, has its own pattern and timing independent of total body growth. Your baby's heart and brain are well developed in the first sixteen weeks, even though the lungs remain nonfunctional for months after that. During the first year, your baby's brain doubles in weight, but increases only 20 percent thereafter. Each organ and tissue needs the nutrients essential for growth and development during intensive growth spurts. Poor dietary intake at one point during your pregnancy might affect the heart, while at another time the nerves might be affected. Luckily, your body is very adaptable and will focus all of its efforts on building a beautiful baby, even if nausea or other pregnancy-related problems keep you from eating perfectly. Your goal during pregnancy is to eat as well as you can, when you can.

Your Diet and the Placenta: Your diet also determines the health of the placenta, which feeds your baby. Consuming enough calories and protein, exercising in moderation and not too vigorously, avoiding emotional

GRAPH 4.1

What Makes Up Weight Gain during Pregnancy?

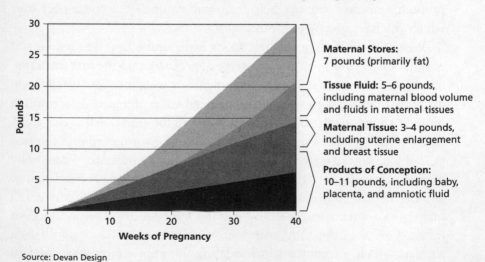

Maternal Stores:
7 pounds (primarily fat)

Tissue Fluid: 5–6 pounds, including maternal blood volume and fluids in maternal tissues

Maternal Tissue: 3–4 pounds, including uterine enlargement and breast tissue

Products of Conception:
10–11 pounds, including baby, placenta, and amniotic fluid

Source: Devan Design

stress, and not smoking are just some of the factors that improve placental growth. In contrast, a poorly developed placenta is associated with an increased risk for high blood pressure, diabetes, heart disease, and blood clotting problems later in your baby's life.

Critical Periods

Nutrition begins at the very foundation of our being—the cell. Organs and tissues are composed of specialized cells. The cells of the brain look, act, and respond differently than the cells of the muscles, liver, eyes, skin, or bones.

The cells of each organ or tissue also have specific times for production and growth that do not correspond necessarily with the organ's growth cycle. For example, in the developing baby's brain there is an early stage when the cells increase dramatically in number. Each time a brain cell divides, it produces two cells that are half its original size. These two cells do not grow but, rather, divide again, producing four smaller cells. During this stage, the size of the brain does not increase, despite a substantial increase in cell numbers. It is only later, when the millions of new cells begin to grow in size while continuing to divide, that the size and number of brain cells increase and the brain grows larger and heavier.

It is during these two critical periods of development—the time of increasing cell number and the time of increasing cell size and number— that the total number of cells in the brain is determined for life. Later still, cell division stops and only the size of the existing cells continues to grow. This third stage, when the total number of brain cells is fixed and only size increases, is when the most intensive growth appears to be happening, but actually, the most important events already have occurred. Because cell division is so rapid, an optimal supply of calories, vitamins, minerals, protein, omega-3 fats, and other essential tissue-building nutrients is needed every second during these critical periods. The importance of having all the essential nutrients available to the brain, or any other organ or tissue, during these critical periods cannot be overemphasized.

The stage of cell division in a particular organ or tissue is a "critical period" because the cell changes occurring at that time can take place *only* at that time. Poor nutrition during a critical period results in reduced numbers of cells in that organ or tissue, such as the heart, brain, or muscles. In contrast, poor nutrition throughout pregnancy results in a reduction in both number and size of cells (and possibly abnormal functioning

of cells) in all the baby's organs and tissues, and in the placenta that nourishes the baby throughout the nine months.

Whatever vitamins, minerals, protein, fats, or other essential nutrients,
as well as calories and other environmental conditions, are needed during
a critical period must be present and supplied in optimal amounts on
time if the heart, brain, muscles, or any other organ or tissue is to reach its
full potential. Granted, nausea and other pregnancy-related problems can
keep you from eating perfectly every day of your pregnancy; however, if
you eat an excellent diet prior to pregnancy so that you enter pregnancy
with nutrient-packed tissues and then eat as well as you can throughout
your pregnancy, your baby should receive all the vitamins, minerals, and
other nutrients needed. Also, regular checkups and routine tests can help
you and your doctor monitor how your pregnancy is progressing. (See
Table 4.3, "Pregnancy Tests: A Sampling.")

What Is an Optimal Intake?

Everyone agrees that nutrition is critical to the outcome of your pregnancy. An optimal supply of calories and all nutrients is needed every
minute, every day, every week, throughout the nine months of your pregnancy. Determining these optimal levels of all the known vitamins, minerals, and other nutrients, however, is a complicated matter.

The Recommended Dietary Allowances (RDAs)—suggested levels of
intake for many of the vitamins and minerals—are the nutrient standards
used in the United States. Established by the Food and Nutrition Board of the
National Research Council, the RDAs provide dietary intake guidelines for

- calories
- protein
- the fat-soluble vitamins A, D, E, and K
- the water-soluble B vitamins and vitamin C
- the minerals, including calcium, phosphorus, iodine, iron, magnesium, selenium, and zinc

An additional table of "safe and adequate daily dietary intakes" provides
ranges of intakes for the B vitamins biotin and pantothenic acid, copper,
manganese, fluoride, chromium, and molybdenum. Estimated minimal
requirements are set for sodium, potassium, and chloride. These recommendations are based on a woman's age, weight, height, and whether or
not she is pregnant or breast-feeding. (See Chapter 3.)

TABLE 4.3

Pregnancy Tests: A Sampling

Test	Who Needs It and When?	What Does It Tell You?
Blood type/ Rh factor	All pregnant women at first visit.	Maternal blood type and whether you're Rh-negative.
Hematocrit/ hemoglobin/ serum ferritin	All; early in pregnancy and at 32–34 weeks.	Check for anemia. Ferritin checks for pre-anemic iron deficiency.
Blood pressure	All; at every visit.	A sudden rise can signal complications.
Urinalysis	All; at every visit.	Protein indicates preeclampsia, glucose indicates gestational diabetes.
Alpha-fetoprotein	All; at 15–20 weeks.	Abnormal levels of AFP indicate Down's syndrome or neural tube defects. Might indicate multiple pregnancy.
Ultrasound	As needed.	Determines due date. Shows rate of growth, etc. Used to detect problems, gender, or to check confirmed conditions or health status of baby.
Amniocentesis	Women with history of birth defects or over age 35. At 14–18 weeks.	Diagnose neural tube defects or Down's syndrome.
Chorionic villus sampling (CVS)	Women with history of birth defects. At 10–12 weeks.	Diagnose chromosomal abnormalities.
Blood sugar	All; at 24–28 weeks.	Glucose in urine indicates gestational diabetes.
Group B strep	All; at 35–37 weeks.	Presence of bacteria that can be passed to baby at birth.
Hepatitis B (HBV)	All; once during pregnancy.	Blood test for virus that can be transmitted to baby at birth.

The RDA for each nutrient is designed to meet or exceed most women's requirement for that nutrient. To ensure the nutritional needs of most people while preventing potential toxicities from overconsumption of a nutrient, the RDA for each nutrient has been set at what the Food and Nutrition Board considers a reasonably high point, to meet or exceed the majority of people's nutrient needs. Theoretically, few women's requirements for any one nutrient would be above this recommendation. For example, the amount of vitamin C known to prevent scurvy is 10 mg, whereas the RDA for this water-soluble vitamin is set at 70 mg.

Since not all functions were considered when the RDAs were set, some nutrition experts question the accuracy of some of the RDAs. For example the role of vitamin E in heart disease was not considered when the RDA was established for this antioxidant nutrient; magnesium's roles in diabetes, hypertension, and heart disease were not included in setting the RDA for this mineral; and no RDA has been established for beta carotene alone, a potent antioxidant suspected to reduce cancer and heart disease risk. The latter is currently lumped with vitamin A, even though there is ample evidence that it often functions independently of its vitamin A activity. Other nutrients, in particular the omega-3 fats, are critical to your baby's development, but no standard amount has been set as optimal during pregnancy.

The RDAs are not perfect, but they are the only guidelines available. They are designed to meet the known nutritional needs of a theoretical "reference" person, that is the average woman or man with an average weight, body fat percentage, nutrient absorption and excretion rate, stress level, and heredity pattern. The "reference woman" is 5'4" to 5'5" tall, weighs between 128 and 138 pounds, requires about 2,200 calories/day, sleeps for 8 hours, engages in 2 hours of light physical activity, sits for 7 hours, stands for 5 hours, and walks for 2 hours each day. No one is that exact reference person. For all practical purposes, the RDAs are simply estimates of your nutrient needs. Many of the RDAs for pregnant women have been approximated from normal women's dietary intakes or from "typical" dietary intakes of pregnant women who appear healthy.

While people who are not pregnant have some room to experiment with different nutrient intakes, requirements of a woman considering or experiencing pregnancy are less flexible. The baby will be eating everything you eat, but is much more susceptible to nutrient toxicities. So during pregnancy erring on the side of moderation is your best bet.

What Should You Do? It is wise to strive for an average weekly dietary intake that meets about 100 percent, but no more than 200 percent, of the RDAs. While a little extra of any one nutrient won't hurt, excessive intake of several nutrients, especially vitamins A and D, is known to be dangerous, can upset the delicate balance between nutrients, and can result in secondary deficiencies of other vitamins or minerals, and even temporary or permanent damage to your baby. Vitamins in large doses act more like drugs than nutrients, and megadoses never should be taken if you are likely to become or already are pregnant.

The discovery of more than 12,000 phytochemicals in fruits, vegetables, whole grains, legumes, nuts, and other real food has forced people to take a hard look at supplements. While you can get recommended amounts of any vitamin or mineral from supplements, never will a pill replace food when it comes to the phytochemicals. Of course, your best bet is to eat your broccoli, whole grains, and legumes along with taking a moderate-dose supplement. Remember, at no other time in life does the well-being of another individual so directly depend on your well-being. When it comes to nutrition, don't settle for adequate. Go for the gold!

Chapter 5

Nutrition during the First Trimester

During the first three months of pregnancy pay attention to:

1. **Nutrition:** Follow the guidelines outlined in the Baby-wise Diet as closely as possible. In the case of serious morning sickness, eat when and what you can, but try to make it nutritious.
2. **Weight:** Try to limit weight gain to approximately two to five pounds (gain more if you entered pregnancy on the thin side, exercise intensely, or are tall, and less if you are short or were overweight and/or sedentary prior to pregnancy.) Do not use this time to begin or continue a weight-loss diet.
3. **Supplement:** Take a multiple vitamin and mineral daily that contains 100 to 200 percent of the Daily Value for all vitamins and minerals, plus at least 400 mcg of folic acid and 18 mg of iron.
4. **Safety:** Do not drink alcohol, use tobacco, or take any medication or drug not approved by your physician during pregnancy, if you have not already adopted this practice prior to conception. Be vigilant against food poisoning.
5. **Exercise:** Discuss with your physician your prepregnancy exercise schedule and adjust as needed.
6. **Medical Checkups:** Make regular visits to your physician to monitor weight and obtain necessary tests.

For some women the first trimester is a snap; for others, severe morning sickness makes it a nightmare. Most women fall somewhere in between with some fatigue, nausea, or changes in food habits. If this is your first pregnancy, you might as well enjoy the hormonal roller-coaster ride as your body generates physical and emotional cues that you might have trouble deciphering. If you've been through this first trimester before, the familiarity might help curb some of the symptoms and help you cope, but still expect surprises.

This is a time to pamper yourself. Take an afternoon nap, whether you are at home or at the office. Leave the dishes in the sink and relax. Let the lawn grow up to your knees while you soak in a warm (not hot!) bubble bath. Your body is adapting to an incredible upheaval in internal chemistry, so don't expect to conduct business as usual. You are producing a new life, so put your feet up when you can and revel in the process!

TABLE 5.1

You're Pregnant!

The first signs that you're pregnant might include:
   A missed period
   Tender breasts
   Increased sensitivity to odors
   Feeling tired
   Slight rise in body temperature (1–2 degrees)
   A metallic taste in your mouth

When and What to Eat and Drink

The guidelines for the Baby-wise Diet are simple and easy to follow. You still can eat your favorite foods, enjoy your favorite recipes, and go to your favorite restaurants; just make sure you first eat the number of nutritious foods in the Baby-wise Diet. You should consume a diet similar to your prepregnancy diet, or have at least:

   2 servings from the Calcium-Rich Group
   5 servings from the Vegetable Group—at least 2 servings should be folic acid–rich choices
   3 servings from the Fruit Group—at least 2 servings should be vitamin C–rich choices
   6 servings from the Grain Group—at least 4 servings should be whole-grain choices

2 servings from the Extra-Lean Meat and Legumes Group—try to
include 2 to 3 servings of fish and 4 to 5 servings of legumes in the
weekly menu

5 servings from the Quenchers Group

Now you can eat all you want, right? Not quite. Your daily energy
needs during the first trimester are the same as they were before pregnancy, with an average of 2,000 to 2,200 calories during prepregnancy
and the first trimester and 2,300 to 2,500 calories for the remaining two
trimesters. (Keep in mind that calorie needs vary greatly from one pregnant woman to the next). Your best indicator of how much you can eat is
the scale; if you are eating the right amount of calories you will gain
weight in a pattern that approximates that in Chart 5.1, "Monitoring Your
Weight Gain," on page 115, while too little food means you'll gain too little weight and too much food will cause too rapid a weight gain.

When it comes to vitamins and minerals, you definitely are eating for
two in the first trimester. During the first three months of pregnancy, you
must consume more nutrients for the same amount of food and calorie
intake, which means every bite counts. That is why the Baby-wise Diet is
packed with nutrient-dense, low-calorie foods; this ensures that every
calorie supplies a whopping dose of nutrients. In contrast, a high-fat or
high-sugar diet that contains too many processed foods supplies few vitamins and minerals per calorie and is called "nutrient poor."

Never has diet been so important. For example, women who eat well
significantly lower their risk for miscarriage in the first trimester, according to a study from the University of Milan in Italy. The dietary habits of
women who gave birth at term to healthy infants were compared to 912
women admitted for spontaneous abortions within the twelfth week of
pregnancy. The risk for spontaneous abortion was inversely related to the
woman's intake of green vegetables, fruit, milk, cheese, fish, and eggs. Risk
was 70 percent lower when mothers ate lots of fruit, 50 percent lower
with adequate cheese intake, 40 percent lower with lots of vegetables and
adequate milk, and 30 percent lower with the addition of eggs and fish.
Diets too high in fatty foods raised abortion risk up to twofold.

The dietary guidelines and menus outlined in this book are just the
beginning if you exercise during pregnancy. You might require calorie
intakes of up to 3,000 calories or more, depending on how often and how
hard you exercise. You should take extra precaution to eat enough food to
maintain a steady weight gain.

Make sure to include fish in your weekly diet. A study from the Netherlands found that intakes of both fish and some B vitamins improved growth in developing babies. While no recommendations for fish oils have been set, researchers at the Canadian Ministry of Health state that pregnant women should consume daily at least 250 mg of the fish oil DHA (the amount obtained from 1 ounce of salmon) on average to ensure adequate supplies for the developing baby and to stockpile this essential fat for breast-feeding. That's the equivalent of two 3-ounce servings of fish in your weekly menu.

Weight Gain and Why

Weight gain during pregnancy is a clear and direct indicator of how you and your baby will fare, and even whether or not your baby will survive. An optimal weight gain in the mother is associated with an optimal weight gain in the baby. If you don't gain enough weight, your baby is likely to be underweight, too.

A small woman is likely to have a small yet healthy baby, so don't be alarmed by that last statement. However, usually the body weight of a full-term baby reflects nutritional health or the nutritional environment in which the baby developed. So a normal-weight baby is most likely to be a healthy baby, while an underweight baby is most likely to be a malnourished one.

Why You Should Take Weight Gain Seriously

Women who do not gain enough weight are more likely to have premature babies. Birth is more likely to be complicated by problems during delivery when the baby is small than if the baby is at least six and a half pounds. Ironically, these low-birth-weight (LBW) babies (also called growth retarded or small-for-gestational-age [SGA] babies to distinguish them from premature babies) also are more likely to battle weight problems later in life, perhaps because the early malnutrition interferes with the development of that portion of the brain that controls appetite and food intake. For example, LBW infants

- often have smaller organs, such as the liver.
- might have abnormal blood sugar regulation, higher blood fat levels, and elevated levels of the stress hormones.

- are more likely to develop heart disease, hypertension, diabetes, learning disabilities, and behavioral problems when they grow up, as well as battle weight problems.
- are at increased risk for mental retardation, cerebral palsy, schizophrenia, and epilepsy, probably because of the reduced availability of nutrients and oxygen to the brain during critical periods of development.
- are more frequently hospitalized for illness.
- have more eye and hearing disorders.

These problems are easily prevented with good nutrition prior to and during pregnancy, adequate weight gain during pregnancy, regular physician visits, and avoidance of the toxic substances also associated with low birth weight, including tobacco smoke, alcohol, and drugs.

Optimal Weight Gain

Optimal weight gain is an individual matter. A normal-weight woman should gain about twenty-five to thirty-five pounds during her pregnancy. Women who gain within this range have babies closer to ideal weight and have fewer complications during delivery compared to women who gain less. Gaining up to forty pounds appears safe, but don't get carried away. You are eating for two, but that second person is a baby not a linebacker. Further weight gain beyond recommended amounts will not make bigger or healthier babies; it will make regaining your figure more difficult after delivery, might prolong labor, and could increase your risk for gestational diabetes and hypertension. In short, if you want that prepregnancy little black dress to fit after pregnancy, stick to a healthy weight gain.

Pace the Gain: Weight gain during the first half of pregnancy is very important to pregnancy outcome. In a study conducted at the University of Michigan in Ann Arbor, researchers found that optimal weight gain at twenty weeks' gestation was positively related to both the length of the pregnancy (these women were less likely to deliver prematurely) and birth weight. One-half of the infants who weighed less than six pounds at birth were born to mothers who had gained fewer than ten pounds by the twentieth week of pregnancy, while there were no LBW infants born to women who gained at least this much weight. Thus, it is not just total weight gain but the pattern of weight gain that is important—with a slow gain in the first trimester of about two to five pounds total (more if you are thin, very active, or tall and less if you are overweight, sedentary, or short), followed by a steady increase to approximately three-quarters to one pound a week in the last two trimesters.

"Total weight gain over the course of pregnancy is not a very clear marker of how the pregnancy is progressing. It's more important that women and their physicians watch for sudden changes in weight, which might alert a physician to other events, such as stress or changes in eating patterns," says Susan Carmichael, Ph.D., researcher for California Birth Defects Monitoring in Emeryville.

So, don't obsess over your weight. Aim for a twenty-five- to thirty-five-pound gain, but don't worry if you fall short or over this mark, as long as you gain steadily and are monitored closely by a physician. "Thirty years ago, women were told not to gain more than twenty pounds during pregnancy; consequently, some women took diuretics before their doctor's visits so they wouldn't be scolded for gaining too much weight. The last thing a woman wants to do is return to the days when weight gain was so restricted that it drove women to these harmful behaviors and created unnecessary anxiety," cautions Dr. Carmichael.

Weight Gain and Athletes: The exercising woman might gain more. "If you are leaner to start with," says Lindsay Allen, Ph.D., professor of nutrition at the University of California, Davis, "expect to gain more weight." Weight-conscious women often are distressed when they gain what they feel is too much weight. "These women shouldn't fight it. The weight gain is perfectly natural and will drop off after a woman stops breast-feeding," says Dr. Allen. According to The National Academy of Sciences and the Institute of Medicine, underweight women should gain approximately twenty-eight to forty pounds depending on their height and degree of leanness prior to pregnancy.

Curb the Cravings: Although you should gain only five pounds or less, your body and baby in the first trimester might scream "I'm hungry now!" How do you curb your overzealous appetite?

- Throw out the three-square-meals idea and instead eat mini-meals and snacks throughout the day. You'll feel like you're eating more and the frequent pit stops will help curb cravings.
- Drink more water, which has no calories but helps fill you up.
- Focus on fiber-rich fruits, vegetables, legumes, and whole grains, which fill you up without filling you out.

- Keep exercising to burn off any extra calories. Women who exercise throughout pregnancy gain about seven pounds less than pregnant couch potatoes.

Should You Diet? Dieting is never recommended during pregnancy, even if a woman is obese. Women who are overweight (more than 25 percent of body weight is fat tissue) should gain no more than fifteen to twenty-five pounds during their pregnancies. Better yet, women who are obese should lose weight prior to conception, since obesity is associated with preterm deliveries and increased health and delivery risks for both the mother and baby. (See "Monitoring Your Weight Gain.")

Supplements: The Right Dose during Pregnancy

Optimal nutrition is important throughout life, but especially during pregnancy. Now is the time to eat really well and supplement responsibly. There are good reasons for many women to take supplements prior to, during, and following pregnancy.

In a study conducted by the U.S. Department of Agriculture, only 6 percent of women consumed RDA levels of vitamin B_6 before and during pregnancy. Babies born to mothers who did not eat well during pregnancy also were low in many nutrients, including vitamins A, E, K, and B_2; folic acid; and the minerals iron, copper, calcium, and zinc. This poor nutritional status predisposes the infant to a variety of illnesses, from tumors, anemia, and poor digestive function to impaired brain function, suppressed immunity, and poor bone formation.

Do You Need to Supplement? National nutrition surveys repeatedly report that women do not get their fair share of many vitamins and minerals. Even women trying to eat well often fall short of optimal for numerous baby-making nutrients, including iron, calcium, zinc, folic acid, and vitamins B_6, D, and E. Bonnie Worthington-Roberts, Ph.D., former professor of nutritional science at the University of Washington in Seattle, says, "There are so many women counting calories that it often is difficult to squeeze in enough of all the nutrients, even if food choices are good. So, play it safe and take a moderate-dose multiple vitamin and mineral."

The stakes are even higher with folic acid. "Many women who have neural tube defect (NTD) babies don't know they are at risk. Rather than take the chance, it is wise to take a 400 to 800 mcg folic acid supplement prior to and during pregnancy," says Dr. Worthington-Roberts.

CHART 5.1   Monitoring Your Weight Gain

The following chart allows you to compare your weight gain during pregnancy to average gains for women who are underweight, normal weight, and overweight at the onset of pregnancy. The right-hand table provides space for you to monitor your weight after each weigh-in during routine physician visits and jot down notes, comments, or thoughts about your weight-gain progress.

Prepregnancy Underweight (·········), Prepregnancy Normal Body Weight (– – –), Prepregnancy Overweight (—————)

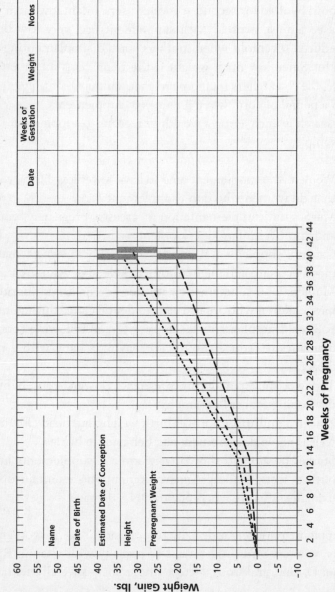

Name

Date of Birth

Estimated Date of Conception

Height

Prepregnant Weight

Weight Gain, lbs.

60
55
50
45
40
35
30
25
20
15
10
5
0
-5
-10

0 2 4 6 8 10 12 14 16 18 20 22 24 26 28 30 32 34 36 38 40 42 44

Weeks of Pregnancy

Date	Weeks of Gestation	Weight	Notes

Reprinted with permission from *Nutrition during Pregnancy and Lactation: An Implementation Guide.* Copyright 1992 by the National Academy of Sciences. Courtesy of the National Academy Press Washington, D.C.

Studies repeatedly show that women who supplement sensibly have a better chance of maintaining optimal nutritional status, avoiding serious pregnancy complications, and giving birth to healthy babies. In a study from the University of Medicine and Dentistry of New Jersey in Stratford, women who took prenatal supplements starting in the first or second trimesters showed a twofold drop in risk of preterm delivery. Very preterm delivery was reduced more than fourfold for first-trimester users and about twofold for second-trimester users. Infant low birth weight also decreased almost twofold with supplement use; very low birth weight was reduced sevenfold when mothers started supplementing in the first trimester. Since low birth weight is the main cause of infant death and disease, the researchers recommend that "an ounce of prevention may be worth a pound of cure" when it comes to supplements.

Research is uncovering a wealth of reasons to supplement responsibly. For example,

- Women who supplement tend to have fewer low-birth-weight infants than do women who don't supplement.
- Magnesium supplementation decreases pregnancy complications and improves infant development.
- Calcium supplementation reduces the incidence of maternal high blood pressure and might improve skeletal development in the baby.
- Mothers who supplement with fluoride or drink fluoridated water have children who are resistant to dental caries throughout life.
- Folic acid supplements taken prior to and following conception can dramatically reduce the risk for having a baby with a neural tube defect.
- Taking a multiple during pregnancy lowers your baby's risk for developing cancer later in life.
- Zinc in a multiple improves birth weight and head circumference, as well as nerve development and behavior in babies.
- Studies on animals show that vitamin E supplements help prevent birth defects, while pregnant women who maintain optimal antioxidant status are less prone to DNA damage.

Supplementation is especially important for some women, including women who are strict vegetarians (especially with vitamin B_{12}, calcium, vitamin D, zinc, and iron), lactose intolerant (especially with vitamin D, calcium, and vitamin B_2), carrying more than one baby, who smoke, or adolescent girls who are pregnant. However, to be on the safe side, most women before, during, and following pregnancy probably would benefit from a well-balanced, moderate-dose multiple vitamin and mineral supplement.

What and How Much to Take: The secret to supplementation is to do it sensibly. For healthy women, a multiple vitamin and mineral supplement is best. A multiple is a convenient, cost-efficient way to supply a balance of nutrients, while avoiding secondary deficiencies that result when you take too much of one nutrient and crowd out another. In general, 100 percent but no more than 200 percent of the Daily Value for a nutrient is sufficient. Do not take more than 100 percent of the Daily Value for vitamin A.

One exception to this rule is iron, which your physician might recommend in amounts up to 60 mg. You and your baby will need an additional 800 to 1,000 mg of iron during the next nine months. Granted, iron absorption increases during pregnancy, almost doubling from the first to second trimesters and almost tripling after that. You still will need to supplement if your serum ferritin levels fall below acceptable amounts (approximately 20 mcg/L).

Large doses of supplemental iron can cause constipation or diarrhea in some women. To sidestep this problem,

- Take an iron supplement that contains both heme iron (iron in the form found in animal sources) and nonheme iron (plant-derived iron), which might have fewer side effects.
- Take iron supplements in small doses throughout the day.
- Start the supplement program by taking a small dose, then gradually increase the amount to help offset digestive-tract problems.

Ideally, take your iron supplements with orange or grapefruit juice, because the vitamin C will help boost the absorption of this mineral. Do not take them with coffee, tea, or milk, which interfere with iron absorption.

Most one-dose multiples don't contain enough calcium or magnesium. Unless you consume at least three servings daily of calcium-rich milk products and lots of magnesium-rich soybeans, nuts, and wheat germ, you might consider an extra supplement of these two minerals. If you choose to take a calcium supplement, you also should increase your intake of magnesium to a ratio of approximately two parts calcium to every one part magnesium (for example, 1,000 mg of calcium and 500 mg magnesium). The mineral is best utilized when divided into several small doses daily, since the body can effectively digest and absorb only approximately 100 mg of magnesium at a time. Take your calcium-magnesium supplement at a different meal than you take your multiple, since calcium will block absorption of the iron in your multiple.

Lead in Supplements: Many calcium supplements on the market contain too much lead. At the University of Florida in Gainesville, the lead content was analyzed in twenty-one calcium formulations, including seven natural (oyster shell), fourteen refined brands, one prescription calcium acetate, and one noncalcium synthetic calcium binder product. The calculations were based on 800 mg and 1,500 mg per day of elemental calcium. Six micrograms/day of lead was considered the absolute dietary limit, with no more than 1 microgram being the goal for supplements. Results showed that four of the seven natural supplements contained about 1 microgram of lead per 800 mg dose and 1 to 2 micrograms for a 1,500 mg dose of calcium. Four of the fourteen refined products had similar lead contents. No lead was detected in the calcium acetate.

Despite these findings, don't stop taking your calcium supplements! Lead is ubiquitous in our environment and in our food supply. According to Dr. Robert Heaney, a calcium expert at Creighton University, a mixed green salad and glass of Chardonnay can contain ten to fifty times the lead in a calcium supplement. You can reduce your risk for exposure, however, by taking calcium carbonate, calcium citrate, or calcium malate and avoiding "natural" calcium supplements, such as bonemeal, dolomite, oyster shell, or chelates, since these often contain up to eleven times more lead. The good news is that calcium reduces lead absorption, so the actual amount of lead that makes it into the body is even less than the little bit of lead in these supplements. Finally, researchers at the University of Georgia in Athens state that vitamin C reduces lead absorption, so it might be possible to further reduce lead exposure by adding more vitamin C–rich foods to your diet.

Don't Overdose: While a moderate-dose vitamin and mineral supplement and extra iron and folic acid might provide nutritional insurance for many women, excessive intake of nutrients is dangerous during pregnancy. Megadoses of some nutrients, such as vitamins A and D, selenium, or fluoride, can produce numerous side effects ranging in severity from mottled teeth to birth defects.

There is always the concern that a supplement will provide a false sense of security, reducing a woman's concern about her dietary practices, which could result in poor food intake and possibly marginal intake of health-enhancing substances not found in supplements. This fear has not been supported by the research, however, which shows that most people tend to eat better, not worse, when they take a supplement. In all cases, consult your physician before taking a supplement during pregnancy. (See Table 5.2, "A Sample Prenatal Supplement.")

The Bugs to Avoid

Prior to this century, the link between diet and pregnancy was based on observations. Only recently has science developed methods for assessing a food's nutritional content. Previously, beliefs about foods were often colored by the emotional and mystical aura surrounding the pregnant state. Salty and bitter foods were discouraged for fear the baby would be born with a "sour" disposition. A woman was told not to eat eggs, because of their similarity to her own fertilized egg or ovum. On the other hand, broth, warm milk, and ripe fruits were thought to soothe the fetus, prepare the uterus for delivery, and ease the birth process. These and other more serious misconceptions about nutrition during pregnancy persist today, so use some common sense when given advice, and ask around if some "words of wisdom" seem suspicious.

Some warnings during pregnancy are well founded, especially when it comes to bacteria and food contamination. Listeriosis, a condition caused by the bacterium *Listeria monocytogenes*, can produce complications during pregnancy, including fever, miscarriage, heartbeat irregularities, and even death of the newborn. A woman considering pregnancy or already pregnant should avoid food sources of this bacteria, including cooked and chilled foods that are inadequately reheated, prepacked salads and coleslaw, uncooked or undercooked meat and poultry, pâté, or raw or unpasteurized milk. You also can reduce risk by:

- Using perishable precooked and ready-to-eat foods as soon as possible.
- Cleaning your refrigerator regularly.

- Using a refrigerator thermometer to ensure the refrigerator stays at 40° F or below.
- Eating hot dogs and other luncheon meats only if they are reheated until steaming hot.
- Avoiding refrigerated smoked seafood, unless it is part of a cooked dish, such as a casserole. The foods to avoid include "nova-style," "lox," "kippered," "smoked," or "jerky" fish such as salmon, trout, whitefish, cod, tuna, or mackerel found in the refrigerated section or sold at deli counters of grocery stores and delicatessens. Canned or fresh fish is fine.
- Avoiding soft cheeses, such as feta, brie, and camembert, or blue-veined cheeses and Mexican-style cheeses, such as *queso blanco fresco*.

TABLE 5.2

A Sample Prenatal Supplement

Three to four tablets daily provide the following nutrients.

Nutrient	Optimal Amounts
Vitamin A	800 RE/4,000 IU*
Beta carotene	10 mg
Vitamin D	5–10 mcg
Vitamin E	60 mg
Vitamin B$_1$	2.0 mg
Vitamin B$_2$	2.0 mg
Niacin	20 mg
Vitamin B$_6$	2.0 mg
Folic acid	400–800 mcg
Vitamin B$_{12}$	2.2 mcg
Vitamin C	100 mg
Calcium	1,000 mg
Chromium	100 mcg
Copper	1.5 mg
Fluoride	2.0 mg[†]
Iodine	75 mcg
Iron	30–60 mg[‡]
Magnesium	320 mg
Manganese	3.0 mg
Molybdenum	100 mcg
Selenium	65 mcg
Zinc	15 mg

*RE: Retinol Equivalents. 1 RE = 1 mcg of retinol or 6 mcg of beta carotene.
†No need for fluoride if your water is fluoridated.
‡Iron, in amounts greater than 18 mg, should be approved by a physician. The amount of supplemental iron often is high because this form of iron is poorly absorbed.

Toxoplasma gondii bacteria are excreted in cat feces and, if ingested, can result in severe problems for the developing baby, including blindness and mental retardation. Treatment of the pregnant mother with antibiotics helps reduce transmission of the infection to the developing baby. However, prevention is the best treatment and includes avoiding contact with anything that might be contaminated with toxoplasmosis, including uncooked or undercooked meat, unwashed fruit and vegetables, and cat feces (avoid the cat box, keep cats off kitchen surfaces, and wear gloves when gardening).

Skin and Hair Changes: Can Diet Help?

Skin and hair are sensitive indicators of your nutritional status. Healthy hair that is shiny, lustrous, firm, not easily plucked, and a healthy scalp and skin that is smooth, slightly moist, and has good color are outward signs of good nutrition. In contrast, dull, brittle, dry, thin and sparse, or easily plucked hair or rough, dry, scaly, pale, or bruised skin are common signals that nutritionally speaking, something is wrong.

Although most of the physical changes during pregnancy happen inside your cells, tissues, and organs, other signs are only skin-deep. In some cases these changes are for the better, as in the case of the pregnancy glow that some women develop, which is caused by increased blood flow to the skin. In other cases, the raging hormones wreak havoc with the skin's oil-producing glands, causing the complexion to take on an adolescent look akin to acne. In addition, other skin and hair changes are a direct result of lifestyle or nutrition, as in the case of pale skin that is a common symptom of iron deficiency or dry, scaly skin that might indicate too little linoleic acid (an essential fatty acid) in the diet.

There is nothing you can do about the hormonal changes and, unfortunately, rubbing vitamin E on your skin has not proved very effective in preventing stretch marks. But you can prevent any skin or hair condition related to a nutrient deficiency and, by maintaining a healthier inside, you will automatically foster a healthier outside.

Nourishing Your Skin from Within

All nutrients, including protein, calories, fat, vitamins, minerals, and water, play important roles in maintaining healthy skin. For example, the skin relies on the bloodstream to supply oxygen and nutrients and to remove waste products of cellular metabolism. Nutrients essential to the maintenance of red blood cells (the oxygen carriers in the blood) and other blood components include protein, iron, folic acid and other B vitamins, copper, vitamin C, selenium, and vitamin E. An inadequate supply of one or more of these nutrients essentially cuts off the skin's supply of oxygen and nutrients, while allowing potentially toxic waste products to accumulate.

Other nutrients directly affect the health of the skin. For example, an essential fat in vegetable oils called linoleic acid helps maintain smooth, moist skin. Skin becomes dry and scaly when the diet is low in this fat. A linoleic acid deficiency might be one reason why women experience dry, itchy skin when on very-low-calorie diets for prolonged periods of time. The condition is reversed within days of adding linoleic acid–rich foods, such as safflower oil, nuts, and seeds, to the diet.

Another example is vitamin C. This vitamin is essential for collagen formation, the "glue" that holds the body's cells together. When vitamin C intake is inadequate, collagen is poorly formed, the body bruises easily, skin loses its elasticity, cuts heal slowly, and the skin does not produce adequate amounts of lubricating oils. A glass of orange juice and a bowl of strawberries each day provides more than the recommended amount of vitamin C. (See Table 5.3, "The Nutrition and Healthy Skin Connection.")

The mask of pregnancy—those patchy brown spots on the cheeks, forehead, and upper lip—is caused by an overproduction of pigment, possibly triggered by hormonal changes during pregnancy. Technically called melasma, this skin condition affects up to 75 percent of pregnant women. Melasma that affects the outer layers of the skin, called epidermal, is sometimes treatable with bleaching creams. Avoiding sun exposure by using hats and sunscreen also helps prevent these dark patches.

Be good to your skin from the outside, too. Warm baths, lotions, and creams can keep your skin moist and soft. However, avoid hot tubs, saunas, and a soak in a hot bath during pregnancy, since this can raise body temperature and increase the odds of having a baby with a defect of the brain and spinal cord. In one study, researchers found that infants born to mothers who had used a hot tub were almost three times more likely to have these defects than babies with no heat exposure.

TABLE 5.3

The Nutrition and Healthy Skin Connection

All nutrients are related to healthy skin. Here are a few examples why.

Nutrient	The Skin Connection	Sources
Protein	Maintains underlying muscles and skin structure, elasticity, resiliency; maintains hormones that regulate skin moisture; regulates skin pigments.	Milk, meat, fish, chicken, legumes
Fat	Essential fatty acid maintains skin moisture. Deficiency results in scaly, dry skin.	Safflower oil, nuts, seeds, whole grains
	Omega-3 fats might reduce skin cancer risk.	Seafood, walnuts, flaxseed
Water	Maintains skin moisture; helps maintain normal oil secretion.	Water
Vitamin B_2	Deficiency causes blisters and cracks at corners of mouth, oily and flaky skin.	Milk, dark green veggies, mushrooms, asparagus
Niacin	Deficiency causes dermatitis.	Chicken, peanut butter, green peas
Vitamin B_6	Deficiency causes itching, dry skin; anemia.	Banana, meat, fish, chicken
Folic acid	Deficiency causes anemia; pale skin.	Dark green veggies; orange juice
Vitamin B_{12}	Deficiency causes anemia; pale skin.	Milk, meat, fish, chicken
Pantothenic acid	Deficiency causes dry, flaky skin.	Milk, chicken, peanut butter, veggies, rice
Vitamin C	Maintains oil-producing glands, collagen, skin elasticity and resiliency; antioxidant against premature aging. and skin cancer.	Citrus fruits, veggies
Vitamin A (beta carotene)	Maintains outer layer of skin; protects against skin cancer and premature aging.	Dark green or orange veggies
Vitamin E	Antioxidant against premature aging and skin cancer.	Safflower oil, nuts, wheat germ
Copper	Prevents anemia.	Oysters, avocado, potato, fish, soybeans
Iron	Prevents anemia.	Dark green veggies, red meat, legumes, dried apricots
Selenium	Antioxidant against skin cancer.	Organ meats, seafood, whole grains
Zinc	Maintains collagen and elastin; might prevent stretch marks; helps heal cuts; deficiency causes dry, rough skin.	Oysters, turkey, pork, wheat germ

Healthy Hair

A low-fat, balanced diet rich in several key nutrients is essential for the growth and life of shiny, strong hair. Hair grows from follicles, which are tiny sacs imbedded in the scalp that are fed by the bloodstream. The blood provides a constant supply of oxygen and nutrients and helps remove waste products from each hair shaft and its follicle. Therefore, a diet packed with the nutrients that promote circulation and hair growth, such as protein and several vitamins and minerals, is the first step in maintaining a healthy head of hair.

Vitamins: Because healthy hair is a reflection of a healthy body, all nutrients are essential for maintaining hair. Vitamin A helps the hair stay supple and the scalp healthy. The B-complex vitamins are crucial for maintaining circulation and hair growth and color. Vitamin C is essential for strong, supple strands of hair that do not break or split. A biotin deficiency also can cause hair loss; however, this is rare and seldom seen in pregnant women.

Minerals: Important minerals for healthy hair include iron, copper, and zinc. For example, the oxygen-carrying capacity of the blood depends on iron and copper. Inadequate amounts of iron can leave the hair and its follicles oxygen starved, while optimal iron intake and red blood cell levels allow a steady and ample supply of oxygen to reach all tissues, including the scalp and hair. Copper also helps in the formation of the hair pigment, while zinc is important in building proteins in the hair and preventing diet-related hair loss. All of these nutrients are supplied in ample amounts in the Baby-wise Diet.

Water: Water is the forgotten nutrient when it comes to both skin and hair. Almost a quarter of the weight of a strand of hair comes from the water locked inside it. This moisture provides suppleness to hair and moisture to the skin. In addition, the bloodstream is a watery medium that constantly needs replenishing to ensure proper circulation of the nutrients and oxygen and to remove the waste products from the scalp, hair follicle, and skin. If you meet your quota for Quenchers in the Baby-wise Diet, you will be getting enough fluid. On the other hand, coffee, tea, and caffeinated soda pop act more like diuretics and dehydrate skin and hair.

How to Take Care of Your Hair: The health of your hair starts from within, but also depends on how the hair is treated from the surface, including washing, drying, and other daily hair-care practices. If you shampoo daily, use warm water and a gentle shampoo that does not contain detergents; use one application; and dilute the shampoo by half. Brushing hair stimulates circulation to the scalp, detangles hair, and distributes beneficial oils from the scalp down the length of the hair. Avoid brushing hair when it is wet and limit the use of hair dryers and curling irons, which can leave hair dull, dry, and brittle.

Hair is susceptible to stress. Emotional stress causes the muscles in the scalp and neck to tense and restrict blood flow, which leaves hair deprived of oxygen and nutrients and interferes with the removal of waste products from the follicle. The stress of pregnancy and the fluctuations in hormone levels may result in hair loss. Don't worry, the loss is usually temporary. Environmental stress, such as sun, wind, or salt water, can leave hair dry, split, and lackluster. Some of these stresses can be avoided, for example, by wearing a hat in the sun, protecting the hair from wind, and washing hair after exposure to salt water. To minimize damage from unavoidable emotional or life-event stresses, it is helpful to improve the blood flow and nutrients available to the hair.

A Nutritional Approach to Common Problems: From Morning Sickness to Fatigue

The first trimester comes with a unique set of problems that can interfere with making the best food choices. Nausea and vomiting sometimes surface in the initial weeks of pregnancy and can foil even the best diet intentions. Chronic or severe fatigue can make even breathing an effort, let alone sitting down to a meal. While you might not be able to avoid these problems altogether, the good news is they usually subside by the end of the first trimester. You also can lessen their severity with a few diet and lifestyle tricks of the trade.

Morning Sickness

At a time when many women should be concerned about eating well for two, they find they cannot even eat poorly for one. The condition is called morning sickness and it affects two out of every three women during pregnancy. At best, it is a nuisance. But in the United States, at least 55,000 women a year experience morning sickness at its worst, with symptoms so severe they result in hospitalization. These numbers, however, might not be accurate, according to Miriam Erick, M.S., R.D., obstetrical clinical dietitian at Brigham and Women's Hospital in Boston and author of *No More Morning Sickness*. "We only record those women who are admitted to the hospital; there are likely many more women who come into the emergency room or who stay home and suffer through it."

Regardless of the exact numbers, the underlying message is that a woman who experiences any degree of morning sickness, from temporary queasiness to severe vomiting, is not alone. More importantly, despite the discomfort and inconvenience, women with mild morning sickness should not be too concerned about how their bouts of nausea will affect the developing baby. "In fact, morning sickness is a marker for a successful pregnancy. It is only the women with severe vomiting and nausea [a condition called hyperemesis gravidarum] who might be at risk and should be watched closely by their physicians," assures Dr. Irvin Emanuel, professor of Epidemiology and Pediatrics at the University of Washington in Seattle.

What Is It and Who Gets It? You don't need to explain morning sickness to most women who have been pregnant. Just mentioning the term can bring back all the miserable sensations. The primary symptom is nausea that may or may not be accompanied by vomiting, cold intolerance, and fatigue. Despite the name, morning sickness can strike any time of the day or night. In severe cases of hyperemesis gravidarum, the severe vomiting can cause dehydration, imbalances in electrolytes, high ketone levels in the urine, and other potentially life-threatening disorders that require hospitalization.

A woman in her first trimester is the most likely candidate, with approximately 40 percent of women reporting that morning sickness stopped suddenly toward the end of the first trimester. However, some women are still nauseated while they are in labor; and some experience nausea with all, some, or none of their pregnancies. The only absolute rule is there are no reported cases of morning sickness lasting after delivery.

What Causes It? Despite four thousand years of recorded reports of nausea and vomiting during pregnancy, this condition remains a mystery. Researchers at Cornell University in Ithaca, New York, suspect that nausea during pregnancy is an evolutionary adaptation, one that causes women to expel and avoid foods that might be harmful to the developing fetus. By avoiding certain foods, a pregnant woman might improve her chances of having a healthy baby, and so pass on the same aversion to the next generation. This theory seems plausible, since the foods women often are repulsed by in the first trimester, especially meat, eggs, poultry, and fish, were once the foods most likely to carry parasites and germs that could harm the developing baby and put the mother at risk. Other common triggers for morning sickness include caffeinated beverages, strong-tasting vegetables such as broccoli and cabbage, and spicy ethnic foods, all of which contain natural toxins that protect plants from pests but that also could have posed a health threat in the days before refrigeration and sanitation. In short, perhaps our age-old genes cause our bodies to respond to what used to be a threat.

Another theory is that morning sickness is brought on by changes in hormone levels, such as human chorionic gonadotropin (HCG), the hormone that indicates pregnancy in blood and urine tests. HCG levels are high during the first trimester, which correlates with the rise and fall of morning sickness in some women. Rising estrogen levels or slowed stomach emptying also have been blamed, while another theory points to the degenerative products given off by the fertilized egg implanting in the uterine lining. Although salt intake and cravings have been blamed for morning sickness, a study from the University of Washington in Seattle discredits this link.

Of course, emotional and psychological factors cannot be ruled out. Stress sets off bouts of morning sickness, while a restful environment often helps curb the nausea. Even hearing about an offensive food can make some pregnant women sick. Some nausea might become a learned response, an idea supported by testimonies from mothers who say they experience the same symptoms of morning sickness, but to a lesser degree, after pregnancy if they listen to music they repeatedly heard when they were pregnant. The knowledge that your body is going to change radically for several months can be distressing if you have worked hard to stay in control of your figure and fitness. For the working woman, the unpredictability and social taboo of nausea and vomiting can be devastating. These stresses add insult to injury.

Regardless of the cause, morning sickness is real; it does not reflect a lack of control, a neurotic personality, or a woman with misgivings about her womanhood, her pregnancy, or her baby. It requires support and encouragement, and a tool kit of strategies for getting through the storm.

Solutions—The Traditional Approach: Many women with morning sickness turn to dry or bland foods. Lindsay Allen, Ph.D., professor of nutritional sciences at the University of California, Davis, recommends "for mild cases of morning sickness, a woman should keep crackers or dry cereal with her or by her bed and nibble before she gets out of bed in the morning and throughout the day. This will help her avoid hunger and keep something in her stomach." Dr. Allen also recommends avoiding coffee, tea, or spicy or acidic foods. Other traditional recommendations include eating small, frequent meals and avoiding fatty or overly rich foods.

Carol Archie, M.D., assistant professor in the Department of Obstetrics and Gynecology at UCLA Medical Center, says "I don't worry about whether a woman gains weight in the first trimester, as long as she stays hydrated." Frequent, small meals that avoid overdistending the stomach might help. Eating when you can and trying to eat nutritious foods when possible also are basic survival skills recommended by all experts. (See Table 5.4, "The Traditional Approach.")

Solutions—Modern Methods: Although the traditional recommendations work for some women, they are not universal truths. Even though seven out of ten women use crackers in an attempt to feel "less horrible," many find little solace. Miriam Erick recommends a more personalized and systematic approach to morning sickness.

"I have women take a good look at what foods sound good at the time and then trust their feelings, no matter how bizarre," says Ms. Erick. During periods when the nausea is at bay (that is, no lower than a 3 on a scale of 1 to 10, with 10 being feeling fine), ask yourself questions such as, "What foods would make the nausea less bad—salty? sugary? liquid? dry? hot? cold? spicy? bland? soft? hard? Would a crunchy food settle my stomach?" If yes, "What color or flavor should it have? What food or beverage, no matter how silly, would have the most appeal right now?"

Also ask yourself what time of day you are most nauseated or whether a situation, person, or place triggers nausea. Then avoid these situations at all costs. (Don't worry about hurting someone's feelings by asking them not to wear that perfume or aftershave lotion or even to ask your partner to curb morning breath by brushing before the first kiss of the day.) Identify what places are most pleasurable to eat and eat there. Finally, when you feel your worst, what food, if presented instantaneously, would help you feel better? The results may surprise you. One woman decided that crunchy, cold, and sour foods sounded good and found she could tolerate raw carrots dipped in vinegar. Once she had eaten this "Band-Aid" food, she then could tolerate eating a few other foods.

Fresh ginger, peppermint, and chamomile also might be helpful, since these herbs/spices have reduced morning sickness in some women. Ginger is especially effective at delaying the onset of nausea and curbing the symptoms. On the other hand, play it safe with herbs in general. Little or no research has been done on the safety of herbs during pregnancy, especially the first trimester when all your baby's organs are forming. Just because herbs are natural doesn't mean they are safe. (See Table 5.5, "Herbal Teas for Two.")

TABLE 5.4

The Traditional Approach

There are no hard-and-fast rules for morning sickness, since effective treatments are as diverse as the women who use them. The first line of defense is to try the traditional approach, which includes the following:

1. Keep crackers, vanilla wafers, or dry cereal (such as shredded wheat bite-size biscuits) by the bed and eat a few before getting up in the morning; nibble on them throughout the day; and keep them handy in office desk drawers, a glove compartment, a purse or briefcase. Eat breakfast after nausea subsides.
2. Eat at least every two hours to avoid hunger and keep something in your stomach at all times.
3. Eat a high-protein snack at bedtime.
4. Avoid overfatigue.
5. Get up slowly (sudden movements can trigger nausea).
6. Have fresh air in the room when sleeping.
7. Avoid offensive cooking odors.
8. Drink beverages and soups in between meals.
9. Use fruit juices mixed with carbonated beverages, such as ginger ale or carbonated water, as fluids to settle an upset stomach between meals.
10. Drink fluids to avoid dehydration. Eat when and what you can.
11. Have someone else cook the meals.
12. Eat before you feel queasy.
13. Take a well-balanced, moderate-dose vitamin and mineral supplement for nutritional insurance.

Always consult your physician if morning sickness is disrupting your normal routine, since some cases of nausea during pregnancy might be a symptom of other medical problems. In addition, some antinausea medications are relatively safe for pregnant women experiencing severe nausea. Consult your physician about the options.

The Sniff Factor: Although many other factors can be trigger events for a bout of nausea—such as loud noises, quick movements, bright lights, hot or humid weather, and low-level claustrophobia—the most common and powerful trigger might be smell. "I found that smells are what drive most women over the edge," says Ms. Erick. If women use smell to their advantage, they can work with the morning sickness to find what breaks the nausea cycle.

TABLE 5.5

Herbal Teas for Two

Herbs are natural, but that doesn't mean they are harmless. Some can trigger allergic reactions, others are toxic, and still others contain active ingredients potent enough to be considered drugs. Take the warning of Varro Tyler, Ph.D., Sc.D., author of *The Honest Herbal,* when he says, "In effect, you're taking an untested drug."

Some herbs are safe and have been used successfully for centuries. For example, red raspberry leaf tea might prevent morning sickness and miscarriage, while helping strengthen and relax the uterine muscles. Gingerroot, lemon balm, and chamomile teas are safe treatments for morning sickness.

On the other hand, avoid:

- Mugwort, which contains thujone, a neurotoxin that might increase risk for abortion.
- Senna, cascara sagrada, and buckthorn, which are potent laxatives.
- Pennyroyal oil, which is said to promote menstruation.
- Juniper, rue, tansy, cotton-root bark, and male fern, which might induce abortion.
- Goldenseal, comfrey, sage (in large amounts), coltsfoot, black cohosh, and blue cohosh.
- Squaw vine tea or slippery elm capsules. Neither fulfills the claims to ease delivery or cure heartburn and indigestion.
- Ginseng, which contains steroidlike compounds.

A woman's "sniff acuity" is heightened during pregnancy, possibly because of elevated estrogen levels, a hormone that regulates smell. She can smell cigarette smoke from the car ahead of her on the freeway and "roasted dust" from the heater. The smell of boiling ham hocks, frying onions, a bathroom in need of cleaning, or mildew can bring her to her knees. The best indicator of both a "hazardous" or a "safe" food is smell. If a food doesn't smell good, it probably won't settle well, while a food that smells good—or at least doesn't smell bad, no matter how unusual—may be the food that stays down. "This is where my recommendations may seem like heresy," says Ms. Erick who gives hospitalized women with severe morning sickness whatever they want to eat. "The traditional bland foods recommended for morning sickness, such as crackers and broth, don't always work. So go with the flow. If spicy spaghetti with meatballs sounds good, give it a try." Keep in mind that what smells or sounds good to one pregnant women may trigger nausea in another, so take all your friends' advice with an open mind and a grain of salt. (See Table 5.6, "From Salty to Cold.")

TABLE 5.6

From Salty to Cold

Weathering nausea during the first trimester might be as simple as identifying what types of foods sound appetizing (or at least tolerable). The following list is a brief summary of the kinds of food characteristics that might soothe your upset stomach.

Salty: Noodles with salted or grated cheese, thin slices of ham, V8 juice, pretzels, salted green apple slices, pickles.

Bitter/Sour: Lemonade, lemons or limes, grapefruit juice, grapefruit, fresh cranberries.

Yeasty/Earthy: Brown rice, pumpernickel bread, hummus.

Crunchy: Baby carrots, celery sticks, cantaloupe, nuts, almonds, taco shells.

Bland: Mashed potatoes, rice, custard.

Soft: Noodles, ice cream, farina, angel food cake, pudding.

Sweet: Candy, sherbet, jam.

Fruity: Fresh fruit, fruit ices.

Wet: Milk, juices, gelatin, broth, bottled water.

Spicy: Salsa, Spicy Carrots (see recipe section, page 308), curried dishes, gingerbread.

Hard: Toasted bagels, frozen jelly beans.

Hot: Baked fruit, soup, cinnamon toast, hot cereal.

Cold: Frozen desserts, potato salad, iced tea.

Acupressure Bands: Another modern treatment for morning sickness that is effective for some women is the "acupressure" wristbands that are used by passengers on planes and boats to prevent motion sickness. A high-tech version of this, called the sensory afferent stimulating (SAS) unit, is worn like a wristwatch and delivers a continuous current directly to the site over which it is worn. Researchers at the University of California, Davis, report that 87 percent of the women they tested reported improvements in symptoms (although 43 percent of the control group who wore a placebo wristband also said they felt better). Some women also report that acupuncture significantly reduces the frequency of morning sickness. Finally, getting plenty of rest, especially afternoon naps, is a big help in curbing nausea.

What about Vitamin B_6? For the tens of thousands of women who battle morning sickness each year, the thought that a cure is as simple as popping a pill seems too good to be true. Since the 1940s, vitamin B_6 has been called the morning-sickness vitamin, although the vitamin's effectiveness is questionable.

The early studies reported that daily doses of vitamin B_6 ranging up to 100 mg curbed nausea and vomiting in pregnant women. Unfortunately, these studies were poorly designed and the effect has since been attributed to the placebo effect (an improvement in a patient's condition resulting from a belief that the treatment will work, rather than properties of the treatment itself). Later studies showed that both vitamin B_6 and a placebo reduced the symptoms of morning sickness.

Granted, vitamin B_6 status declines in the pregnant woman, and it takes two to five times normal intakes to keep blood levels at prepregnancy concentrations. On the other hand, it is questionable that the pregnancy state should match the nonpregnancy state, while the amount theorized to prevent morning sickness is fifty, not five, times recommended amounts.

Meanwhile, limited evidence shows that a multiple vitamin and mineral supplement that includes a moderate dose of vitamin B_6 might help sooth nausea. Andrew Czeizel, M.D., director of the Department of Human Genetics and Teratology at the National Institute of Hygiene in Budapest, reports that women who take multiple-vitamin supplements during early pregnancy show better weight gain, report better appetite, and have fewer bouts of nausea and vomiting compared to women who don't supplement. Another study found that women who began supplementing before the sixth week of pregnancy had the lowest risk for developing morning sickness. In the research, the supplements didn't eliminate morning sickness, but they reduced the frequency and severity of symptoms.

The issue remains controversial. The American Medical Association's Council of Drugs found no scientific evidence that vitamin B_6 is effective in the treatment or prevention of morning sickness. Some physicians disagree and find vitamin B_6 somewhat useful. According to Carol Archie, M.D., at the UCLA Medical Center, "Vitamin B_6 (given in 50 mg doses twice a day) is effective, not for your 'garden variety' nausea, but for women with severe and persistent nausea and vomiting." A woman considering vitamin B_6 first should consult with her physician, since large doses taken for long periods of time can cause nerve damage and possibly affect the growing baby's nutritional status.

The most important message for all pregnant women experiencing morning sickness is this: You aren't crazy, strange, or neurotic, and, except for extreme cases, morning sickness will not hurt your baby. Although a nutritious diet is important to you and your baby, this might not be a time when you can stomach many of the foods in the Baby-wise Diet. Don't feel guilty if a bag of potato chips soothes your nausea or sniffing lemons gets you through the day. The most important thing is to feed your taste buds at the moment and worry about optimal nutrition when the dust settles and you regain control of your appetite.

Food Cravings

Don't be surprised if your taste buds during the first trimester behave as if they're possessed. As many as 85 percent of women report craving foods or combinations of foods they never would have eaten prior to pregnancy. A woman who has always eaten whole-wheat noodles suddenly craves only refined egg noodles. You might swear off sugar, but find yourself possessed by a desire for fudge-ripple ice cream. Prepregnancy spinach salads might be replaced with frozen macaroni-and-cheese dinners. One woman might crave foods she ate as a child; another woman will eat egg-salad sandwiches at every meal. Commonly craved foods include sweets, fruits and fruit juices, sour fruits, salty or spicy foods, and hard or chewy foods.

Cravings also might be accompanied by aversions. That delicious cup of French roast coffee now smells and tastes repulsive. You no longer can prepare your favorite bean soup because the smell sends you running from the kitchen. Italian food or pizza, once your favorite foods, now hold no appeal. A metallic taste in your mouth could make foods or beverages, such as tea, taste different and distasteful. If you found cigarette smoke annoying prior to pregnancy, you probably will find that during pregnancy, even a hint of smoke turns off your appetite for hours.

Occasionally, these cravings and aversions are based on an underlying nutritional need. This is true of an iron deficiency–related condition called pica, where a woman craves nonfood items and will eat clay or dirt, baking soda, laundry starch, chalk, or even ice. Cravings for salty foods—for example, pickles—might reflect increased needs for this substance as blood volume expands. Aversions often develop toward things you should not be consuming during pregnancy, such as coffee, alcohol, and cigarettes.

However, more often than not, the craving is driven by scrambled messages to your appetite center in the brain, caused by changing hormones.

What Can You Do? Most cravings and aversions are more interesting than serious and, for the most part, can be indulged in moderation. A healthful diet is one that meets your nutritional and your emotional needs, as well as your preferences. So don't fight a healthy craving or aversion.

- If you crave carbohydrate-rich donuts, try substituting more nutritious carbohydrate-rich foods, such as a bagel, English muffin, or apple cinnamon muffin.
- If you can't stand the sight of fish or chicken, try other protein-rich foods, such as tofu, or try disguising the food by mixing small amounts in a casserole or stir-fry dish.
- If beta carotene–rich dark green leafy vegetables are on your aversion list, try eating more beta carotene–rich fruits, such as peaches or apricots.
- If the sweet taste is your weakness, try using sweet-tasting flavorings and spices, such as vanilla, nutmeg, spearmint, cinnamon, and anise.

Other crave-control tips include eating breakfast that contains at least one serving of whole grain and one serving of fruit, since skipping breakfast will escalate food cravings later in the day. If you can, plan your cravings. Set aside a calorie allotment to accommodate a small sweet snack and make it low-fat—for example, nonfat frozen yogurt, fruit ices, vanilla wafers, or fig bar cookies. Abstinence leads to binge eating, while allowing small servings of your favorite food helps curb the crave attacks.

Exercise and Hugs: Remember to exercise daily. While couch potatoes are likely to make regular trips to the refrigerator and struggle with their weight, women who regularly exercise maintain a more constant weight and are less prone to bingeing and cravings. Women who exercise throughout pregnancy most often choose walking, swimming, or aerobics as their activity du jour. Finally, don't confuse emotional needs with nutritional needs. You might be more sensitive and emotional during the first trimester and this ebb and flow of emotions can cause you to turn to food, when what you really need is a hug.

Constipation

Before your tummy begins to bulge, your digestive tract could be doing tailspins. Along with altered taste and food preferences comes a slowing of your digestive tract and reduced digestive secretions in the intestines. The female hormone progesterone is partially to blame, since it decreases the tone and motility of the smooth muscles that line the digestive tract.

Constipation is only one symptom. You might begin regurgitating your food (heartburn becomes more common later in pregnancy) and find it takes longer to digest a meal. The relaxed muscles allow waste products to linger in the intestines, with more water being reabsorbed; constipation results. Later in pregnancy, the enlarged uterus puts pressure on the abdominal and back muscles and also can contribute to constipation. Not drinking enough water, eating low-fiber foods, or not exercising daily aggravate the condition. If constipation is allowed to persist, hemorrhoids can develop.

What Can You Do? Follow the Baby-wise Diet guidelines. This will ensure that you consume lots of fiber-rich fruits, vegetables, whole grains, and legumes and enough water. Use laxatives only as a last resort and then only sparingly and with medical supervision. Frequent use of these medications aggravates the condition and leads to a dependency on the laxative.

Fatigue

If during the first trimester you feel as though you are running on fumes, rather than a full tank of supreme, you're not alone. Nine out of ten women feel tired to flat-out exhausted during the first few months of pregnancy. Many are tired from the moment they open their eyes in the morning and, often, rest does little to energize them. Many of these women have never experienced fatigue until now. The good news is that fatigue is usually followed by a burst of energy during the second trimester.

What Causes It? Although the exact cause of first-trimester fatigue is poorly understood, there are a few commonsense theories. The rapid and unique storm of physiological changes that sets in within minutes to weeks after conception diverts your body's resources and probably leaves little energy leftover for normal chores. For example, it takes a tremendous amount of energy to set up the nutritional processing plant—the placenta—for your baby.

Progesterone, the female hormone responsible for many of the physical changes during early pregnancy, also has a sedative effect. Finally, sleep disturbances, nausea, vomiting, and mood swings also contribute to fatigue. Granted, a wanted pregnancy and a positive attitude probably help more than hinder energy levels, but fatigue is not necessarily caused by deep-seated confusion about having a baby. Fatigue happens to the most willing and eager mothers, while some women with unwanted pregnancies sail through the first trimester with little change in their energy level. In other words, don't let anyone tell you "it's all in your head." In fact, preliminary evidence shows that the fatigue is often related to nausea and psychological changes triggered by hormones, including depression, anger, anxiety, and confusion.

What Can You Do? There are no magic pills for fatigue, but you can curb the energy drain by eating well, exercising when possible, and listening and responding to your body's needs. Not surprisingly, one study found that women who entered pregnancy in good physical condition and with good stamina, regardless of age, reported less problems with fatigue in early pregnancy.

To fuel your energy, rather than your fatigue, avoid sugary foods and caffeinated beverages, which are temporary quick fixes and usually leave you feeling even more tired in the long run. Instead, try to eat every four hours, include a whole grain and a fruit or vegetable at each meal or snack, always eat breakfast, and drink lots of fluids. In addition, take an afternoon nap (even if you have to close your office door or take the phone off the hook), go to bed early, and pamper yourself whenever possible. If your fatigue lingers beyond the first trimester, is accompanied by pallor or dizziness, or seriously affects your daily routine, consult with your physician about a blood test for iron status.

The Bottom Line

The daily calorie goal for the first trimester of pregnancy for most women is approximately 2,000 to 2,200 calories (or a calorie intake that maintains a desirable prepregnancy weight). While the baby's calorie needs are small during this time, the nutrient needs are high.

Morning sickness during the first trimester might mean eating what you can, when you can. Try to stick to the menus and the guidelines for the Baby-wise Diet as closely as possible or divide the food intake into small meals that you can eat when your stomach settles. (Worksheet 5.1, "My First Trimester Daily Checklist," will help you monitor your diet.) A moderate-dose supplement will help cover your nutritional bases if food intake is too erratic during these first few weeks.

Worksheet 5.1   My First Trimester Daily Checklist

Copy this master sheet to complete daily.

Food Groups	Minimum Servings	Actual Intake
Calcium-rich foods	2	_____
Vegetables (at least 2 folic acid–rich choices)	5	_____
Fruits (at least 2 vitamin C–rich choices)	3	_____
Grains (at least 4 whole-grain choices)	6	_____
Extra-lean meats and legumes	2	_____
Quenchers	5	_____

Did I reach my goals? Why or why not? _____

_____

What needs improvement? _____

What will I do differently next week? _____

Chapter 6

Nutrition during the Second Trimester

During the second trimester of pregnancy take care of:

1. **Nutrition:** Follow the guidelines outlined in the Baby-wise Diet.
2. **Weight:** Try to limit weight gain to approximately 0.7 to 1.4 pounds a week for a total of 9 to 19 pounds (more if you entered pregnancy on the thin side, exercise intensely, or are tall, and less if you are short, or were overweight and/or sedentary, prior to pregnancy).
3. **Supplement:** Take a multiple vitamin and mineral that contains 100 to 200 percent of the Daily Value for all vitamins and minerals plus at least 400 mcg of folic acid and 18 mg of iron.
4. **Safety:** Continue to avoid alcohol, tobacco, and any medication not approved by your physician. Practice good sanitation habits in the kitchen.
5. **Exercise:** Exercise daily, but adjust the routine, intensity, or duration as needed.
6. **Medical Checkups:** Make regular visits to your physician to monitor weight and obtain necessary tests.

Weight Gain and Why

A steady weight gain continues to be important in the second trimester. Women who gain at least the minimum recommended weight each week are most likely to carry their babies to term and are at lowest risk for spontaneous preterm delivery. According to a study from the University of Alabama, their babies also are more likely to develop at a normal rate and are less prone to growth retardation or low birth weight. On the other hand, excessive weight gain during the second trimester makes it more difficult to regain your prepregnancy weight after the baby is born. Your best bet is to gain just enough, but not too much during the fourth through sixth months.

What's a normal weight gain? By the beginning of the fourth month of pregnancy, you should notice a gradual increase in weight that approaches approximately a half to one and a half pounds a week. The average rate of weight gain during the second trimester usually is slightly greater than during the third trimester; a slowing of weight gain or even a slight weight loss is common in the final weeks before delivery.

These weight-gain goals are merely estimates. A healthful weight gain for each woman will depend on her weight and health status prior to pregnancy, her activity level, and a rate that is natural and normal for her. In short, the experiences of many pregnant women are unlikely to fit exactly onto a standardized weight-gain grid. One concern, however, is any rapid gain of more than two pounds in one week, which could signify excess fluid retention and the onset of a serious medical condition called preeclampsia (discussed later in this chapter).

When and What to Eat and Drink

Many women finish the first trimester still wearing their regular clothes, but by the fourth or fifth month are beginning to show the outward signs of baby making. While cell and tissue diversity was your baby's goal during the first trimester, increases in cell, tissue, and body size become more pronounced in the second and third trimester. That means your baby will be demanding more energy for growth, which equates to about a 300-calorie increase in food intake above the first trimester, for a total of about 2,500 calories a day (more if you exercise).

As always, the Baby-wise Diet forms the basis of your eating plan, with the following minimum number of daily servings from each list:

3 servings from the Calcium-Rich Group
6 servings from the Vegetable Group (at least 2 servings should be folic acid–rich choices)

4 servings from the Fruit Group (at least 2 servings should be vitamin C–rich choices)

7 servings from the Grain Group (at least 4 servings should be whole-grain choices)

3 servings from the Extra-Lean Meats and Legumes Group (try to include 2 to 3 servings of fish and 4 to 5 servings of legumes in the weekly menu)

6 servings from the Quenchers Group

Why Do I Feel So Tired? Marginal Nutrient Deficiencies

While many women report experiencing a burst of energy during the second trimester, the increased demands of pregnancy leave other women feeling not up to par. It is easy to blame low energy or mood swings on pregnancy or the stress of a busy lifestyle, but fatigue could be a simple matter of not getting enough nutrients from your diet.

Just because you don't have anemia or other signs of clinical nutrient deficiencies, that doesn't mean you are well nourished. Nutritional depletion progresses from mild to severe over the course of days, weeks, months, or years, much like other disorders from the common cold to heart disease. In essence, each person's nutritional status fluctuates along a continuum. Marginal deficiencies are the middle ground on this continuum, bordered by either increasingly better health on one end or advancing clinical deficiencies on the other.

Symptoms of Marginal Deficiencies: The problem with a marginal deficiency is that the symptoms, if any, are vague. "The definition of a marginal deficiency is still very imprecise," says Douglas Heimburger, M.D., associate professor and director of the Division of Clinical Nutrition at the University of Alabama at Birmingham. "Often the effects of a marginal deficiency have nothing to do with how a person looks or feels." If there are symptoms, they may be something as vague as "feeling under the weather." A marginally nourished person also might feel tired, stressed, or irritable; have trouble concentrating or remembering where she put her keys; or be more prone to colds and the flu. For example, suboptimal intake of vitamin B_1 produces feelings of depression or anxiety even in otherwise normal, healthy people. Complications following surgery or birth also are more common in marginally nourished women. The nutritional demands of pregnancy can be all it takes to push a woman over the edge from adequate nutritional status to a marginal deficiency.

Fatigue as a Symptom of Marginal Deficiency: Fatigue can result from a host of factors, not the least of which is diet and, in particular, iron intake. As mentioned in Chapter 1, iron is a component of hemoglobin in red blood cells and myoglobin within the muscles and other tissues. These iron-dependent molecules are responsible for oxygen transport from the lungs to all of the cells and utilization within the cells. When dietary intake of iron is low or when iron absorption is poor, iron in the tissues is released to make up deficits in the blood. The cells slowly suffocate from lack of oxygen and inefficiently burn carbohydrates for energy. Consequently, a woman experiences everything from sluggishness to poor concentration. These symptoms occur as the tissue stores are drained, even when there are no signs of anemia. Symptoms worsen as the deficiency progresses to anemia.

Women—especially those who exercise, are or have been pregnant within the past two years, or consume diets of less than 2,500 calories—are at particular risk for iron deficiency. Rather than allow your energy level to crumble or accept fatigue as a normal part of pregnancy, take the offensive by having your iron levels checked. That means:

1. Consume ample amounts of iron-rich foods in the Baby-wise Diet.
2. Ask for a serum ferritin test rather than only the typical hemoglobin or hematocrit.
3. Request an iron supplement if your serum ferritin level is below 20 mcg/L and/or your total iron binding capacity or TIBC is greater than 450 mcg/L.

Colds and Infections: The immune system, the body's natural defense against everything from the common cold to cancer, is dramatically influenced by suboptimal amounts of numerous vitamins and minerals. Consuming a little but not enough copper, iron, selenium, zinc, vitamin A and beta carotene, vitamin E, vitamin C, and/or the B vitamins, especially folic acid, vitamin B_6, and pantothenic acid, can have far-reaching effects on your ability to fend off infection and disease.

Preterm Delivery, Pregnancy Problems, and Marginal Deficiencies: Folic acid is another nutrient that, when low, can interfere with your pregnancy. Women with low blood levels of folic acid in their second trimester, even with no overt signs of deficiency, are at a twofold greater risk of preterm delivery and giving birth to a low-birth-weight baby compared to women who maintain optimal blood levels of this B vitamin. As you'll read later in this chapter, even many of the most serious complications of pregnancy, such as preeclampsia, might be at least in part caused by marginal deficiencies.

Mood Swings: Some mild emotional problems, from depression to irritability, can result from marginal intake of one or more vitamins or minerals. But even more likely causes of emotional ups and downs during pregnancy are the fluctuations in hormones and the experience of pregnancy itself.

Your body is undergoing a total makeover, which is exciting and wonderful in one way, but possibly upsetting for other reasons. As your breasts enlarge, your waistline disappears, and your graceful walk transforms into a waddle, you may have mixed feelings about what is happening to your body. There will be days when you feel fat or wonder if you will ever regain your figure. These feelings are perfectly normal. Exercise can help you feel good about yourself, while following the Baby-wise Diet and gaining enough, but not too much, weight will help you stay healthy during your pregnancy and will make it easier to regain your "old self" after the baby is born.

What Can You Do? Marginal deficiencies are almost always a result of not eating well enough to support the demands you place on your body from pregnancy to exercise and stress. Preventing a deficiency or at least treating it in the early stages is your best bet, just as identifying and treating abnormal cell changes of the cervix from a routine Pap smear has an almost 100 percent cure rate, as compared to the poor prognosis when cervical cancer has progressed to advanced stages. Even if the deficiency doesn't progress, why settle for feeling average when you could feel good or great?

While there are no inexpensive and reliable tests to assess nutritional status for every vitamin and mineral, following the Baby-wise Diet prior to and during pregnancy will improve your chances of getting everything you need to feel your best. Granted, the vague symptoms attributed to marginal deficiencies also result from a host of other factors, from the genes you were born with to the hormone storms of pregnancy. Regardless, setting your nutritional sights on optimum improves your stamina and well-being, while a healthy body is more resilient to the problems of daily living. Consuming enough—not just a little—of all nutrients could make the difference between feeling under the weather and at your best.

The Stress of Pregnancy

Stress comes packaged in many of life's most wonderful experiences. While daily tensions or the loss of a loved one can cause negative stress or distress, even positive experiences such as a promotion at work or pregnancy can upset normal routines and increase your stress load. Muscle tightness, headaches, sleep problems, a quicker heart rate, or frequent irritability are red flags of stress.

Pregnancy adds its own set of stresses to a woman's life. Not only do the profound physical changes that accompany pregnancy require many adjustments, but the psychological and emotional changes as a woman anticipates the birth of her baby can add additional layers of stress. You also might worry about the delivery, birth defects, and the pain of labor. Most of these worries can be minimized by talking to your physician, who can give you the facts about what to expect in each phase of pregnancy.

Unrelieved stress can increase a pregnant woman's susceptibility to health problems, which then affect the developing baby. In studies on animals, pups born to overly stressed mothers were less active and showed signs of reduced nerve and organ development. Unhealthy coping habits, such as cigarettes, alcohol, or drugs, aggravate the situation and increase the risk for birth defects. In addition, chronic high stress might increase a woman's risk for premature labor and having a low-birth-weight baby.

We also eat terribly when we're under stress. In a study from the University College of London, people's dietary intakes were monitored during periods of high and low stress at work. The highest-stress times coincided with the greatest intakes of sugary foods, calories, and saturated fat. Even when not stressed, Americans consume their weight in sugar every year; sugar makes up to 16 percent of our total calories every day, which is considerably more than the 6 to 10 percent recommended by nutrition experts. Soft drinks top the list, supplying a third of our sugar, followed by baked goods, fruit drinks, sugary dairy foods, and candy. It goes without saying that sugar is not the stuff on which babies are made!

You should make every effort to avoid or successfully cope with the stress of pregnancy by focusing on eating well, adopting a positive attitude, developing a realistic expectation of the pregnancy process, and taking charge of each stressful situation to find a reasonable solution. You might need to lessen the workload on the job, reduce noise at home or at work, avoid long periods of standing or sitting, take time during the day for a short nap, or let go of superwoman expectations that you can do it all. Prioritizing your time and efforts and developing an assertive communication style to effectively ask for what you need are two essential skills you must acquire. In addition, spend time with people who understand and are supportive of you during your pregnancy, and take time to exercise and rest or meditate daily.

The Importance of Exercise

The second trimester comes with a unique set of challenges and experiences. This is the time best suited for maintaining your exercise program, since the morning sickness and fatigue of the first trimester has waned, while your body still moves relatively easily. On the other hand, as morning sickness subsides other health issues might surface, such as heartburn, constipation, preeclampsia, gestational diabetes, and high blood pressure, all of which should be prevented when possible or closely monitored if they develop.

Exercise: How Much of What?

Don't take a maternity leave from the gym. While in the past a pregnant woman wasn't supposed to lift a finger, let alone walk a mile, today some women are running the entire nine months.

Exercise is very important for both you and your baby. Not only does exercise ensure a big, healthy baby, but a study published in the *Journal of Pediatrics* found that babies born to exercising moms might even have higher IQs! Other studies show that women who exercise before and during pregnancy have half the risk of delivering prematurely; are better able to handle the stress pregnancy puts on the body; have fewer backaches, constipation, ankle swelling, fatigue, and excess weight gain; and report feeling better and emotionally more positive than do pregnant women who don't exercise. The American College of Obstetricians and Gynecologists (ACOG) has published guidelines acknowledging that a woman entering pregnancy in good physical condition usually can maintain a higher degree of exercise performance throughout pregnancy, and she will recover from pregnancy and delivery faster than can a sedentary woman. (See Table 6.1, "Exercise Guidelines for Pregnancy.")

For example, a woman who has exercised routinely at 75 percent of her maximum exertion prior to pregnancy, may drop down to 57 percent by the twentieth week of pregnancy, and to 47 percent by the thirty-second week, but she is still in excellent physical shape and will return to prepregnancy fitness quickly after delivery. In short, exercise is beneficial during pregnancy as long as women keep in mind the shift in gravity and weight distribution that comes in the second and third trimester as their bellies expand, and they exercise with reasonable caution.

TABLE 6.1

Exercise Guidelines for Pregnancy

The following guidelines are proposed by the American College of Obstetricians and Gynecologists (ACOG) and are intended for women who do not have any additional risk factors for adverse maternal or perinatal outcomes.

1. Women can continue to exercise during pregnancy and will experience health benefits even from mild to moderate activity. Regular activity—at least three times a week—is preferable to sporadic activity.
2. After the first trimester, a woman should avoid any exercise that requires lying down in the supine position (on the back). This position reduces cardiac output (blood flow from the heart). Long periods of motionless standing also should be avoided.
3. Because there is typically decreased oxygen available for aerobic activity, a woman should adapt all exercise to accommodate this shift in oxygen supply. She should stop exercising if she feels fatigued and should not exercise to exhaustion. Non-weight-bearing activities, such as swimming or cycling, help minimize the risk of injury; however, even weight-bearing activity, such as jogging, can be continued with modification under many circumstances and with physician approval.
4. Any activity that poses a threat of abdominal trauma or the loss of balance and risk to the mother or infant's well-being should be avoided.
5. Women who exercise will require up to 300 additional calories to sustain normal body functioning and a gradual weight gain.
6. To counter any increase in body temperature, a pregnant woman should drink plenty of fluids, wear appropriate clothing, and avoid exercising in hot climates.
7. Many of the physical changes of pregnancy persist six to eight weeks after delivery, so exercise routines should be resumed gradually based on a woman's physical capability.

What If I've Never Exercised? Even sedentary women have the go-ahead to move during pregnancy. Just start slowly, increase gradually, and keep your heart rate below 65 percent of maximum or at a mild to moderate level that allows you to talk while moving. Walking and swimming are perfect exercise starters during pregnancy.

Intensity and Duration: Always let perceived exertion be your guide. Pregnant women, in general, cannot exercise at the same intensity and duration as they did prior to pregnancy. In addition, conventional methods for measuring exercise intensity, such as pulse, might not be accurate because of the increase in a pregnant woman's resting heart rate from the first to the third trimester. Instead, focus on your level of exertion; exercise at whatever level makes your body feel the same as it did before you were pregnant. Don't force yourself to do anything that doesn't feel right. If running no longer feels good, try walking or swimming. Aim for a level that is moderate to somewhat hard, as long as you don't become breathless. (See Table 6. 2, "When Not to Exercise.")

TABLE 6.2

When Not to Exercise

According to the American College of Obstetricians and Gynecologists (ACOG), several medical or pregnancy-related conditions are contraindicators for exercise or at least will impose important limitations to an exercise program, including:

1. Intrauterine growth retardation
2. Pregnancy-induced high blood pressure
3. Premature rupture of membranes or placenta previa
4. Persistent bleeding during the second and third trimester
5. Preterm labor, either during the current or a previous pregnancy
6. Incompetent cervix/cerclage (a surgical procedure that closes the cervix to keep the fetus intact in the uterus)
7. A history of chronic high blood pressure; active thyroid, cardiovascular, or pulmonary disease; or miscarriage
8. More than one fetus, i.e., twins, triplets, etc.
9. Asthma

Exercises to Avoid: Increased body mass, a relaxing of the ligaments around the joints, fatigue, and increased cardiovascular demands also affect how much you can do. After the fourth month of pregnancy, you should avoid exercising while lying on your back, since the expanding uterus can compress the vena cava, the main vein that carries blood back to the heart. This could interfere with normal blood flow to the uterus. Also, don't do crunch exercises or any activity that causes you to hold your breath.

Weight training is fine, but use light weights to avoid straining, and avoid diving, water skiing, or any activity that poses harm to you or your baby.

Your Balance: Your center of gravity has shifted, which upsets your balance. Consequently, it is best not to begin a new activity that requires balance or the risk of a fall, such as aerobic dance, roller skating, step exercises, or even cycling, during pregnancy. These limitations are hardly an excuse not to exercise, but they require some changes in how hard, how long, or even what type of exercise you choose during pregnancy.

Body Temperature: The American College of Sports Medicine (ACSM) recommends that pregnant women monitor their body temperature during exercise, since even a moderate elevation to 102.5°F or higher could create problems for the developing baby. The research is incomplete on what effects elevated body temperature might have on the developing baby, while limited evidence shows that women who engage in strenuous work, prolonged standing in the third trimester, or heavy weight lifting are more prone than other women to preterm deliveries.

Your body temperature might rise more rapidly during exercise than it did prior to pregnancy, so you will need to relearn your body's signals by keeping a close eye on any changes. On the other hand, body temperature, called core temperature, seldom increases more than 2.7°F in women who exercise at a comfortable or constant moderate pace during pregnancy, so you don't need to worry if you break a sweat. To be safe, always consult your physician before beginning or continuing an exercise program during pregnancy.

Unfortunately, a safe upper limit for exercise has not been established. This probably has more to do with a woman's individual fitness and pregnancy status than with a standard for all women. Some sports, however, seem to be made for pregnancy. Swimming is a perfect example.

The Advantages of Swimming: Swimming is an aerobic activity that keeps your blood circulating, improves the flow of oxygen to your baby, increases your strength and endurance, and decreases the risk for developing high blood pressure, edema, varicose veins, and hemorrhoids. Like other sports, swimming also might help you shorten your labor and reduce overall risk for pregnancy complications. But unlike other sports such as jogging, which can jar and stress your already strained back, joints, and legs, swimming and other water activities are weightless and gentle to your body. Your body is supported by the water while you exercise all the major muscle groups. It also improves your upper body strength, which is likely to be useful in the months following delivery when you need to tote around your bundle of joy.

Food Additives: Which Ones Are Safe?

Most food additives are hardly essential nutrients, but they also probably won't harm you or your baby. Because government regulatory agencies, such as the U.S. Food and Drug Administration (FDA), require stringent testing of any new substance before it enters the food supply, our food supply is safer than it has ever been in recorded history. Consequently, most additives used to preserve, treat, or improve foods are safe. When a substance is found harmful, such as cyclamates and Red Dye No. 2, which produce by-products damaging to a baby, it is banned from the United States food supply.

The Ones to Avoid: A few additives should be avoided if possible during pregnancy. The preservative BHT, which is added to some ready-to-eat cereals, instant mashed potatoes, and other processed foods, produced behavioral problems in pups born to female mice who consumed this additive during pregnancy. Monosodium glutamate (MSG) is a flavor-enhancing additive that is too high in salt (sodium) to be a safe bet during pregnancy. Some people are sensitive to MSG and develop headaches, nausea, vomiting, dizziness, or sleep disturbances after eating it. Hydrolyzed vegetable protein is another food additive that contains MSG. Avoid this additive whenever possible.

High concentrations of additives called sulfites found in some dried fruits and wines (which you aren't drinking anyway) also might cause adverse reactions in 5 to 10 percent of women with asthma who are sensitive to sulfites. The FDA has banned the use of sulfites from salad bar ingredients and now requires labeling on foods that contain sulfites, such as some processed potatoes, beer, wine, and golden raisins.

Sugar Substitutes: Sugar substitutes, such as saccharin and aspartame, appear relatively safe, but it is probably a good idea to limit intake to moderate amounts during pregnancy. That is not to say that sweetened soda pop is nutritionally equivalent to orange juice, because nothing could be further from the truth. However, nutritious foods sweetened with aspartame, such as sugar-free yogurt and low-sugar instant oatmeal, can be a safe alternative to sugar for women with diabetes and are probably safe for most pregnant women when consumed in moderate amounts, such as two to three sweetened foods a day.

Waxes and Pesticides: Waxes and pesticides on fruits and vegetables are another source of unwanted additives in the pregnant woman's diet. Waxes formulated from plants and petroleum sources are used to replace the natural waxes removed during washing and to retain moisture during shipping. They also improve the appearance of vegetables and fruits by reducing bruising and the growth of molds and other pathogens. Waxes may or may not be used on a variety of produce, including apples, peppers, cucumbers, eggplants, lemons, melons, oranges, peaches, pineapples, sweet potatoes, and tomatoes.

Wax coatings have been approved by the FDA as safe additions to foods. However, a few wax coatings are made from animal products and would not be suitable for people following vegetarian or kosher diets. Another concern is not the wax, but the pesticides and fungicides sealed in with the waxes. Since federal law requires wax labeling by shippers and retailers, you can ask your grocer for information on which fruits and vegetables at your store have been treated with wax. Don't let a little wax scare you! You still need lots of produce during your pregnancy! (Are you getting enough? Take Quiz 6.1 at the end of this chapter.)

Although the evidence is not conclusive, you probably are better off avoiding excessive amounts of pesticides in food if possible, especially when you're pregnant. The Environmental Protection Agency (EPA) reports that approximately seventy pesticides now in use are "probable" or "possible" cancer-causing agents. Several studies suggest, but do not prove, that exposure to low levels of pesticides for long periods of time can be harmful. For example, researchers at the Mount Sinai School of Medicine and the New York University Medical Center analyzed blood samples for women with and women without breast cancer. They found that women who had the highest levels of DDE in their blood, a breakdown product of the pesticide DDT banned from use more than a decade ago, were four times as likely to develop breast cancer as women with low levels of the pesticide residue.

Regulations on pesticide use are somewhat enforced in the United States and our food supply is growing increasingly more safe. For example, potentially toxic pesticides, such as DDT, dieldrin, heptachlor, and chlordane, are suspended from use and other pesticides, such as alar and EDB, are tightly regulated and monitored. However, in other countries regulations, if any, may or may not be enforced. Consequently, produce coming into the United States from other countries can contain illegal residues or levels of pesticides not allowed in this country. These foreign-grown foods are the ones to limit or avoid, if possible. Many herbal supplements also contain small amounts of heavy metals, such as lead and arsenic, and organochlorine pesticides, such as DDT, that have been banned in the United States.

Despite the unanswered questions about pesticides, people should be eating more fruits and vegetables. For one thing, the permissible residue levels already include hefty margins of safety, so they are likely to be protective even if studies show some produce might contain too much. To limit your pesticide exposure,

- Purchase certified organic produce or locally grown produce when possible.
- Peel all waxed produce.
- Thoroughly wash all other produce.

Keep in mind that pesticide residues also are found in meat, poultry, fish, butter, grains, and other foods. You can cut down on your risk by removing the fat from meats, since that's where some pesticides concentrate. Dried beans and peas have very low levels of pesticides and are a fat-free, nutritious alternative to meat.

Mercury: This metal is toxic to nerves, especially those of developing babies. Mercury released into our lakes, rivers, and oceans accumulates in tissues of fish, which is why recreational fishing is restricted today in many states. As discussed in Chapter 2, pregnant women should avoid the types of fish most likely to contain unacceptable levels of mercury, including large tuna, shark, and swordfish. However, a study from the University of Rochester School of Medicine found no adverse effects on mental function at sixty-six months of age in babies whose mothers consumed fish daily during pregnancy. Whether adverse effects might be noted later in life is unknown. Your best bet is to eat fish known to have relatively little or no mercury during pregnancy. (See Chapter 2, page 42, for a list of these fish.)

Food Poisoning
Food poisoning from food eaten at a restaurant might make the headlines, but home kitchens are the worst offenders when it comes to tainted food. Since no one from the local health department inspects your kitchen, you must be your own inspector. Careless food storage and handling not only

increases the risk for food poisoning, it also results in loss of nutrients and good taste from foods. The four basic rules are

- always wash your hands in hot, soapy water before preparing food and after using the bathroom, blowing your nose, petting the dog, etc.;
- wash your kitchen towels and rags often and replace sponges regularly;
- thaw foods in the microwave or in the refrigerator, never on the kitchen counter;
- separate raw meats and produce—use separate cutting boards, wash the meat board in the dishwasher after use, use paper towels to wipe away blood from meats, and wash hands with soap after handling meat.

Fish: Eat only cooked seafood and avoid sushi, raw oysters, sashimi, and seviche. See above and Chapter 2 for more on seafood.

Meat, Poultry, and Eggs: Cook meat until done. Check "sell dates" on packages of processed meats and meat spreads, since *Listeria* also has been detected in these products. Cook eggs until whites and yolks are firm, and avoid foods that contain raw eggs, such as Caesar salad, homemade ice cream, and homemade mayonnaise. Use a liquid egg substitute in recipes calling for uncooked eggs.

Vegetables and Fruit: Wash produce to remove bacteria, dirt, and surface pesticides. Peel produce to remove surface pesticides. Avoid farmstand apple ciders and unpasteurized bottled juices that might contain *E. coli*, a harmful bacteria killed by the high heat used in pasteurization. In addition, refer to Table 6.3, "Safe Keeping," for more ways to minimize food contamination in your kitchen. See Chapter 5, pages 119–21, for guidelines on reducing food poisoning from milk products.

A Nutritional Approach to Common Problems: From Heartburn to Eclampsia

Some women sail through the second trimester with hardly a care in the world, while others battle minor problems. A few pregnancy-related conditions, including preeclampsia and gestational diabetes, can be potentially serious and the early warning signs should be taken seriously. Routine medical checkups throughout pregnancy are critical to early discovery and treatment of these conditions, which otherwise can progress undetected.

TABLE 6.3

Safe Keeping

To keep your kitchen free of harmful bacteria, follow these steps:

- The refrigerator door does not stay as cold as the rest of the refrigerator. Store highly perishable foods (especially milk) in the coldest part of the refrigerator.
- Keep beverage containers closed. Orange juice loses vitamin C when exposed to air and milk loses riboflavin (vitamin B$_2$) when exposed to light.
- The egg holders built into refrigerator doors are not cold enough to safely store eggs. Do not wash eggs before storing, and throw away any eggs with cracked shells.
- Butter and margarine absorb smells from other foods if left uncovered and turn rancid if left unrefrigerated. Rancid fats are a source of free radicals, those highly reactive compounds associated with many degenerative diseases and premature aging.
- Vegetables keep best and stay moist when stored in the crisper drawer or in plastic bags on the lower shelf of your refrigerator.
- Whole grains and wheat germ are susceptible to rancidity and insect infestation and should be kept in the refrigerator.
- Avoid stale peanuts. Aflatoxin, a mold that contaminates peanuts and some grains, is a potent cancer-causing substance that is harmful to both the mother and the developing baby. It is wise to avoid stale peanuts, cornmeal stored in open bins at the health-food store, or rice products of questionable quality or freshness. Do not grind your own peanut butter at your local store by using their bulk nuts. Instead, purchase brand-name peanut butters and corn or rice products from well-known manufacturers.
- Do not freeze meats, poultry, or fish in the see-through plastic wrap in which they were purchased. Rewrap them in foil or freezer wrap.
- Hot foods packed in large containers are a breeding ground for bacteria, since it takes hours for the center to cool enough to retard bacterial growth. Instead, divide large portions into several small freezer containers.
- Do not store foods under the sink. Cleaning products often stored there may leak. Leaking pipes can rust cans and damage boxes. Openings in the walls for pipes give insects and rodents easy access to the foods.
- Store seldom-used pots and pans above the stove. The temperature in this area is too hot for safe storage of foods, including packaged and canned foods.
- Never use pottery with a lead-based glaze for drinking hot beverages, storing acidic juices such as orange juice, or cooking.
- Avoid using warm tap water for drinking or cooking if it has been exposed to lead pipes (as was customary in homes built before 1930) or lead-soldered pipes (as was customary in homes built between 1978 and 1988). Have your water tested if you have any doubt about its lead content.
- Refrigerated foods should be kept at 40°F and the freezer temperature should be at or below 0°F.
- Test the refrigerator and freezer doors by closing a dollar bill in the door. You should not be able to pull out the bill if the seal is tight.

Heartburn

The term *heartburn* is a misnomer, since this condition has nothing to do with your heart and a whole lot to do with your digestive tract. As many as 80 percent of all pregnant women struggle with heartburn or a full or burning feeling in the chest, especially after a meal. Heartburn can start as early as the first trimester, but usually is more troublesome by the fifth month and increases in frequency or severity in the third trimester.

The hormones of pregnancy—estrogen and progesterone—are responsible for much of the discomfort. For one thing, progesterone, either alone or with estrogen, decreases the tone and motility of smooth muscles that line the digestive tract and decreases the pressure of the sphincter that usually blocks the stomach contents from moving upward into the esophagus. This results in regurgitation into the esophagus, decreased emptying time of the stomach into the small intestine, and reversed peristalsis (food moves backward instead of flowing in a constant downward motion).

In addition, the pressure of the enlarging uterus crowds the adjacent digestive tract, especially the stomach. With this crowding, the stomach contents after a meal, now semiliquid, move up into the esophagus rather than down into the intestines, causing a burning sensation from the gastric acid mixed with the food. Increased gastric acidity during pregnancy also contributes to heartburn.

Heartburn is aggravated by large meals, foods that produce gas such as beans and cabbage, and fatty or spicy foods. You can avoid the discomfort, or at least reduce the frequency and severity, by dividing the day's food intake into several small meals and snacks, drinking liquids between rather than with meals, eating a light dinner at least three hours before bedtime, and chewing and eating slowly. Other foods that might aggravate heartburn and should be avoided include coffee, chocolate, salami and other processed meats, rich pastries and fried foods, alcohol, and carbonated beverages.

The heavier you are, the more pressure you place on the esophagus and the more likely you will experience heartburn. Consequently, a moderate weight gain of twenty-five to thirty pounds is less likely to cause heartburn than is a weight gain of forty pounds or more. Other heartburn remedies include the following:

- Wear loose-fitting clothes. (If your waistband or panty hose leave a ring around your growing tummy, your clothes are too tight!)
- Sit up while eating.

- Walk or sit after eating; avoid lying down right away.
- Don't exercise for two hours after eating.
- Keep your head elevated when in bed.
- Avoid stooping or bending.
- Avoid stress during the day and tension when eating.
- Chew gum or suck on a sour lemon drop (this will stimulate saliva, which helps neutralize the acid in the esophagus). A study from the University of Alabama found that women who chewed an average of 4½ sticks of gum every day suffered less heartburn than when they didn't chew gum.

Sodium bicarbonate should be avoided as a treatment for heartburn, since it can upset the normal acid-base balance in the body. Discuss the use of antacids with your physician. Overuse of antacids can interfere with iron absorption, so take supplements at opposite times of the day if you use antacids.

Constipation

Progesterone not only contributes to heartburn, it also slows the movement of food in your intestine, which leaves more time for the absorption of water and nutrients and increases the likelihood of constipation. Another hormone called motilin, which normally stimulates movement of food through the intestines, also is in short supply during pregnancy. The pressure of the growing baby on your intestines and rectum can aggravate this problem. Iron supplements also cause constipation in some women (other women develop diarrhea as a result of iron supplementation). Most women report improvement or even alleviation of constipation when they drink plenty of fluids, eat lots of fiber-rich whole grains, fruits, vegetables, and legumes as recommended in the Baby-wise Diet, exercise daily, and avoid caffeine, which acts like a diuretic and can cause further fluid loss. Following this dietary and exercise advice also will lessen your chances of developing hemorrhoids by avoiding constipation.

If the Baby-wise Diet does not remedy constipation, try adding a little wheat bran or flaxseed meal to the diet. Start with one teaspoon on your morning cereal and gradually increase the dose until you find a level that works for you. Too much fiber might increase intestinal gas, which can be uncomfortable at any time but especially during pregnancy. So take it slow with any concentrated fiber product. In all cases, never take a laxative unless prescribed by your physician, since frequent use of laxatives can aggravate the condition and result in a dependency on the medication.

The same diet and exercise recommendations for constipation also are useful in the prevention and treatment of intestinal gas (flatulence). In addition, eat small, frequent meals, rather than gorging. Chew slowly and thoroughly and don't gulp your food, which will cause you to swallow air. This captured air forms painful pockets of gas in your intestines. Stay relaxed while eating, which lessens the chance of swallowing air and will help avoid digestive-tract discomfort. Identify and eliminate from the diet any foods that cause you gas, such as fried foods or sugary items including cookies and pies. If nutritious foods, such as Brussels sprouts, broccoli, and cooked dried beans, peas, and lentils, cause more trouble than they are worth, then make sure you find other nutritious foods to take their place.

Diarrhea

While some women struggle with constipation during pregnancy, others are troubled by diarrhea. A hormone called relaxin that is released from the placenta quiets smooth muscle contractions, which can relax the digestive tract and allow food to pass through too quickly. In addition, switching too quickly from a low-fiber diet to the high-fiber Baby-wise Diet could cause temporary flatulence as your body adapts to the new eating style. This can be avoided by making dietary changes gradually, rather than all at once. On the other hand, diarrhea can be a sign of infection, food poisoning, or other digestive tract disorders, so always check with your physician if symptoms are severe or persist.

Gum and Tooth Problems

More gum and tooth problems occur during pregnancy than at any other time in the childbearing years and probably result from changing hormone levels. Gingivitis is more common in the first half of pregnancy. Some women also develop reddened, fingerlike protrusions of inflamed gum tissue between teeth called pregnancy tumors, which are not cancerous and usually disappear after the baby is born. X rays are usually necessary if the growths do not subside, so wait until after pregnancy to have them surgically removed. You can lessen the risk or the symptoms of all gum disorders by entering pregnancy with well-cared-for teeth and rigorous dental hygiene, including frequent professional cleaning, during pregnancy.

High Blood Pressure

Your doctor will be keeping a close eye on your blood pressure during pregnancy, since blood pressure can be an early sign of a serious condition called pregnancy-induced hypertension (PIH), or can be a complication of pregnancy without the link to PIH. Elevated blood pressure (a systolic blood pressure of 140 mmHg or greater and/or a diastolic blood pressure of 90 mmHg or greater, or a rise in systolic blood pressure of 25 mmHg or more and/or a rise in diastolic blood pressure of 15 mmHg or more before conception or in the first trimester) is an unwelcome event. In addition to its links with PIH, high blood pressure can reduce blood flow to the placenta and baby, resulting in a diminished supply of oxygen and nutrients, and necessitating an early delivery. Also, as the blood pressure of hypertensive mothers rises, so does the death rate of their infants. Fortunately, most cases of elevated blood pressure during pregnancy are not related to PIH, and most women with this problem can complete pregnancy and give birth to healthy babies, as long as they are monitored closely by their physicians.

Mild to moderate hypertension usually requires that you limit your activity and rest frequently, since inactivity is one way to reduce blood pressure. In addition, while your physician may recommend limiting salt if intake is very high, in almost all cases some salt (sodium) is needed in the pregnant woman's diet.

The Salt Issue: In past decades, women were told to restrict salt to prevent PIH or eclampsia. While this belief has lingered, most experts now agree that a pregnant woman needs some salt in the diet. In fact, many women crave pickles, chips, or other salty foods during pregnancy, which probably reflects their bodies' need for more salt. About 60 percent of the expanding tissues in the mother's body is water, and sodium is needed to regulate this fluid in the cells and tissues.

Fluid balance in the body is maintained, in part, by how much sodium is outside and how much potassium and chloride are inside the cells. In essence, water follows sodium. Just as water moves out of the cells of a tomato when you sprinkle salt on it, sodium outside of body cells draws water out of these cells, while the potassium and chloride prevent too much fluid from escaping. It is this balance of potassium, chloride, and sodium that ensures your cells do not go limp from excessive water loss and your blood does not become too concentrated from excessive water moving into the cells.

Some people overrespond to sodium so that a high salt intake results in too much water leaving the cells. The blood volume expands, placing greater pressure on the heart and blood vessels to pump this expanded blood volume. The result is high blood pressure. On the other hand, the blood volume naturally expands during pregnancy by up to 50 percent (even more for multiple births), so slightly more sodium, potassium, and chloride are needed to maintain the extra fluid volume. The cells also hold more water during pregnancy, so a little bit of swelling is normal starting in the second trimester and especially in the last few weeks of pregnancy. This mild edema should not be treated with salt restriction or diuretic medications (also called water pills), since you need a little extra fluid. Abnormal accumulation of fluid in the cells, however, is called edema and often is associated with a medical condition that requires physician monitoring.

What to Do: Pregnant women with high blood pressure fare better when they consume normal (not excessive) amounts of salt, because it helps maintain the blood volume of the mother and that of the developing baby. So unless otherwise advised by your physician, continue to salt foods to taste, but avoid wasting calories on highly salted, high-fat snack foods. You will consume ample amounts of potassium when you follow the Baby-wise Diet recommendations to eat plenty of fruits and vegetables. If you struggle with cravings for salty foods, drink a can of V8 juice or dunk a cup of raw vegetables in a fat-free, salty dip, which will meet one serving of your vegetable needs and has some added salt.

Edema

Edema is a sign of PIH or preeclampsia, but not all women with edema develop the more serious disorder. In fact, as many as one out of every two pregnant women will develop some degree of edema during pregnancy without ever developing preeclampsia. Women with edema can gain as much as 9½ quarts of fluid and still have normal pregnancies and give birth to healthy babies. The difference between normal fluid retention and edema associated with preeclampsia is the rate of fluid retention. A rapid increase in fluid accumulation is a sign of preeclampsia, while a gradual gain in fluid is not abnormal.

So just because your feet and ankles swell after a long day does not mean you should worry. Sitting or lying down and putting your feet up might be all it takes to reduce swelling. In addition, drink plenty of fluids, wear comfortable clothing, and avoid wearing tight panty hose, slips, or pants. If you have a sudden weight gain, haven't been following the

Baby-wise Diet, and don't feel up to par, or any unusual symptoms have developed including headaches or blurred vision, you should contact your physician immediately. Early treatment of preeclampsia and regular physician monitoring will reduce the seriousness of the disorder and avoid harming your baby.

Pregnancy-Induced Hypertension (Eclampsia)

Up to 30 percent of women experience some elevation in blood pressure. One-third to one-half of these women have essential hypertension, or elevated blood pressure of unknown cause. In some women, this elevated blood pressure signals a more serious condition called pregnancy-induced hypertension (PIH). PIH includes gestational hypertension, preeclampsia, and eclampsia. (See Table 6.4, "Defining the Terms of Pregnancy-Induced Hypertension.")

Once called toxemia, PIH is a general term for a serious condition that develops in middle to late pregnancy and is characterized by edema, protein in the urine, and high blood pressure. The condition can occur anytime after the twentieth to twenty-fourth week of pregnancy, but it is most common in the later months, has an unpredictable onset, and develops in stages.

TABLE 6.4

Defining the Terms of Pregnancy-Induced Hypertension

Term	Symptoms and Signs
Hypertension	Blood pressure > 140/90 mmHg
Severe Hypertension	Systolic blood pressure > 160mmHg or Diastolic blood pressure > 110mmHg
Gestational Hypertension	Hypertension only (also called "transient hypertension")
Preeclampsia	Hypertension with protein in urine or edema
Eclampsia	Preeclampsia with seizures

Source: American College of Obstetricians and Gynecologists

The Stages of Eclampsia: In the first stage, called preeclampsia, a woman might experience edema (swelling caused from fluid retention), high blood pressure, a sudden weight gain of two or more pounds in one week, and protein loss in the urine. In the second stage, a woman can develop vision problems, severe headaches, and abdominal pain. If allowed to progress to the final stage (called eclampsia), convulsions, lapsing into a coma, and even death can result. High blood pressure prior to pregnancy or transient high blood pressure without accompanying protein in the urine or edema is not part of the toxemia condition. Also, don't worry if your only symptom is a headache—it may be just that!

What Causes Eclampsia? While preeclampsia/eclampsia is one of the most serious obstetrical complications, there is little agreement on its cause. Some physicians believe that gaining too much weight might be a factor, although there is no scientific evidence to support this theory. Others once thought eclampsia resulted from excessive salt intake, so salt-restricted diets were prescribed. One theory gaining increasing support is that eclampsia is related to a problem with the placenta, or more specifically with constricted blood vessels in the placenta that reduce blood supply to the developing baby. Another theory is that preeclampsia might be caused by abnormal attachment of the placenta to the uterine wall, which triggers widespread problems in most of the mother's major body systems. Hormonelike compounds called prostaglandins also have been blamed. It is likely that preeclampsia results from a variety of interconnecting factors that include age (teenage women and women over thirty-five are more prone to preeclampsia), parity (first pregnancies are more frequently associated with preeclampsia than subsequent pregnancies), socioeconomic factors, and nutritional deficiencies. In addition, women at highest risk of developing this disorder are those with mothers or sisters who developed preeclampsia during their first pregnancies, have existing high blood pressure or diabetes, or are carrying more than one baby.

The most prevalent belief today is that preeclampsia can be prevented or at least the symptoms can be lessened by improving the quality of the diet, not by salt or weight restriction.

Calcium: Calcium supplementation shows promise in preventing preeclampsia or reducing the severity of these disorders when they occur. While calcium supplementation lowers blood pressure in both pregnant and nonpregnant women, the women who derive the greatest benefits are those pregnant women with low blood calcium levels.

In a study from McMaster University in Ontario, researchers reviewed results from 14 randomized trials involving 2,459 women. They found that high blood pressure rates dropped 70 percent in women who consumed or supplemented their daily diets with 1,500 mg of calcium; preeclampsia rates dropped 62 percent. The researchers concluded that physicians should routinely recommend milk products and calcium supplements to pregnant women. Other studies have found similar bene-fits with calcium. Up to 2,000 mg of calcium taken daily might signifi-cantly reduce the incidence of both hypertension and preeclampsia. Favorable effects on blood pressure are often noted within weeks of beginning the calcium supplements.

How calcium lowers hypertension and PIH risk is poorly understood. Altered calcium metabolism has been noted in hypertensive patients, while red blood cell calcium concentrations are elevated and urinary cal-cium levels are low in women at risk for preeclampsia. Changes in how the kidneys handle sodium also might affect calcium metabolism. Regard-less of the mechanism, maintaining an optimal calcium intake before and during pregnancy might be important to the prevention of preeclampsia.

Magnesium: Magnesium supplementation might help prevent both hypertension and the seizures associated with preeclampsia. However, limited evidence shows that increased magnesium intake might aggravate low calcium levels unless calcium also is increased in the diet. In other words, increasing your intake of magnesium-rich foods, such as legumes, wheat germ, green vegetables, and whole grains, or taking a moderate-dose supplement that contains magnesium should be accompanied by increases in calcium-rich foods, such as low-fat milk and dark green leafy vegetables or a moderate-dose calcium supplement. If you choose to sup-plement during pregnancy, make sure you select a supplement that con-tains both magnesium and calcium in a ratio of one to two; for example, 250 mg of magnesium for every 500 mg of calcium. You automatically will consume a diet rich in both of these minerals if you are following the Baby-wise Diet. Never self-treat the symptoms of preeclampsia; this dis-order is very serious and at the first signs should be monitored and treated by a physician. Regular physician visits throughout pregnancy are the only means of early detection, since preeclampsia can progress unnoticed to the later, more serious stages.

Dietary Fats: If prostaglandins contribute to the onset or progression of PIH, then building blocks for these hormonelike substances might be ben-eficial in the treatment of PIH. Preliminary evidence suggests that evening primrose oil, fish oils, or linoleic acid (a type of fat in safflower oil) might help prevent preeclampsia or edema associated with preeclampsia. In con-trast, trans fatty acids in processed fats might increase risk.

Antioxidants: Vitamins E and C also show promise in lowering risk. In a study of 283 women at high risk for preeclampsia, those who took these two vitamins between the sixteenth and twenty-second weeks of their pregnancies had a 76 percent lower risk of preeclampsia than those who took placebos. Researchers suspect that free radicals damage cells in the placenta, thus contributing to the initiation and progression of preeclampsia. If this proves true, antioxidant nutrients would help offset that effect.

Other Vitamins: Increased intake of vitamins B_6 and B_{12} and folic acid showed some benefits in curbing the risk for preeclampsia in a study from the University of Washington. However, other studies have found no link between these vitamins and preeclampsia, so no recommendations can be made at this time.

What Can You Do? Women with preeclampsia who do not respond to nutrient-dense, moderate-salt diets plus bed rest might need to be hospitalized or their physicians might recommend antihypertensive medications, such as diuretics, as a last resort. That latter option reduces the total blood volume, but with any medication, there is the risk of side effects, which are especially worrisome prior to the sixteenth week of pregnancy. However, your physician will know which medications carry the least risk while providing the greatest benefits to normalizing your blood pressure. Also discuss with your physician some of the above-mentioned nutrients when tailoring your nutritional plan for pregnancy. At this time, no proven preventions for preeclampsia exist. But with careful monitoring by a physician, the condition can be successfully treated.

Diabetes: Gestational and Insulin-Dependent

Diabetes during pregnancy, called gestational diabetes, is a high-risk situation. However, diabetic women who are closely monitored by their physicians and who commit to taking extra care during their pregnancy have a 95 percent chance of having a successful pregnancy and a healthy baby.

What Is Diabetes? Diabetes is a disorder of the pancreas. More specifically, it is a disorder in the amount or effectiveness of insulin secreted by the pancreas. Problems with insulin activity upset the blood sugar regulating systems in the body, resulting in an inability to use and metabolize dietary carbohydrates. Consequently, blood sugar levels are elevated (hyperglycemia) and there is an abnormal amount of sugar in the urine. In the diabetic, blood sugar cannot enter the cells at the normal rate. The body cells are starved for energy, while blood sugar levels reach abnormally high levels and sugar spills into the urine through the kidneys.

Diabetics are at increased risk for other life-threatening diseases, such as heart disease, blindness, stroke, and gangrene. Adult-onset diabetes, also known as noninsulin-dependent diabetes mellitus (NIDDM), often responds favorably to improved dietary habits and weight loss, while diabetes that begins early in life, called juvenile-onset diabetes or insulin-dependent diabetes mellitus (IDDM), usually requires supplemental insulin therapy. Women who enter pregnancy with diabetes have an increased risk for spontaneous miscarriage and giving birth to infants with birth defects.

A woman can either enter pregnancy with diabetes or develop the disorder as a result of the pregnancy, a condition called gestational diabetes. In the first case, the disorder will persist after delivery, while in the latter case, the diabetes usually disappears after the baby is born. Women who are diabetic before pregnancy usually know of their condition and have made appropriate dietary changes and/or are taking insulin. Attaining a desirable weight and good metabolic control of the condition prior to conception reduces the risk for birth defects and lowers the incidence of pregnancy complications.

Gestational diabetes is less difficult to control and is generally associated with fewer complications than insulin-dependent diabetes; however, it still requires careful physician monitoring and adherence to a good diet to ensure a healthy pregnancy, since it can be associated with preeclampsia and urinary tract infections. The risks of congenital abnormalities and spontaneous abortion are also higher in these women. Diabetic women often deliver a large baby, which can complicate delivery and traumatize the infant or increase the risk for delivering cesarean. In addition, there is a greater risk in the baby for hypoglycemia (low blood sugar), increased bilirubin in the blood (jaundice), and respiratory distress syndrome.

A physician will individualize the diabetic's pregnancy care based on her health history, existing complications, and physical needs with the goal of maintaining tight controls on blood sugar (since both too high and too low a blood sugar can have serious effects on the developing baby) and preventing diabetes-related disorders, such as hypertension, excessive fluid surrounding the baby, and premature birth. Complications of diabetes, such as eye and kidney disorders, can intensify during pregnancy, so physicians monitor closely any changes.

A Cultural Link? Most women in the developed world experience some loss of carbohydrate (glucose) tolerance during pregnancy; however, only two to three out of every one hundred pregnant women develop gestational diabetes each year. Oddly, many women in underdeveloped countries show no fluctuation or even experience a slight drop in blood sugar during pregnancy, suggesting that either genetics or lifestyle play a role in pregnancy-induced changes in blood sugar.

A Dietary Link? Gestational diabetes is associated with increased loss of nutrients, including loss of chromium, magnesium, potassium, and vitamin B_6. A marginal deficiency of any one or more of these nutrients increases the risk for abnormal blood sugar regulation because each of these nutrients is essential in pancreatic insulin production. So the condition is a catch-22 scenario that might mean women with gestational diabetes require higher amounts of these nutrients to offset escalating losses. The birth defects associated with diabetic pregnancy are suspected to be at least partially caused by increased free-radical damage to the developing tissues. Although this suspicion has not been proven, it does suggest that antioxidant nutrients in fruits and vegetables might be especially important during pregnancy. Discuss supplementation of any or all of these nutrients with your physician.

Tests for Diabetes: In developed countries, gestational diabetes usually occurs during the second half of pregnancy and might be related to hormones secreted by the placenta that oppose the normal metabolism of insulin. If the pancreas cannot meet the extra demands of pregnancy, gestational diabetes develops, but subsides after delivery. Since many women with gestational diabetes develop no signs of the disorder, a routine test that measures blood sugar levels in response to a test dose of sugar often is used between weeks twenty-four and twenty-eight to determine the presence of diabetes. Up to 20 percent of women do not develop gestational diabetes until week thirty-two, so a woman should be retested if there is any suspicion that hyperglycemia (high blood sugar) has developed.

What Can You Eat? Ideally, a woman with diabetes who wants to have a baby should first achieve the best possible glucose control before conception. The diet of a pregnant woman with diabetes is similar to the Baby-wise Diet and is high in complex carbohydrate–rich foods, such as whole-grain breads and pasta, legumes, and vegetables; moderate in protein (20 percent of total calorie intake); and low in fat (25 to 30 percent of total calories with fewer than 10 percent coming from saturated fat). Energy is often distributed into three meals and three snacks with 17 to 18 percent of calories consumed at breakfast, 30 percent each at lunch and dinner, and 30 grams of carbohydrate and one protein exchange (7 or 8 grams of protein) for an evening snack. These foods also will supply the added fiber, chromium, and magnesium needed to help regulate blood sugar levels, as well as the vitamin C, vitamin E, and other nutrients associated with diabetes control, while maintaining a calorie intake that allows moderate weight gain. Snacks and spacing meals will be important, as will daily exercise and plenty of rest. Sugars and sweets should be eliminated. Suggestions for making simple changes in your diet can be found below.

TABLE 6.5

Simple Changes

Overwhelmed by how many changes you need to make in your diet just to break the ceiling on adequate? Even small, sometimes even tiny, changes or additions to your diet can make a difference in your health, energy level, and pregnancy.

1. **Drink a small glass of orange juice with breakfast.**
   A six-ounce glass of orange juice every morning reduces your risk for stroke, lowers the "bad" cholesterol called LDLs, and boosts the good cholesterol called HDLs, thus reducing heart disease risk, lowering colon cancer risk, and reducing blood pressure. A glass of orange juice supplies up to 140 mg of vitamin C, potassium, folic acid, and a phytochemical called d-limonene that detoxifies cancer-causing substances.
2. **Chomp on a carrot.**
   A carrot a day could slash stroke risk by 68 percent, according to a study from Harvard on almost 90,000 female nurses who ate carrots at least fives times a week. Carotenes in carrots and other orange veggies also lower cancer and heart-attack risks. Other options: Munch on baby carrots, add grated carrots to a salad or burrito, or add frozen carrots to canned soups.
3. **Switch from iceberg to romaine lettuce.**
   Iceberg is fine, if you like crunchy water. But if you want to get the best nutritional bang for your buck, you can double your nutrients for no extra calories by switching to romaine or other leaf lettuces. Romaine has twice the fiber, B vitamins, folic acid (a B vitamin that lowers heart disease and cancer risk and prevents birth defects), calcium, potassium, and trace minerals as iceberg. It has seven times the vitamin C and vitamin A.
   If you want to do yourself an even bigger favor, switch to spinach salads. A salad made with two cups of spinach supplies half your day's need for folic acid and vitamin C, all of your requirement for vitamin A, and more than 25 percent of your day's need for vitamin E, magnesium, and potassium. An equal amount of iceberg doesn't make a dent in your day's requirements.
4. **Eat nuts.**
   Not only are nuts a good source of protein, magnesium, vitamin E, and B vitamins, but recent research shows that a handful of nuts as a snack several times a week lowers heart-disease risk by 35 percent and cancer risk. The fat in nuts

is heart-healthy monounsaturated fat. Nuts are high in fat, yet adding them to the daily diet helps with weight loss after the baby is born.

5. Cook in cast iron.

Throw out that expensive cookware and return to Grandma's cast iron. The iron leaches out of the pot into the food, boosting iron content severalfold, especially in acidic foods such as Chunky Spaghetti Sauce, in the Appendix, and tomato-based soups, such as SouthWest Tuscany Soup, also in the Appendix.

6. Drink your decaf tea and coffee between meals.

These beverages contain compounds called tannins that reduce iron absorption by somewhere between 60 and 94 percent. Herbal teas do the same: Peppermint blocks iron by up to 84 percent, chamomile and others by half.

7. Switch from white to whole-wheat bread.

Order your turkey sandwich on whole-wheat instead of white bread and you'll boost your intake of just about every vitamin and mineral, plus add a few grams of fiber to your daily routine. Whole-wheat bread has four times the fiber, magnesium, and chromium (a mineral that helps regulate blood sugar), and lots more zinc, copper, vitamin E, and vitamin B_6 than white bread. And, while refined grains are on the hot seat for aggravating diabetes risk, whole grains lower your risk for diabetes, stroke, and colon cancer.

8. Chew gum while cooking.

Women unconsciously chow down on hundreds of calories while cooking meals. They taste the sauce not once but several times. Chew sugarless gum when cooking or drink ice water to keep your fingers out of the food and to satisfy your need to munch.

While most women are discouraged from restricting calories or "dieting" during pregnancy, obese women with gestational diabetes benefit from a moderate calorie-restricted diet of 1,600 to 1,800 calories a day. Normal blood sugar is maintained, excessive weight gain is avoided, and the infant's birth weight is closer to "normal" when calories are restricted to less than 2,000 calories a day in these women. Blood sugar responses to a diet and/or exercise prescription will vary from one person to the next, so all eating plans should be validated with blood glucose monitoring to ensure that the optimal mix of carbohydrate at each meal and snack is maintaining a steady blood sugar level. Your physician and a dietitian can work with you in developing a meal plan that suits you.

What about Exercise? Daily exercise is a useful addition to good eating in the management of gestational diabetes. Moderate weight training at home using two-pound cans or sacks of flour or sugar and a moderate aerobic activity such as walking are a good starting point.

Second Trimester Nutrition

The second trimester of pregnancy is considered by some women to be the "golden months." Often the inconveniences of the first trimester, such as morning sickness and fatigue, have subsided, yet the growing baby has not become so cumbersome as to interfere with eating or exercise. This is the time to make up for any nutritional transgressions during the early stage of pregnancy and to foster optimal eating habits that will fuel the growth of a beautiful baby. Use Worksheet 6.1 at the end of this chapter, "My Second Trimester Daily Checklist," to monitor your food intake for the next three months.

Quiz 6.1   Are You Getting Enough? Fruits and Vegetables That Is . . .

Be honest. Are you religiously gobbling your daily ten servings of fruits and vegetables? Or, are you cutting corners, fooling yourself, downright avoiding the produce section? Take the test below and see.

1. My breakfast resembles:
   a. a cup of decaf coffee and a quick glance at the paper.
   b. bacon and eggs or a Starbucks muffin.
   c. a bowl of whole-grain cereal, sliced banana, nonfat milk, and a glass of orange juice.
2. My midmorning snack typically includes:
   a. if anything at all, a quick jaunt to the vending machine.
   b. a doughnut, muffin, or bagel.
   c. a piece of fruit or a box of raisins.
3. My lunch typically includes:
   a. a trip through the drive-through for a hamburger, fries, and cola.
   b. a sandwich, chips, and milk.
   c. a low-fat entrée, tossed salad, piece of fruit, and milk.
4. At a salad bar, I go for the:
   a. meats, pastas, and cheese with a light helping of lettuce.
   b. iceberg lettuce, tomatoes, creamy dressing, and croutons.
   c. spinach or romaine lettuce, heaps of plain vegetables, and low-fat dressing.
5. My midafternoon snack typically includes:
   a. a can of soda pop.
   b. a bag of chips or a cookie.
   c. baby carrots, apple, or yogurt with berries.

6. My dinner typically includes:
   a. meat and potatoes.
   b. pizza or other takeout.
   c. a plate heaped with vegetables, a salad, and small servings of lean meat and/or beans.
7. My dinner vegetable typically is:
   a. the thin slice of onion on my pizza.
   b. potatoes, french fries, corn, and/or iceberg lettuce.
   c. a dark green or yellow vegetable, cruciferous vegetable (cabbage, broccoli, asparagus, brussels sprouts, etc.), or other deeply colored selection.
8. Other than nonfat milk or soy milk, I typically drink:
   a. soda pop.
   b. water, apple juice, or other fruit drinks or ades.
   c. 100 percent fruit juice, such as orange juice, grapefruit juice, pineapple juice, carrot juice, tomato or V8 juice, or prune juice.
9. At restaurants, I typically order:
   a. steak or hamburger and fries.
   b. pasta with meat or fish sauce.
   c. grilled chicken or fish, salad, steamed vegetables, side order of fruit.
10. I order my pizza topped with:
    a. extra cheese and sausage, bacon, or pepperoni.
    b. chicken or beef.
    c. extra peppers, mushrooms, and other vegetables, along with a side salad.
11. In my gym bag, you'll usually find:
    a. a pair of dirty socks only.
    b. a granola or energy bar.
    c. a banana or other fruit, along with other snacks and a water bottle.
12. My typical after-dinner treat is:
    a. chocolate chip cookies, cake, or candy.
    b. popcorn or chips.
    c. berries or other fresh fruit with or without ice cream or frozen yogurt.
13. I typically include _____ vegetable(s) and/or fruit at every meal:
    a. If you don't count French fries, I'm a perfect zero.
    b. one.
    c. two or more.
14. The last time I tried a new fruit or vegetable was:
    a. when I was a toddler and my mother forced me to try peas.
    b. within the past year.
    c. I am constantly trying new vegetables and fruit and new ways to prepare them.

Scoring:

C was your most common choice:
Good work! You're probably including the recommended eight to ten servings of fruits and vegetables in your daily menu.

B was your most common choice:
You're trying to eat healthfully, but you probably are falling far short of your allotment for produce. Aim to include at least one fruit or vegetable, other than fries, iceberg lettuce, and apple juice, to each meal and snack.

A was your most common choice:
You've got a little work to do. You are at or below the national average of three servings a day. Skip the fries and include at least one citrus and one dark green leafy vegetable every day.

Worksheet 6.1 My Second Trimester Daily Checklist

Copy this master sheet to complete daily.

Food Groups	Minimum Servings	Actual Intake
Calcium-rich foods	3	_____
Vegetables (at least 2 folic acid–rich choices)	6	_____
Fruits (at least 2 vitamin C–rich choices)	4	_____
Grains (at least 4 whole-grain choices)	7	_____
Extra-lean meats and legumes	3	_____
Quenchers	6	_____

Did I reach my goals? _____

What needs improvement? _____

What will I do differently next week? _____

Chapter 7

Nutrition during the Third Trimester

During the third trimester of pregnancy your concerns will be:

1. **Nutrition:** Follow the guidelines outlined in the Baby-wise Diet.
2. **Weight:** Try to limit weight gain to approximately 0.7 to 1.4 pounds a week for a total of 9 to 19 pounds. Don't be surprised if weight gain slows slightly in the final two to three weeks.
3. **Supplement:** Continue to take a multiple vitamin and mineral that contains 100 to 200 percent of the Daily Value for all vitamins and minerals, plus at least 18 mg of iron each day.
4. **Safety:** Continue to avoid alcohol, tobacco, and any medication not approved by your physician as safe during pregnancy.
5. **Exercise and Rest:** Exercise daily, but adjust the routine, intensity, or duration as needed. Balance exercise with rest, by putting your feet up and taking an afternoon nap.
6. **Medical Checkups:** Make physician visits weekly now to monitor weight and obtain necessary tests.

Weight Gain and Why

During the third trimester your baby gains a considerable amount of weight, stretching your abdomen to its maximum. Some women eat less during this time because their stomachs cannot find room for large meals. Others cut back on their food intake because they think they look or feel heavy. This is not a time to limit weight gain.

Weight gain in the last trimester is just as critical during the previous six months, if not more so.. Women who restrict calories at this time could jeopardize the birth weight, health, and mental development of their babies. The placenta, head circumference (a measurement of brain development), and birth length of your baby depend on optimal intake of calories, protein, carbohydrates, and some fats. In fact, some evidence shows that the mother's weight gain in the third trimester is the most important indicator of the baby's birth weight. Studies from both the University of California at Berkeley and the University of North Carolina at Chapel Hill found that a slow steady weight gain during the later part of pregnancy was especially important to the mother and baby, while inadequate weight gain during the final trimester was closely associated with an increased risk for preterm delivery.

The effects of weight gain carry over from one generation to the next. A woman whose mother restricted calories in the third trimester and was a low-birth-weight baby can also pass on this heritage to her baby. Consequently, your mother's weight gain throughout, and especially in the third trimester, might affect your baby's birth weight, just as your weight gain during pregnancy could influence the birth weight of your grandchildren! However, it cannot be overemphasized that the sins of our ancestors can be, to a great extent, corrected by taking good care of ourselves before, during, and after pregnancy.

Not the Time to Binge! Encouraging weight gain during the last trimester does not give you a license to gorge! (Excessive weight gain, or more than two pounds a week, could be a sign of pregnancy-induced hypertension, or PIH, and should be checked by your doctor.) Also, limit the number of times you weigh yourself to once a week. Your weight is likely to vary during this last trimester because of water retention and fluctuations in rate of gain, so daily weigh-ins could give you a false reading.

How Much Weight Should You Gain? Much of your weight gain in the second trimester was caused by your expanding tissues, including the placenta, your fat stores, breast tissue, and blood volume. In contrast, weight gain in the third trimester is your baby, and to a lesser extent the placenta and amniotic fluid. Your baby will double in size during the last three months of pregnancy. Your breast tissue and other body tissue are gearing up for breast-feeding, too. That means you'll be gaining between 10 and 18 pounds during the last three months of pregnancy, with an emphasis on pacing the gain—that is, about 1 to 1½ pounds per week. In general, women who entered pregnancy already overweight should gain less and women who were underweight prior to pregnancy should gain more.

Can't Eat Enough? If you are having trouble eating enough, try dividing your food intake into several small meals and snacks so that you eat every three hours. Drink liquids between meals, rather than at mealtime so that you can save every bit of your small stomach for food. If you aren't gaining enough weight, reevaluate your eating habits. Are you following the Baby-wise Diet guidelines or are you falling short of one or more essential servings? Are you forgetting to include several nutritious snacks throughout the day? If you are eating only three meals a day, chances are you aren't consuming enough calories or nutrients.

Are You Gaining Too Much? Check with your physician to make sure there are no health issues related to your weight gain if you are gaining more than 1½ pounds a week. Also consider the following:

- Check your fat intake. Have extra salad dressing, fried foods, gravies, creamy desserts, or other hidden fats crept into your menu plans?
- Are you choosing foods that give you the most nutrient "punch" for the least calories? That means concentrating on nonfat milk not whole milk for your calcium-rich servings; strawberries not dried apricots for your fruit servings; and broccoli not corn for your vegetable.
- Are you cheating? Even an extra hundred calories can add an extra pound in one month, so stick closely to the Baby-wise Diet.
- What's up with exercise? Have you stopped walking every day or cut back? Although the intensity and duration of your exercise might decrease in the third trimester, you can still exercise in several short sessions during the day to maintain a good level of fitness and burn extra calories.

When and What to Eat and Drink

While your baby is putting on the pounds (at a rate of an ounce or two a day in the ninth month!) during this trimester, the infant brain is also developing rapidly. The brain increases in size and in the number of mature nerve cells it contains. These metabolically active cells account for only 2 to 3 percent of body weight, but are now consuming up to 20 percent of the baby's entire energy intake. Your baby is also storing nutrients, in particular iron and calcium. You are now transferring more calcium to help calcify your baby's bones and iron to help build his or her iron stores and protect against anemia in the first few months of life. So you must make sure you eat enough or the supply will go to the baby, leaving you feeling tired and mentally sluggish.

Your calorie intake should average approximately 2,500 calories a day (more if you exercise). As always, the Baby-wise Diet forms the basis of your eating plan, with the following minimum number of servings from each list:

3 servings from the Calcium-Rich Group
6 servings from the Vegetable Group (at least 2 servings should be folic acid–rich choices)
4 servings from the Fruit Group (at least 2 servings should be vitamin C–rich choices)
3 servings from the Extra-Lean Meats and Legume Group (try to include 2 to 3 servings of fish and 4 to 5 servings of legumes in the weekly menu)
7 servings from the Grain Group (at least 4 servings should be whole-grain choices)
6 servings from the Quenchers Group

This is the time to keep cheating in check. A piece of chocolate cake might taste good, but it is a poor source of the vitamins and minerals that your baby needs right now. So, make sure you've eaten your quota of nutritious foods before diving into the cheesecake! Be a shrewd cheater. If you want a cookie, make it a more nutritious oatmeal-raisin, rather than a chocolate sandwich cookie. A slice of Glazed Blueberry-Lemon Bread or a serving of Apple Bread Pudding (from the recipe section of this book) might satisfy the sweet tooth and either is more nutritious than pound cake with icing, while a frozen fruit ice or Frozen Frappacino (also from the recipe section) can satisfy a craving for something sweet and cold without spending the extra calories on ice cream.

Carbohydrate-Rich Foods: Your diet should continue to be rich in carbohydrates, such as fruits, vegetables, whole grains, and cooked dried beans and peas. These foods help avoid constipation and fatigue and supply ample amounts of all the vitamins and minerals, while being low in fat, and thus helping to regulate weight gain. (See Table 7.1, "Love Those Veggies.")

TABLE 7.1

Love Those Veggies

After trying some of these suggestions, you'll have no excuse for not eating your seven a day.

1. Open a bag of preshredded cabbage. Mix with a little light coleslaw dressing (chopped apples or canned pineapple chunks are optional).
2. Add grated carrots or zucchini to spaghetti sauce.
3. Mash green peas into guacamole. It reduces fat without changing taste or texture.
4. Add chopped fresh tomatoes and cilantro to bottled salsa as a quick dip for chips, baby carrots, or pita bread, or pile it on as dressing for salads, tacos, burritos.
5. Make pumpkin pie with fat-free canned milk and low-fat crust.
6. Add lots of leaf lettuce, red onion, and thick tomato slices to a turkey sandwich.
7. Pop frozen blueberries or grapes into your mouth for a sorbetlike treat.
8. Top your morning cereal with dried plums or cranberries or a handful of fresh berries.
9. Drink a travel-size box of orange juice on the way to work.
10. Stir fresh peaches or berries into frozen yogurt.
11. Add canned mandarin oranges to your spinach salad.
12. Skewer more vegetables (cherry tomatoes, carrot slices, mushrooms, eggplant, onion, squash, sweet potato, etc.) than meat on your shish kebabs.
13. Add frozen green peas to canned chicken noodle soup.
14. Never, *and I mean never,* leave the house without a snack stash (i.e., banana, orange, apple, baby carrots, raisins, grapes, and/or jicama).
15. Puree fresh fruit, sweeten with concentrated apple juice, and freeze into ice cubes or pops. Add cubes to club soda for a refreshing drink.
16. Add fruit to your milkshake.
17. Make fruit or vegetable salsa and sauces with mango, papaya, peaches, or pineapple and use in place of creamed sauces on meats, fish, and chicken.
18. Purchase nonfat plain yogurt and sweeten with fruit.
19. After dinner, place a platter of cut-up fruit on the dinner table for evening snacking.
20. At the restaurant, order entrées that feature vegetables (grilled vegetable sandwich, salad, vegetable soup).
21. Ask your waiter to hold the potato and instead bring two side orders of vegetables (steamed) with your order.
22. Add grapes, mandarin oranges, or cubed apples to chicken salad.
23. Skip syrup, and top pancakes, waffles, or French toast with fresh fruit.
24. Puree vegetables, such as cauliflower, carrots, or broccoli, and add to soup stock and sauces.

TABLE 7.1 continued

25. Add dried fruit to stuffings and rice dishes.
26. Double your normal portion of any vegetable (except French fries or iceberg lettuce)!
27. Cut sweet potatoes into ½-inch strips and roast for a tasty alternative to French fries.
28. Stuff an almond into each of five pitted dried plums for a sweet, chewy, crunchy snack.
29. Plan your dinner around the theme of "meat and three veggies."
30. Toss a bag of frozen stew vegetables (large hunks of carrots, potato, celery, and onion) with a tablespoon of olive oil, dash of salt and pepper, and a few sprigs of fresh rosemary. Roast at 425° for thirty minutes.
31. Toss chopped tomatoes, corn, red onion, salt, and rice vinegar for a quick and filling snack or lunch salad.
32. Add cilantro, chopped tomatoes, corn, grated carrots, or other vegetables to tacos and burritos.
33. When flying, ask for tomato or orange juice for your in-flight beverage.
34. Once a week, have a meal salad for dinner, such as Cajun salmon caesar salad or grilled chicken spinach salad with mandarin oranges.
35. Take advantage of precut vegetables, prepackaged salads, supermarket salad bars, and exotic specialty produce.
36. Grill extra vegetables at dinner to use in a quick wrap for tomorrow's lunch.
37. Fill a halved cantaloupe with lemon-flavored yogurt.
38. Skip the fruit drinks, blends, and ades; go for the 100 percent orange, grape-fruit, prune, and pineapple juices.
39. Add flowers, like dandelions, violets, daylilies, clover, and oxalis, to salads.
40. Add steamed asparagus or green beans to your favorite pasta dish.
41. Top pizza with extra quartered artichoke hearts (canned in water), roasted red peppers, red onions, sliced zucchini, and fresh tomatoes.
42. Order deli sandwiches with extra tomatoes.
43. Whip steamed, chopped collards or chard into mashed potatoes
44. Buy produce at various stages of ripeness to avoid spoilage.
45. Stock up on frozen plain vegetables for last-minute meals.
46. Keep dried fruit on hand for a quick snack.
47. Plant a pear or apple tree, row of blueberry bushes, or vegetable garden in the backyard.
48. When eating out, order off the menu, ask for two sides of vegetables, or split an entrée and complement with a salad.
49. At parties, sip on orange juice, tomato juice, or Blood Mary mix.
50. Take a low-fat cooking class and share vegetable recipes with friends.

Protein-Rich Foods: Protein requirements also are at an all-time high in the last trimester. Protein is the building block for the baby's muscles and tissues, which are growing at record rates. Extra protein also is needed as you get ready for labor, delivery, and breast-feeding. However, typical American diets are already high in protein, so, unless you are following a strict vegetarian diet or are eating few protein-rich foods, your intake of this nutrient is probably more than adequate. The Baby-wise Diet supplies at least 70 grams of protein daily, which is more than the 60 grams recommended for pregnant women. In addition, your protein needn't come from expensive cuts of meat, such as lamb chops, steak, or roast prime rib. Cooked dried beans and peas, tofu, chicken without the skin, low-fat milk, and fish are also sources of quality protein.

Vitamins and Minerals: Other nutrients that become increasingly more important as you approach labor and delivery are all those related to immune function, including vitamin A, copper, zinc, and the B vitamins; the antioxidant system including beta carotene, vitamin C, vitamin E, and selenium; and circulation, including protein and iron. All these are needed in moderate amounts for optimal healing of tissues after delivery. In addition, several of these nutrients also function directly in the healing process.

Vitamin C is especially important in wound healing and recovery from delivery. Skin, blood vessel walls, and all body tissues are "glued" together by connective tissue, of which collagen is a major component. Repairing tissues includes producing and laying down new connective tissue and collagen, and vitamin C is a critical factor in collagen formation. Slow wound healing and poorly formed scars that break open, scaly skin, and tender joints are symptoms of vitamin C deficiency. Make sure you include those seven vegetables and four fruits, and focus on colorful ones, such as strawberries, citrus, and broccoli.

Zinc, vitamin E, and several B vitamins, including pantothenic acid, are important in healing wounds and speeding recovery after surgery. Vitamin A is essential for maintaining and repairing the delicate tissue that lines the vaginal and uterine walls, called epithelial tissue. Optimal intake of this vitamin helps restore these tissues after the baby is born. Marginal intake of these nutrients has been reported in pregnant women, while deficiencies are common during times of stress, illness, or hospitalization. (See Chapter 2 for sources of these nutrients.)

Most people know that folic acid is essential for preventing neural tube defects in the weeks surrounding conception, but the vitamin might be just as important in the third trimester, according to state researchers at the University of Medicine and Dentistry of New Jersey. When average folic acid intakes in pregnant mothers were measured and compared to pregnancy outcomes, the researchers found that women with low daily folic acid consumption (i.e., less than 240 mcg/day) and/or low blood folic acid levels had a twofold increased risk of preterm delivery and low-birth-weight babies. Make sure you include at least two dark green leafy vegetables in your daily diet.

Pregnant women who consume less than 1,100 mg of calcium in the third trimester produce milk that is low in this essential mineral compared to women who consume higher levels of calcium during pregnancy, which suggests that babies breast-fed by mothers who consume calcium-poor diets during pregnancy might receive suboptimal amounts of calcium. In a study from the University of Tennessee in Memphis, women who previously consumed calcium-poor diets and then boosted their daily intakes to about 2,000 mg of calcium during the second and third trimesters delivered babies with increased bone densities compared to women who didn't supplement. Calcium supplementation had no additional benefits for women already consuming optimal amounts of calcium prior to and during pregnancy. (See Table 7.2, "Sneaking More Calcium into Your Diet.")

Vitamins and minerals also are important to offset the stress from carrying a growing baby and from labor and delivery. A study from the University of California at Davis found that long labors and stress to the mother and baby during labor and delivery interfered with the initial stages of breast-feeding after the baby was born. Ensuring that you are rested and well nourished prior to labor can help curb this stress and ease the transition from pregnancy to parenthood.

By following the Baby-wise Diet, you are assured of obtaining all the nutrients you need to meet the added stress of the third trimester and of labor and delivery. If you have chosen to take a vitamin and mineral supplement, keep in mind that moderation is the rule. For example, although increased intake of zinc either through dietary or supplemental sources is recommended for helping improve healing and recovery from injury, caution should be used in overdosing with this trace mineral. Intakes in excess of 50 mg could result in secondary deficiencies of other trace minerals, such as copper.

TABLE 7.2

Sneaking More Calcium into Your Diet

Tired of drinking four glasses of milk every day? Does the thought of another cup of yogurt put a damper on your appetite? You can obtain ample amounts of calcium without even knowing it. Try the following tricks for adding calcium to your diet:

1. Make creamed soups and cream sauces with evaporated nonfat milk instead of cream.
2. Cook your brown rice, oatmeal, or noodles in nonfat milk or calcium-fortified soy milk.
3. Add nonfat dry milk powder to recipes for muffins, breads, pancakes, milk-shakes, or even meat loaf.
4. Drink calcium-fortified orange juice or use calcium-fortified bread.
5. Substitute low-fat cheese for meat in lasagna, ravioli, or stuffed shells.
6. Use undiluted evaporated nonfat milk in mashed potatoes.
7. Use canned salmon with the bones.
8. Blend nonfat milk or calcium-fortified soy milk with fresh fruit to make a fruit shake.

Water: The Most Important Nutrient

Water is one of the most important nutrients in your diet, and you can undermine your energy and mood during pregnancy if you let it go in short supply. Water constitutes half of your body weight, or ten to twelve gallons. You need this essential fluid to digest and absorb other nutrients, remove waste products from the body, regulate body temperature, and perform the millions of metabolic processes essential to life. You also lose about two to three quarts of water every day through perspiration, urination, and other wastes. Consequently, dehydration can set in quickly if you aren't replacing these fluid losses. Weight gain during pregnancy and milk production during breast-feeding place an added demand on your body's fluid supply; you must consume ample amounts of water and other fluids to meet this need.

Many women fall far short of optimal when it comes to drinking enough water. Since thirst is a poor indicator of need, your best bet is to drink at least twice as much water as it takes to quench your thirst, with a minimum of at least six to eight glasses of fluids each day. If you exercise regularly, you'll need even more.

Mood Changes

There is nothing quite so permanent as having a baby. You can change jobs, move to a new city, and get a divorce, but you can't stop being a parent. So, it's not surprising that while pregnancy is one of the best times in a woman's life, it also can have its not-so-good moments when fears, worries, or doubts surface. Don't worry if you have a few mixed feelings as the due date approaches. Most women experience at least a little ambivalence; it's just that until recently many women kept their feelings to themselves. Now, we are becoming much more vocal about our experiences. Many women report problems with memory loss during pregnancy. One study found that recall, recognition, and memory were impaired in pregnant women compared to nonpregnant women; however, there is no evidence that any loss of memory persists longer than a few weeks after the baby is born. Follow these basic rules for managing your mood during this final stage of pregnancy:

- View your mood swings as natural, not pathological. In fact, emotional ups and downs can result from changes in hormones, such as prolactin, a hormone that stimulates milk production and mood swings, and is being produced in increasing amounts in the last trimester.
- Recognize that any emotional high or low is probably a phase that will pass. So revel in the highs and wait out the lows.
- Share your feelings with someone you can trust and who can provide understanding: a spouse, a friend, a parent, or even your physician. A support network is critical for getting the help, advice, and hand-holding that every mother-to-be needs.
- Be honest with yourself about your fears (Will I be a good parent? Can I juggle work and a family?). Also, be realistic; you don't have to be perfect to be a good parent.

Food and Mood

Besides the normal emotional ebb and flow of pregnancy, what a woman eats, even at a single meal, could affect whether she is happy, sad, irritable, calm, absentminded, or clear-thinking.

It is no coincidence that people turn to pasta, desserts, and other carbohydrate-rich foods when they feel down in the dumps. Carbohydrates have a profound effect on numerous body chemicals that regulate how a woman feels and acts.

Carbohydrates stimulate the release of the hormone insulin from the pancreas, which in turn lowers blood levels of all amino acids, except tryptophan. Normally, tryptophan must compete with other amino acids for entry into the brain, but with reduced competition, tryptophan levels rise. The brain then converts tryptophan into serotonin, a neurotransmitter that sends messages between nerve cells. Serotonin helps regulate sleep, reduces pain and appetite, alleviates irritability, and elevates mood.

Interestingly, several conditions associated with depression and fatigue also are linked to increased cravings for carbohydrate-rich foods, suggesting that people unknowingly self-regulate their moods with the foods they eat. The carbohydrate-rich snack alters brain chemistry and provides temporary relief from mild depression or tension. In contrast, a high-protein diet, by supplying more of the competing amino acids, reduces tryptophan and serotonin levels in the brain. Consequently, carbohydrate-sensitive women who eat a high-protein breakfast might experience fatigue or mood swings and crave a carbohydrate-rich midmorning snack in an effort to raise brain serotonin levels and "feel better."

Often people are less alert, have trouble concentrating, make more mistakes, and feel sleepier after a carbohydrate-rich meal compared to a protein-rich meal. Consequently, the time of day you grab a bagel or chow down on a plate of pasta also could affect your mood. Pasta for dinner might leave you feeling relaxed, while the same meal for lunch could make you sluggish.

Sugar Cravings: Mood swings and depression also might be linked to your sugar or caffeine intake. Depression and fatigue often vanish when sugar (and caffeine) are removed from the diet. In essence, using sugar to self-regulate mood is a temporary fix. In the long run, it could create a vicious cycle. "The person suffering from depression who turns to sugary foods may relieve the fatigue and feel better for a short while, but the depression and fatigue return," says Larry Christensen, Ph.D., at the University of Southern Alabama. The person then must either reach for another sugar fix or seek help elsewhere. As opposed to the temporary sugar high, eliminating sugar and caffeine from the diet is a permanent solution.

So What Can You Do? Carbohydrate cravers cannot "will away" their cravings, so they should work with them instead. Make sure every meal contains some complex carbohydrate–rich foods, such as bread, cereals, crackers, or other starches. In addition, carbohydrate cravers should plan a carbohydrate-rich snack during that time of the day when they are most vulnerable to snack attacks, and they should choose whole-grain breads and cereals. People who know they are sensitive to sugar should avoid sweets or eat them in small doses and always with other, more nutritious foods.

Make changes gradually. Any dramatic change in normal eating patterns can alter brain chemistry. Cutting calories, bingeing on sweets, skipping meals such as breakfast, or other unusual eating habits affect neurotransmitter levels and, consequently, mood and behavior. In contrast, the Babywise Diet that contains at least 2,200 calories from fresh fruits and vegetables, whole-grain breads and cereals, cooked dried beans and peas, nonfat milk products, fish, poultry, and extra-lean meats provides ample amounts of all the nutrients associated with mental and physical health. Consuming several small meals or snacks throughout the day, rather than two to three big meals, helps maintain steady blood sugar and neurotransmitter levels.

Regular exercise, effective coping skills, and a strong social support system also are important considerations. Chronic depression and fatigue can be symptoms of other problems and can affect the outcome of your pregnancy, so always consult a physician if emotional problems persist or interfere with the quality of your life and your pregnancy.

Gearing Up for Delivery

In the games of life and birthing, there are no guarantees. Every woman's experience giving birth is different and even varies from one pregnancy to the next. Even a pregnancy nourished on whole grains, dark green leafies, and brisk walks cannot promise a two-hour, pain-free labor. However, good nutrition and daily exercise prior to and during pregnancy improve your odds for an easier pregnancy and delivery, and reduce the time it takes to get your figure back. Feeling good and fit also pumps up your self-esteem, helps you tolerate labor pains, and boosts your endurance during the hard work of birthing a baby.

The fluid and nutrient needs of a woman in labor have been compared to the needs of a competition athlete. Consequently, depriving yourself of food and fluids before, and possibly during labor, could affect the labor progress and outcome. Researchers at St. Louis University Medical School speculate that consuming ample amounts of carbohydrate-rich foods (or carbohydrate loading) the week before labor onset—the same dietary practice used by athletes prior to a marathon—might increase tissue glycogen stores and help supply extra energy for labor and delivery.

To Eat or Not to Eat during Labor: Most physicians recommend restricting food and/or fluids during labor because of the possibility of vomiting or problems with aspiration if anesthesia is required. On the other hand, not eating throughout a lengthy labor is similar to fasting all day. Blood sugar and muscle glycogen (energy) stores, the major sources of energy for both the laboring mother and the baby, are depleted during a fast, and this could affect the baby's well-being. Babies of mothers who did not eat anything for several hours prior to and/or during labor are less active than babies born of mothers who periodically replenished energy stores by drinking fruit juice or eating small snacks. When blood and muscle stores of sugar are depleted, the body turns to fat tissue. As a result, large quantities of fat fragments, called free fatty acids, are partially broken down for energy, causing an increase in blood levels of ketones. The accumulation of these fat fragments is called ketosis. It is unclear whether or not ketosis is harmful to the mother or infant. There is some evidence that ketosis is associated with prolonged labor, but it is uncertain which comes first.

As ketone levels rise in the mother, they cross the placenta and rise in the baby's blood, increasing the acidity of the blood. Babies apparently have a relatively high tolerance for this fluctuation in the normal acid-base balance. On the other hand, women who consume some carbohydrates, in the form of juice or other clear liquids, during labor lower their ketone levels and decrease the babies' exposure to these breakdown products as well. Levels of essential amino acids, the building blocks of protein, also drop after only twelve hours of food deprivation.

Despite the lingering belief that women should not eat during labor, more recent evidence shows that eating something periodically could be beneficial. In one study of forty laboring women, those women who ate light meals of toast, ice cream, yogurt, or fresh fruit required less pain relief and their labors were shortened by an average of ninety minutes, as compared to women who were allowed only toast and tea at the onset of labor and sips of water thereafter. In addition, Apgar scores (an indicator of a baby's physical condition a few minutes after birth) of babies in the well-fed group were higher than in the food-restricted group. Of course, chances are, once labor progresses, you won't be very hungry anyway.

Acupuncture and Delivery: Some women call their acupuncturist at the same time they call their physicians—when the labor contractions start. An ancient Chinese medical practice that uses hair-thin needles for the treatment of pain and stress, acupuncture might be useful for labor, especially to stimulate contractions, dilate the cervix, and relieve pain.

Moxibustion (using herbs to stimulate acupuncture points) also shows promise in preventing or treating breech presentation of the baby in the week prior to the onset of labor, according to a study published in the *Journal of the American Medical Association.*

In the weeks prior to your due date, you should discuss all of your labor plans with your physician, including who you want as part of your delivery team and how you will nourish yourself prior to and during the birthing process. (See Table 7.3, "Delivering Your Baby.")

TABLE 7.3

Delivering Your Baby

Whom do you want to deliver your baby? Here are a few options.

Family practitioner: A physician who attends to your entire family's health needs and also delivers babies.
Obstetrician: A physician who specializes in the care of women and pregnant women, including delivering the baby.
Perinatologist: A physician who specializes in high-risk pregnancies.
Nurse-midwife: A registered nurse with additional training and certification in caring for pregnant women and delivering babies either in a hospital, birthing center, or in your home. Usually only women at low risk for complications choose midwives outside of a hospital setting.

Premature Labor and Delivery

Premature labor occurs when a woman begins labor more than three weeks before the due date. Uterine contractions cause the cervix—the mouth of the uterus—to open sooner than normal, which can result in the birth of a premature baby who is at risk of developing serious complications, including problems with breathing, eating, and body temperature regulation. Understanding the early signals of premature labor can help you prevent your baby from being born too soon.

Premature labor often is not painful, but can be accompanied by uterine contractions that occur every ten minutes or more frequently. A woman might experience some menstrual-like cramping in the lower abdomen that comes and goes or stays constant. These cramps are the uterine wall tightening and you can feel it tighten or harden during the contraction and soften after the contraction stops. Other symptoms of premature labor include intermittent or constant dull aches and pains in your lower back below the waistline, some pressure in the pelvic area as if the baby were pushing down, and a sudden increase in vaginal discharge. While most women experience some "false alarm" contractions during pregnancy, called Braxton Hicks' contractions, these harmless cramps are irregular. In contrast, call your doctor right away if you experience regular contractions or more than five contractions in one hour with or without any of the other symptoms. Medications are available that can stop premature labor if it is caught in the early stages.

A Nutritional Approach to Common Problems: From Hemorrhoids to Insomnia

The last trimester comes with its own set of ups and downs. Some you might have encountered in the second trimester, such as constipation; others, such as insomnia or leg cramps, might develop for the first time in the last months or weeks of pregnancy. In many cases, there is something you can do to prevent or at least lessen the symptoms.

Constipation

If constipation wasn't a problem during your second trimester, it might develop now. Try drinking plenty of water—at least six to eight glasses of water and other fluids every day. If you are following the Baby-wise Diet, your intake of fiber-rich fruits, vegetables, legumes, and whole grains should be sufficient to keep constipation at bay. Try prunes, prune juice, or figs, or adding a little extra bran to your breakfast if you need an added fiber boost. Eating regularly also helps, since it keeps your body on a schedule that might help regular bowel movements. Daily exercise also is important. As mentioned before, do not take laxatives without physician approval. (See Chapter 6, pages 154–55, for more on constipation.)

Hemorrhoids

Hemorrhoids are varicose veins that swell in small lumps around the anus. They usually develop from the uterus putting pressure on these veins or from straining associated with constipation. Although the pressure of the expanding uterus and weight of the baby alone can cause hemorrhoids, often these painful, swollen veins around the rectum develop as a result of constipation. Straining during bowel movements and having very hard stools only make the situation worse. Always check with your physician before self-medicating with over-the-counter preparations. In addition, the Baby-wise Diet contains plenty of fiber-rich foods to help prevent constipation and, combined with daily exercise and at least six to eight glasses of water a day, can go far in preventing hemorrhoids. Warm baths, ice packs, and lying down periodically can help relieve hemorrhoids. The associated itching and burning can be treated with topical ointments or a physician-approved safe suppository.

Frequent Urination

The expanding baby and uterus put pressure on your bladder, especially after the baby drops lower into the pelvic space in preparation for delivery. This might increase the need to urinate during the day and throughout the night. Even though your bladder can be almost empty, the pressure places the same sensation of fullness as if the bladder were filled to capacity. Do not cut back on your fluid intake! However, you might try drinking most of your fluid allotment in the early part of the day and cutting back in the evening hours. When you are resting, lie on your side so that the uterus is not pressing on the kidneys and bladder, interfering with their proper function.

If the pressure of the uterus on the bladder causes urine to leak between visits to the bathroom, you can practice Kegel exercises to strengthen the muscles that surround the urethra (the tube that carries urine from the bladder out of the body). Your doctor or nurse can help you learn the proper technique for doing Kegels correctly. Basically, you contract the muscles in the vaginal, urethra, and anal areas as if you were stopping the flow while urinating. Contracting these muscles for three seconds, then relaxing and repeating this exercise twelve to fifteen times in a row, at least six times a day should help you hold your urine and will help strengthen the vaginal walls after delivery.

Insomnia

Irregular sleep habits, an inability to fall or stay asleep, or frequent awakenings are all symptoms of insomnia, which can develop in the last trimester of pregnancy. Your abdomen has grown so large that a comfortable position is hard to find, plus the anticipation of the new baby might keep you awake at night. Pregnant women are most likely to have trouble falling asleep and are likely to wake up more frequently in the middle of the night, often because of the increased need to urinate. In contrast, after the baby is born, new mothers report they have no trouble falling asleep, but either do not sleep soundly or are awakened frequently in the middle of the night by you-know-who. Either way, many women yearn for mornings when they awaken refreshed, energized, and free from fatigue.

Many people assume that insomnia refers only to chronic sleeplessness. They're wrong. Insomnia is any sleep problem, from occasional difficulties falling asleep or waking up in the middle of the night to awakening too early or sleeping too lightly. While insomnia is a complex issue with numerous causes, sometimes the answer to your sleep problems might start at the dining table.

While most women cut back or eliminate coffee and other caffeinated beverages during the early months of pregnancy, they sometimes resume drinking colas later in pregnancy. Not only are these soft drinks a source of caffeine, but they could contribute to sleep problems. "People eat chocolate or drink a caffeinated soda pop during the day and then wonder why they can't sleep at night," says Robert Sack, Ph.D., professor of psychiatry and director of Adult Sleep Disorder Medicine at the Oregon Health Sciences University in Portland. "Even small amounts of caffeine can affect sleep architecture, especially in caffeine-sensitive people."

Light Dinners: What and how much you ate for dinner could be at the root of your insomnia. Big dinners make you temporarily drowsy, but they also prolong digestive action, which keeps you awake. Instead, try eating your biggest meals before midafternoon and eat a light evening meal of 500 calories or less. Small, low-fat meals also help curb the heartburn that can trouble you during the last trimester. Include some chicken, extra-lean meat, or fish at dinner to help curb middle-of-the-night snack attacks.

Cut Out Spicy Foods: Spicy or gas-forming foods also might be contributing to your sleep problems. Dishes seasoned with garlic, chilies, cayenne, or other hot spices can cause nagging heartburn or indigestion, while the flavor enhancer MSG (monosodium glutamate) causes vivid dreaming and restless sleep in some people. Gas-forming foods or eating too fast causes abdominal discomfort, which in turn interferes with sound sleep. Try avoiding spicy foods at dinnertime. Limit your intake of gas-forming foods to the morning hours and thoroughly chew food to avoid gulping air.

The Evening Snack: The evening snack might be the best alternative to sleeping pills. A high-carbohydrate snack, such as crackers and fruit or toast and jam, triggers the release of a brain chemical called serotonin that aids sleep. "According to our preliminary studies," comments Gary Zammit, Ph.D., director of the Sleep Disorders Institute at St. Luke's Hospital in New York City, "a light carbohydrate-rich snack [before bedtime] may not influence how fast you fall asleep, but it may help some people sleep longer and more soundly." On the other hand, a glass of warm milk or a protein-rich beverage probably doesn't affect serotonin levels, but the warm liquid soothes and relaxes and provides a feeling of satiety, which might facilitate sleep.

Stress, Exercise, and Sleep: The stress of pregnancy or the anxiety associated with the approach of labor and delivery can cause insomnia. Often solving tensions and anxieties eliminates sleep problems. In addition, a major difference between good sleepers and poor sleepers is not what they do at bedtime, but what they did all day. Good sleepers exercise and use every opportunity to move. Physical activity helps a woman cope with daily stress and tires the body so it is ready to sleep at night. In addition, try a warm bath before bedtime, and when sleeping, try lying on your side with a pillow supporting your abdomen and another supporting your legs.

Muscle Cramps

Some women suffer from leg cramps, especially at night when they are tired, during the last trimester. In the past, some people mistakenly thought that too little calcium caused muscle cramps; however, there is no evidence that dietary calcium is a factor in pregnancy-related leg or muscle cramps. Many cramps probably develop because of poor circulation and the pressure of the growing baby on your bladder, ribs, lungs, blood vessels, nerves, stomach, and intestines.

Pain in the pubic area and in your thighs could be caused by the baby's pressing against the nerves or by the pelvic joints as they soften in preparation for labor. Women who carry their babies low are most prone to twinges and cramps in the pelvic area that may be relieved by wearing maternity support pantyhose or an elastic maternity belt that helps brace and support this area. Serious discomfort in the pubic area could come from oversoftening of the cartilage, called the symphysis pubis, that holds the pelvic bones in place. Discuss any problems and possible solutions with your physician.

Although the exact cause of leg cramps is unknown, often moderate exercise, such as walking, and flexing your feet toward your knees is helpful. In addition, stretching your legs before going to bed can help relieve cramps. Avoid pointing your toes while stretching or exercising, since this added tension can trigger toe cramps. Wearing support hose during the day and elevating your legs several times throughout the day helps eliminate leg cramps.

Fatigue

The renewed zest you felt during the second trimester might wane as your due date approaches. Diet cannot completely wipe out that burned-out feeling. However, fueling your body with all the nutrients and calories it needs to function at its best will minimize unnecessary fatigue and help cope with the stresses of pregnancy.

Make sure you exercise daily, get enough rest (including an afternoon nap), and follow the guidelines outlined in the Baby-wise Diet. Don't turn to candy bars and doughnuts for a quick energy fix; they'll only aggravate your fatigue in the long run. Turn instead to nutritious snacks that include at least one whole grain, fruit, or vegetable and one protein-rich selection, such as low-fat milk or yogurt, beans and peas, a slice of chicken breast, or peanut butter. Don't push through the fatigue; rather, take advantage of these last few weeks before your baby is born to nurture yourself.

Third Trimester Meals and Snacks

The biggest obstacles to eating well in the third trimester are a limited capacity, caused by the enlarged uterus pressing against the stomach, and heartburn. If you cannot eat large meals, especially in the evening, try dividing your food intake into several small meals and snacks so that you eat approximately every three hours. This means your snacks will be more like mini-meals and your meals will be more like large snacks. Also, drinking enough fluids remains very important, but try drinking fluids between meals to save more room in your crowded stomach for food. (You can watch your diet by using Worksheet 7.1, "My Third Trimester Daily Checklist.")

Worksheet 7.1 My Third Trimester Daily Checklist

Copy this master sheet to complete daily.

Food Groups	Minimum Servings	Actual Intake
Calcium-rich foods	3	_____
Vegetables (at least 2 folic acid–rich choices)	6	_____
Fruits (at least 2 vitamin C–rich choices)	4	_____
Grains (at least 4 whole-grain choices)	7	_____
Extra-lean meats and legumes	3	_____
Quenchers	6	_____

Did I reach my goals? _____

What needs improvement? _____

What will I do differently next week? _____

Chapter 8

Nutrition and High-Risk Pregnancies

1. **Nutrition:** If you are a teenager or a woman carrying more than one baby, you will need more food, more calories, more protein, and more vitamins and minerals than other women. The Baby-wise Diet should be supplemented with additional servings of nutrient-packed foods.

2. **Weight:** A normal weight teenager should gain at least thirty-five pounds, more if she is underweight prior to pregnancy and less (approximately twenty pounds) if she enters pregnancy over-weight. Multiple births require weight gains between thirty-five and sixty-eight pounds, depending on prepregnancy weight and whether you are carrying twins, triplets, or more.

3. **Supplement:** Take a multiple vitamin and mineral that contains 100 to 200 percent of the Daily Value for all vitamins and minerals, plus at least 25 to 30 mg of iron each day.

4. **Safety:** Avoid alcohol, tobacco, and any medication not approved by your physician as safe during pregnancy. Mature women should avoid birth control pills in the months prior to conception.

5. **Exercise and Rest:** Exercise daily, adjusting the routine, intensity, or duration as prescribed by your physician. Balance exercise with rest, by putting your feet up and taking afternoon naps.

6. **Medical Checkups:** Physician visits are very important throughout high-risk pregnancies to monitor weight and progress and to obtain necessary tests. Mature women might require additional tests, such as amniocentesis, to rule out birth defects.

Every woman's dream is to have a problem-free pregnancy and give birth to a healthy, bright baby. Most women's dreams come true as far as having a healthy baby, although they might have a few minor ups and downs, such as nausea or heartburn, on their way to delivering. Even teenage girls and women in high-risk situations who battle the odds against having a healthy baby often can reach their goals with medical attention, good nutrition, and a healthful lifestyle.

Some of the factors that contribute to a high-risk pregnancy are beyond a woman's control, including age; teenagers and women over thirty-five years old are at higher risk of pregnancy complications and health problems in the newborn than are other women. Multiple births—that is having twins, triplets, or more—also have their own set of complications. Certain medical conditions, such as diabetes (discussed in Chapter 6) or certain infections, also can stack the odds against a pregnant woman. However, just because you are in a high-risk category does not mean you will have problems, especially since you can control most of the other contributing factors, including what you eat, when and how often you exercise, and the quality of your medical attention before, during, and following your pregnancy.

Pregnant Teenagers

Teenaged pregnancies are on the decline in the United States. The most recent statistics show a more than 17 percent drop since peaking in 1990. Today's averages are below 97 pregnancies for every 1,000 young women between the ages of fifteen and nineteen years old. That still accounts for roughly 880,000 pregnancies each year, including the 334,400 infants born to mothers younger than seventeen years old. The rates vary from state to state and from country to country. For example, Washington, D.C., has more than five times the rate of teenage pregnancies compared to North Dakota, while teenage pregnancy rates continue to rise in England and Wales, with more than 90,000 conceptions per year and 2,200 pregnancies in girls younger than fourteen years old.

Biologically speaking, a "mature" woman is at least eighteen years old. By this age, her body has matured enough to handle the physically demanding job of building and delivering a healthy baby. Realistically, however, women between eighteen and twenty-five years old are in an in-between zone, since the most successful time for pregnancy is between twenty-five and thirty-four years old.

These teens are taking on one of life's most serious, intense, and important tasks at a time when their own bodies are teetering between childhood and adulthood. For example, often the uterus is not structurally or functionally fully developed and does not respond to ovarian hormones in the same way a mature organ does. So, teenage pregnancy comes with its own set of challenges.

The Risks: A mother less than fifteen years old who does not eat well or obtain regular medical care is twice as likely to have a preterm or low-birth-weight infant compared to a woman in her mid to late twenties. Pregnant teens are at high risk for eclampsia, anemia, lung disease, and renal disease. Babies born to teenage mothers often weigh less at birth than babies born to older women and are more likely to require intensive care or die at birth or within the first twenty-eight days of life. For those babies that live, low birth weight increases the risk for numerous complications, from infection to reduced intelligence. Many of these babies never catch up as they mature and require special attention, schooling, and health care.

To complicate the issue, many health problems are related to insufficient nutrient intake. The nutritional needs of a teenager's body are at an all-time high. To support the accelerated growth during this stage of life, teenagers need as much as 50 percent more nutrients, such as calcium, iron, magnesium, protein, and zinc, compared to older women. Because of the increased energy demands, the recommended intake for the B vitamins increases. Vitamin D is important in the formation of longer bones, and the recommendation for many nutrients, such as folic acid and vitamins A, C, E, and B_6, for the first time reach adult levels.

Couple these high nutrient needs with the added nutritional demands of pregnancy and you have a situation where the mother's growing body fights with the baby's developing body for each calorie and every nutrient. Often, both end up getting less than they need. For example, the competition for nutrients can:

- decrease uterine blood flow during the period of maximum growth in the baby (the third trimester),
- reduce availability of nutrients in the mother's blood, and
- limit transmission of nutrients from the mother to the baby, all of which can interfere with infant development and birth weight. (See Table 8.1, "Daily Food Guide for the Pregnant Teenager.")

TABLE 8.1

Daily Food Guide for the Pregnant Teenager

Food Family	Servings Each Day
Calcium-Rich Group	4–5
Vegetables	6–7
Fruits	4–5
Whole Grains	8–9
Extra-Lean Meats and Legumes	4–5
Quenchers	6–8

Sample Menu

Breakfast: Oatmeal cooked in nonfat milk and sprinkled with brown sugar and wheat germ; 1 percent low-fat milk, canned peaches, and a glass of orange juice.

Snack: Low-fat fruited yogurt, a whole-wheat bagel with peanut butter, an apple, and water.

Lunch: Cheeseburger, milkshake, carrot-raisin salad, and tomato juice.

Snack: Baby carrots, grilled chicken drumstick, and 1 percent low-fat milk.

Dinner: Two bean-and-cheese burritos, brown rice, tossed salad with low-calorie dressing, steamed broccoli, and fruit juice or water.

Snack: Ice cream topped with fresh berries, and a glass of water.

Teens' Diets: In contrast to older women, teenagers' diets mimic what their friends are eating. They are more likely to fill up on soda pop, French fries, and snack foods than on nonfat milk, steamed broccoli, and grilled chicken. Pregnant teens nibble often on sweets, desserts, soda pop, chips, and other snack items while watching television (for up to five hours) each day. According to researchers at the University of Pennsylvania School of Medicine, teens who consume highly sweetened and processed diets are at high risk for delivering low-birth-weight infants who, in turn, are at elevated risk for disease and even death.

Teens also are likely to have irregular eating habits: As many as one in five teenagers skips breakfast and another 50 percent eat nutritionally poor breakfasts. So when her needs and those of her baby's body are at their nutritional peaks, the pregnant teenager is eating at her worst.

In fact, national nutrition surveys show that the diets of most teenagers fail to meet even their own nutritional needs, let alone the added needs during pregnancy. Only one out of every one hundred teens in this country eats a well-balanced diet, according to the National Cancer Institute in Bethesda. Only 30 percent consume enough fruit, grain, meat, and milk, while most don't eat enough vegetables. To make matters worse, teens are consuming too much fat and sugar. A study from the University of North Carolina found that adolescents' diets are too high in fat, salt, and protein and too low in fiber and nutrients.

It is not surprising that half of all teenage girls consume less than two-thirds of their requirements for calcium and up to 70 percent have depleted tissue iron stores; 30 percent are in the final stages of iron deficiency and are diagnosed as anemic. (Iron-deficiency anemia escalates to 55 percent of teenage mothers after the baby is born.) Magnesium, zinc, vitamin C, vitamin A, and other nutrients also are low. These marginal intakes are likely to affect the outcome of pregnancy, while teenagers who eat nutrient-packed diets and supplement their diet with well-balanced vitamin and mineral supplements show improvements in their health and the health of their babies.

Young mothers can eat well and can give birth to healthy, full-term, robust babies. It just takes planning and dedication. If you are under age eighteen and pregnant, you must eat enough nutrient-packed foods to fuel both your growth and the growth of your baby. Both your body and your baby's body are growing twenty-four hours a day, so you must space your food intake so that you eat at least every four hours in order to ensure a constant supply of nutrients and calories. If you skip meals, you are more likely to come up short nutrient-wise and are more likely to deprive your baby of essential nutrients needed for growth and development.

Weight Gain for Teen Pregnancy: A teenager who is of normal weight should gain approximately thirty-five pounds during pregnancy; more if she entered pregnancy underweight and less (approximately twenty pounds) if she entered pregnancy overweight. It is also important to space the gain. Teens who gain little weight in the first six months of pregnancy (less than ten pounds by week twenty-four) are more likely to give birth to low-birth-weight babies, even if they make up the weight gain by delivery time. Gaining less than a pound a week in the last trimester also increases the chances of having a premature baby or a low-birth-weight baby. So put aside the "thin is beautiful" mystique and think more about having a healthy baby. Don't worry; most teenagers return to their prepregnancy weight within forty weeks after having their babies (and many well before this).

Can't Gain Weight? If you are eating all the foods outlined on page 192 and still are having trouble gaining sufficient weight, boost your calorie intake by snacking on ice cream, milkshakes made with Instant Breakfast, nuts, cheese, and other high-calorie snacks. Avoid the high-calorie junk foods, such as potato chips, candy, and French fries. Instead, nibble on dried fruits, baby carrots, cherries, frozen blueberries, and other nutrient-packed nibble foods.

Quick-Fix Meals: Keep in mind that even if you are pressed for time, preparing a nutritious meal takes no more than five minutes.

- For breakfast, you can put two slices of cheese in a flour tortilla and microwave it for one minute and top it with salsa.
- Peanut butter mixed with honey and toasted wheat germ and spread on whole-wheat bread takes five minutes at the most.
- Even nutritious convenience foods, such as a granola bar, oven-baked tortilla chips, individual-size containers of chocolate soy milk, or cold pizza, are great quick-fix snacks.
- Take nutritious foods with you, such as fresh fruit, whole-wheat bagels, boxed 100 percent fruit juice, or packaged cheese and crackers.
- Snack on yogurt mixed with cereal, trail mix, cottage cheese with fruit and crackers, or fresh apple or pear slices topped with grilled cheese.

The challenges of teen pregnancy aren't over when the baby is born; the quality of the baby's life is now a major consideration. A teenage mother faces numerous conflicting issues, including social, financial, legal, educational, vocational, and other difficulties. An unplanned or unwanted baby is at even higher risk for problems related to mental, emotional, and physical development. Optimal nutrition continues to be essential, but adopting a healthful diet is most successful only if these other lifestyle issues are also addressed. (See Table 8.2, "Vitamins, Minerals, and Other Nutrients in the Pregnant Teenager's Diet.")

Mature Women and Pregnancy

While the pregnancy rate has dropped for women in their twenties, it has skyrocketed for women past the age of thirty-five. The rate of births in women over thirty years old has more than doubled in the past few years. Today, it is common for a woman to have her first baby or start a second family when she is in her forties. While the risks associated with pregnancy and childbirth are higher in this age group than for younger women, at the same time these women often have planned their pregnancies and are more willing and ready to accept the responsibilities of parenthood than they would have been in earlier years. These women are more mature, better educated, financially more secure, and more settled and patient than they were in their teens and twenties—all factors that make for good parenting. In short, they are willing to accept the slight increase in risk for the even higher benefits that having babies will add to their lives.

TABLE 8.2

Vitamins, Minerals, and Other Nutrients in the Pregnant Teenager's Diet

Nutrient	Recommended Amount
Calories	at least 2,500 to 3,000
Protein	76 grams
Vitamin A	5,000 IU
Vitamin D	15 mcg
Vitamin E	20 mcg
Vitamin B_1	2 mg
Vitamin B_2	2 mg
Niacin	16–17 mg
Vitamin B_6	2.4–2.6 mg
Folic acid	800 mcg
Vitamin B_{12}	4 mcg
Vitamin C	80–100 mg
Calcium	1,600 mg
Iodine	175 mcg
Iron	30–60 mg
Magnesium	450 mg
Zinc	20 mg

Health Risks for Older Women: The first challenge faced by the mature woman is getting pregnant, since infertility increases with age. This results possibly from the aging reproductive system's reduced efficiency, the increased frequency of disorders such as endometriosis and pelvic inflammatory disease, or the escalating risk of diabetes and obesity in this age group. Uterine function and receptivity as well as ovarian hormone levels also decline with age, while the risk for spontaneous abortion rises. (See Chapter 1 for more information on fertility.)

Once a woman conceives, the next hurdle is to avoid other health risks. The mature woman who becomes pregnant is slightly more likely to develop high blood pressure (especially if she is overweight), diabetes, and other pregnancy-related conditions than a younger woman, and she is at a slightly greater risk for a miscarriage. Older women are at even higher risk of delivering low-birth-weight babies if they smoke cigarettes. However, most of these conditions are not related to postponing pregnancy until late in the reproductive years, but are linked to preexisting conditions that worsen with age. There is no evidence that low-birth-weight rates, premature delivery, or the labor and delivery experience are any different for the younger or older woman, although there is a higher rate of cesarean section in older women. Other health conditions of concern to the mature pregnant woman are an increased risk for having a Down's syndrome baby and the possibility of finding a breast lump while pregnant. These issues should be discussed with your physician, but are not directly related to diet and nutrition.

The importance of lifestyle cannot be overemphasized when it comes to having an uncomplicated pregnancy and healthy baby in the middle years. In essence, advanced age does not automatically place a woman at high risk, while a lifetime of smoking, drinking alcohol, eating poorly, being sedentary, having chronic stress, and maintaining other unhealthful habits does take a toll. An older mother who eats well, exercises regularly, avoids tobacco and limits alcohol, and takes good care of herself cuts years off her pregnancy profile and can reduce her risk of pregnancy complications to that of a younger woman. Numerous studies show that women past thirty-five years old who take good care of themselves have no more serious maternal complications than women between twenty and thirty-four years of age. In fact, one study showed that their babies had lower rates of prenatal death and were less likely to be of low birth weight. In essence, women in their thirties and forties who want to get pregnant should:

1. Avoid using birth control pills, since these drugs might delay conception even after they are discontinued.
2. Avoid cigarette smoking and alcohol consumption before and during pregnancy, since these can increase the rate of miscarriage and birth defects.

3. Undergo an amniocentesis (a routine screening test for all mothers-to-be who are more than thirty-five years old) to detect early the presence of Down's syndrome or other congenital abnormalities.
4. Seek professional assistance if pregnancy does not occur within six months or so, since the sooner you or your partner begins treatment for infertility the better.

The dietary recommendations for mature pregnant women are the same as for women in their twenties and thirties. See the Baby-wise Diet recommendations for gearing up for pregnancy (Chapter 1), during the three trimesters (Chapters 5, 6, and 7), and after pregnancy (Chapters 9 and 10).

Multiple Births

More women today are having twins and triplets than ever before. In 1995, there were more than 100,000 twin births in the United States, the highest number ever recorded. Twin births have increased by 68 percent, and triplet and "higher-order" births (like quadruplets and more) have increased by 357 percent in the past few years. This increase is partially due to the use of ovulation-induction drugs. (The reported incidence of multiple births while using these drugs ranges from 25 to 50 percent.) The growing number of women older than age thirty-five who are getting pregnant also is a factor in the increased rates. Regardless of cause, less than one-tenth of one percent of all births are triplets or higher-order births and only 2.5 percent of births are twins. So while all pregnant women are special, there is something superspecial about a multiple birth.

High-Risk Pregnancies: Although advances in pre- and postnatal medical care in the last ten years have improved the outcome of these pregnancies, multiple births still remain a high-risk condition that can result in premature labor and delivery and low birth weights. These babies have higher risks for disease and death than do single births and are more likely to show delayed growth while in the uterus, called intrauterine growth retardation (IUGR), especially from week thirty-two to term. IUGR is partially related to inadequate calorie and nutrient intake and/or tobacco use, but also is strongly related to reduced blood supply to the placenta and the degree to which the uterus can expand, as well as genetic makeup and the woman's prepregnancy condition and age.

A woman carrying twins or triplets also is less likely to have a full-term pregnancy (the averages are 37 weeks for twins, 33.8 weeks for triplets, and as little as 31 weeks for quadruplets versus the normal 40 weeks). Women carrying more than one baby are thirty-three times more likely to give birth to preterm, low-birth-weight, or very low-birth-weight infants. For example, the average birth weight for triplets is a little more than 4½ pounds, with an average hospital stay of twenty-nine days. The average weight of quadruplets is only 3½ pounds. This high incidence of low birth weight is a major contributing factor to the increased risk for health problems in these babies. Consequently, the most important contributing factor in producing healthy twins and triplets is reducing the rate of low birth weight.

Triplets and higher-order multiple births also are more prone to nervous system problems, including cerebral palsy and mental retardation. The good news is that healthy twins and triplets who are not of very low birth weight at delivery show little or no differences in nerve and sensory development by one year of age and at school age compared to single-birth babies.

Complications for the mother include postpartum hemorrhage, probably because of the inability of the overdistended uterus to contract effectively after delivery; increased risk for developing pregnancy-induced hypertension (PIH); and an increased risk for birth trauma if the babies are born vaginally. (See Box 8.1, "Bed Rest Survival Kit.")

BOX 8.1   BED REST SURVIVAL KIT

Remember the old adage, "Be careful what you wish for, you might get it." While most women dream of the chance to put up their feet, lie in bed all day, and enjoy a little stress-free time, for the woman carrying triplets or quadruplets assigned to her bed for months during the second and third trimesters, bed rest can be as stressful as cabin fever.

A physician will prescribe bed rest for a variety of reasons, including pregnancy-induced hypertension, multiple fetuses, premature labor, or intrauterine growth retardation (IUGR). Whatever the reason, if you are assigned to bed for more than a few days, you need to develop some strategies for making it a pleasant experience.

1. Set up your makeshift bedroom in an area of the house where you can live and visit with family, such as a family room or a room off the

kitchen. (One woman even had a hospital bed brought to her office and continued working from bed until her eighth month!)

2. Surround yourself with the essentials—soft pillows; a telephone; a television with a remote control; a mini-refrigerator or ice chest filled with fruit, chopped vegetables, ice water, fruit juice, and other nutrient-packed items; a table with nutritious snacks, such as rice cakes, peanut butter, nuts, and dried fruit; an intercom system; and any medications for constipation, heartburn, or other pregnancy-related problems.

3. With the help of your physician, identify exercises you safely can do, such as arm exercises using weights (even soup cans will work) or isometric exercises, and do them regularly.

4. Be creative. Take this time to read, keep a diary, write letters, balance your checkbook, write shopping lists for your family, complete a puzzle or crossword puzzle, take up knitting or cross-stitching, listen to books on tape, or give yourself a facial.

5. Be industrious. Volunteer to do phone work for a fund-raiser. Call elderly shut-ins to check on their health. Take a correspondence course. Learn a foreign language. Plan your finances or retirement. Start your Christmas shopping by using catalogs. Plan a flower or herb garden.

Diet, Weight Gain, and Multiple Births

If you are carrying more than one baby, you can improve your chances of having bigger, healthier babies by careful selection of what and how much you eat. For one thing, how much weight you gain has a lot to do with how much weight your babies will gain. You need more food, more calories, more protein, and more vitamins and minerals than a woman carrying a single baby. However, a study from Brigham and Women's Hospital in Boston found that women carrying more than one baby ate about the same amount of food as women with just one baby. In short, they were eating for two rather than three or more, so the babies were forced to split their meals.

Weight Gain Guidelines: Additional babies means additional weight gain, not only from the baby but because the placenta(s), the amniotic fluid surrounding the babies, the blood volume, the uterus, and other support tissues also expand. An approximate weight gain of thirty-five to forty-five pounds above your prepregnancy weight (unless already overweight) best improves chances for birthing healthy twins. Women carrying healthy twins should gain at least forty-four pounds by week thirty-seven of pregnancy.

Even the rate of gain is different for multiple births. Weight gain is more rapid and earlier for mothers carrying twins, with increases in weight beginning as early as the eighth week. Underweight women entering a multiple pregnancy should strive to gain at least one pound a week before twenty weeks and one and a half to two pounds a week after that. A low rate of gain early in pregnancy, even if weight gain is optimal later, is associated with an increased risk for poor growth and higher rates of health problems in the infants.

There is not enough research on triplets and higher-order pregnancies to establish an ideal weight gain. Limited evidence shows that a weight gain of forty-five to sixty-eight pounds by weeks thirty-one to thirty-three is not uncommon. At least thirty-six pounds gained by week twenty-four is needed to ensure higher birth weights and optimal outcomes for triplets.

Nutrient Needs: No guidelines have been developed for women with twins, triplets, or higher-order pregnancies. A woman carrying two babies does not need twice as many calories or twice as much nutrients and a mother carrying triplets doesn't need three times the nutrition, but these women do need more than a woman carrying only one baby.

The recommendations for multiple births are at best guesstimates based on the increased weight gain, with a proposed 50 to 100 percent increase in the Recommended Dietary Allowances (RDAs) advised for normal pregnancies. To ensure optimal nutrient intake, a woman carrying more than one baby should seriously consider taking a moderate-dose multiple vitamin and mineral supplement, if she is not already taking one. (See Table 8.3, "Nutrient Needs for a Woman [at Least Age Twenty-five] Carrying Twins.")

A high-calorie, nutrient-packed diet can have profound effects on improving a woman's chances of having healthy twins. In one study, women who consumed additional calories and protein after week twenty gave birth to bigger babies. They also had lower risks of having low-birth-weight and very low-birth-weight infants (25 percent and 50 percent lower, respectively) and were less likely to have preterm infants compared to women carrying twins who did not eat the higher calorie and protein diets. In addition, the well-nourished mothers had lower rates of pre-eclampsia and gestational diabetes. In general, a mother of twins should strive for 3,000 to 3,500 calories a day. A woman carrying triplets should aim for 4,000 calories a day and quadruplets can raise calorie needs above 4,500. (See Table 8.4, "What Does a 3,000-Calorie Diet Look Like?")

TABLE 8.3

Nutrient Needs for a Woman (at Least Age Twenty-five) Carrying Twins

Nutrient	Normal Pregnancy	Twin Pregnancy
Calories	2,500 calories	3,000+ calories
Protein	60 mg	90–120 mg
Vitamin A	800 mcg	1,000 mcg
Vitamin D	5 mcg	10 mcg
Vitamin K	65 mcg	97 mcg
Vitamin B$_1$	1.4 mg	3.0 mg
Vitamin B$_2$	1.4 mg	3.0 mg
Niacin	18 mg	25 mg
Vitamin B6	1.9 mg	4.0 mg
Folic acid	400–800 mcg	800 mcg
Vitamin B$_{12}$	2.6 mcg	4.0 mcg
Vitamin C	70 mg	100+ mg
Calcium	1,000 mg	1,800 mg
Chromium	50–200 mcg	200 mcg
Copper	1.5–3.0 mg	3 mg
Fluoride	3.0 mg	3.0 mg
Iodine	175 mcg	175 mcg
Iron	30–60 mg	50+ mg
Magnesium	350 mg	450 mg
Selenium	65 mcg	100 mcg
Zinc	15 mg	30 mg

Iron also is a concern for multiple pregnancies. The extra demands on the mother's iron reserves from the larger placenta and the need to provide a greater blood volume to the two or more babies increases the likelihood that these mothers will develop anemia. In fact, up to 35 percent of these mothers are anemic, which implies that many more are iron deficient (the stage prior to anemia). These women must combine an iron-rich diet with iron supplements to make sure they maintain their tissue iron stores and should continue this regimen for at least one year after the babies are born. Even with the best diet, babies born prematurely usually have not had time to accumulate iron in their tissues and are more

TABLE 8.4

What Does a 3,000-Calorie Diet Look Like?

Most women have spent their lives cutting calories. The thought of packing in 3,000 or 4,000 calories seems as alien as walking on water. Here's a brief look at what feeding several growing babies at once, plus yourself, should look like.

Breakfast:

3 packets instant oatmeal cooked in 1 cup low-fat milk and topped with toasted
    wheat germ, brown sugar, raisins, and crushed walnuts
½ cantaloupe
1 cup orange juice

Snack:

large apple
water

Lunch:

Chicken salad sandwich on whole wheat
1½ cups carrot-raisin salad
1 cup ice cream

Snack:

1 cup low-fat milk
5 small cookies

Dinner:

5-ounce broiled steak
baked potato with 2 tablespoons butter
2 cups steamed broccoli
10 sauteed mushrooms (in olive oil and garlic)

Snack:

1 cup low-fat milk
5 small cookies

Nutrition Score: 3,028 calories; 32 percent fat (109 g: 37 g saturated), 47 percent
    carbohydrates (360 g), 21 percent protein (163 g), 35 g fiber, 1,945 mg calcium,
    948 mcg folic acid, 39 mg iron.

susceptible to anemia in the first few months of life. Your pediatrician can help monitor your babies' iron status and may recommend supplements if iron levels drop below normal.

A diet of 3,000 calories or more might seem like a lot and you may wonder how you can eat this much food. However, it's really quite an easy task.

- Stick to basics. Follow the Baby-wise Diet, which forms the foundation for your nutrition plan.
- Boost calories: You need an extra 500 to 1,500 calories over and above what other pregnant women need. You can add more of the same foods, such as more milk (some evidence shows women carrying more than one baby should drink the equivalent of six glasses of milk each day), fruits, vegetables, or grains; or you may choose to splurge and add a few calorie-dense items to make up the difference in energy without adding too much bulk. Adding a little butter to your toast, choosing whole milk instead of nonfat, or snacking on a few cookies in the evening might be all it takes to pump up your calorie intake.
- Eat often. Divide your food intake into five or six meals and snacks throughout the day, so that you eat at least every three to four hours during waking hours.
- Drink water. Dehydration can trigger uterine contractions, which could result in premature labor. Strive for at least eight to ten glasses daily, but drink it between meals so that you don't fill up on fluids when eating.
- Take a supplement. Supplement your diet with a moderate-dose multiple vitamin and mineral that contains extra folic acid and at least 30 mg of iron.

(See Table 8.5, "Special Considerations for Women Pregnant with Twins, Triplets, or More.")

AIDS and Pregnancy

Human immunodeficiency virus (HIV) infection is in epidemic proportions in many countries around the world. Heterosexual intercourse is now the leading mode for the spread of HIV in women in the United States. Consequently, prior to pregnancy, any woman considering pregnancy should be tested for HIV, which is responsible for the AIDS complex.

(Keep in mind that an antibody test for the virus can show up negative for up to three months after infection and no test is 100 percent accurate.)

TABLE 8.5

Special Considerations for Women Pregnant with Twins, Triplets, or More

1. Seek out a physician with extensive training in managing multiple pregnancies.
2. Schedule more frequent visits with your physician than if you were pregnant with only one baby.
3. Cut back on physical activity. Rest during your lunch hour or immediately upon returning home from work. Take a leave of absence from work after week twenty-four. Take two-hour naps in the afternoon.
4. Know the signals of premature labor and other potential complications.

More than likely there will be no symptoms of infection in the first few years after exposure to HIV; however, since pregnancy affects the immune system, it may trigger the onset of AIDS in a woman who is antibody positive to HIV but previously had no symptoms. It also is possible to become infected with HIV during pregnancy or for symptoms of AIDS to develop soon after the baby is born.

HIV infection can be transmitted from the mother to the baby and is associated with high rates of disease and death in infants and children. In fact, AIDS in children represents 2 percent of all AIDS cases; AIDS is now as prevalent as cancer in children and is in the top ten leading causes of death in children under the age of eighteen. In babies, 80 to 90 percent of the time the HIV infection is caused by transmission of the virus from the mother to the developing baby or newborn. Transmission of the virus to the unborn happens 13 to 50 percent of the time in infected mothers, and might occur during pregnancy, at birth, or after birth if the baby is breast-fed.

Babies born to HIV-infected women always have antibodies to the virus. However, a baby born to a healthy HIV-infected woman may lose the antibodies after six to eighteen months. But it may take a year or more of repeated testing before it is certain a baby is or is not carrying the virus. Slightly less than one in four HIV-positive newborns actually develops AIDS. The incidence climbs to 66 percent in women who already have given birth to an infected infant. The risk is even higher for a woman with AIDS. A baby infected in the womb can have birth defects that include a characteristic facial appearance with a very small head, box-shaped forehead, flat nose, widely spaced blue eyes, and full lips.

Several studies report that babies born to HIV-positive women are more likely to be low birth weight, and a report from Baltimore concluded that babies who are infected with the virus are small for gestational age compared to noninfected infants born to infected mothers. However, many of these women used illicit drugs during their pregnancies, so the low birth weights could have resulted from the exposure to drugs or a combination of the HIV infection and drug exposure.

The Bottom Line: Women who test HIV-positive should think seriously about pregnancy and the potential harm to the baby if the virus is transferred. Women who discover they are HIV-positive after they have become pregnant should make sure they eat an excellent diet. In addition to the immunological consequences of HIV infection, there are several nutritional deficiencies associated with AIDS, including poor intake and blood levels of vitamin A, beta carotene, vitamin E, vitamin C, vitamin B_6, vitamin B_{12}, calcium, magnesium, selenium, and zinc. Preventing these deficiencies could help slow the progression of the disease and help protect the developing baby.

These women also should not use tobacco, drugs, and alcohol; get plenty of rest and avoid becoming overly stressed; discuss the condition with their physicians and obtain regular medical checkups and monitoring; and generally obtain and maintain their highest level of health. They also will be advised to formula-feed their infants, rather than breast-feed. On the other hand, if you are not infected, breast-feeding provides additional benefits in preventing infection in your baby. Note that banked human milk is pasteurized to destroy the HIV virus, but retains properties that could be helpful to infants of HIV-positive mothers.

After a High-Risk Pregnancy

Women who have experienced complications during pregnancy and have delivered healthy babies sometimes have new issues to face after the baby is born. Women who experience complications, such as diabetes or pregnancy-induced hypertension, during their pregnancies are more likely to be overprotective and overly concerned about their children's health and safety for years after delivery compared to women who had normal pregnancies. They are more likely to keep their children indoors, call the doctor more often, or worry about daily nuisances such as the sniffles. If you find yourself overly worried about your child, discuss your concerns with your physician to make sure you are not dragging past worries into the present.

Chapter 9

❦

Nutrition and Nursing Your Baby

If you choose to breast-feed, be concerned about:

1. **Nutrition:** Follow the guidelines outlined in the Baby-wise Diet. Include two to three servings of fish or other omega-3-rich foods in the weekly diet.
2. **Weight:** Don't attempt weight loss for the first six weeks postpartum, then aim for no more than a two-pound loss per month.
3. **Supplement:** Continue to take a multiple vitamin and mineral that contains 100 to 200 percent of the Daily Value for all vitamins and minerals, plus at least 18 mg of iron each day.
4. **Safety:** Continue to avoid alcohol, tobacco, caffeine, and any medication not approved by your physician as safe when nursing.
5. **Exercise and Rest:** Exercise daily, but adjust the routine, intensity, or duration as needed. Purchase a sports bra to provide extra support.
6. **Medical Checkups:** Seek help if you suffer from postpartum depression.

Pregnancy is more than the nine months of developing a baby. The baby-making process began months before you ever conceived, and if you choose to breast-feed, plan on having another baby, or want to regain your prepregnancy figure, it can continue for up to a year after the baby is born. For women who choose to breast-feed their babies, the nutritional link between mother and child remains as important as it was during pregnancy. While you provide your baby with the best that nature can offer, you also must make sure you eat a good diet to replenish nutrient stores.

When and What to Eat and Drink When You Are Nursing

Your intake should average approximately 2,200 to 2,700 calories a day (more if you exercise). As always, the Baby-wise Diet forms the basis of your eating plan, with the following minimum number of servings from each list:

  3 to 4 servings from the Calcium-Rich Group
  6 servings from the Vegetable Group (at least 2 servings should be folic acid–rich choices)
  4 servings from the Fruit Group (at least 2 servings should be vitamin C–rich choices)
  3 servings from the Extra-Lean Meats and Legume Group (include 2 to 3 servings of fish and 4 to 5 servings of legumes in the weekly menu)
  9 servings from the Grain Group (at least 4 servings should be whole-grain choices)
  8 servings from the Quenchers Group

You have a little more leeway because of the extra 500-plus calories needed to produce breast milk. If you want to splurge every so often, now's the time to do it. That is, unless you are trying to gradually lose weight, in which case you still can eat more than ever, but should limit your choices to nutritious foods within the Baby-wise Diet.

Breast-Feeding Twins or Triplets

Common sense alone says if you are feeding more than one baby you will need to consume more nutrient-packed foods than the average nursing mom. You will be secreting daily 420 to 700 calories per child, which means you will need, on average, an additional 500 calories for each baby. For twins, the average nursing mother should consume 2,200 calories plus 1,000 calories for a total of 3,200 calories or more daily. For triplets, the total intake is approximately 3,700 calories. You will need more fluids, protein, calcium, trace minerals, and vitamins, which means additional servings of whole grains, nonfat milk products, protein-rich beans or animal products, and more fruits and vegetables.

Breast Milk: The Best for Your Baby

"My baby will look up every so often while nursing. Our eyes meet and she breaks into the sweetest grin. It makes me weak in the knees."
"My baby boy would gently stroke my side as he nursed. It was the most heavenly massage I've ever had."
"Even though I love my sleep, I wouldn't give up those peaceful middle-of-the-night nursings. Often my baby and I fell asleep while nursing and woke up in the morning rested and ready to nurse again."

Although breast-feeding went "out of fashion" for a while, women are returning to it, with about 60 percent of new moms opting to nurse rather than bottle-feed their babies. Unfortunately, few women nurse their babies as long as the American Academy of Pediatrics recommends—at least for the first twelve months of life.

Breast-feeding is the ideal option when it comes to feeding your baby. It's cheap, convenient, and requires no equipment. You can feed your baby on demand anywhere, from the car or a department store fitting room to the park or a clean women's lounge.

Almost all women can breast-feed their babies, regardless of age, breast size, or work schedule. Even health conditions, such as diabetes or lupus, are not deterrents to nursing as long as the woman consults a physician. Nursing remains the option of choice even for a woman with silicon breast implants. While having an epidural for pain relief during labor might temporarily affect some babies' ability to latch onto the nipple and feed, this is overcome by keeping the baby with you during the hospital stay (including at night), frequent skin-to-skin contact between mother and baby, and feeding your baby when she is ready to feed, not on a schedule. Breast-feeding is a learned skill, not a natural one, so make sure you locate a breast-feeding specialist at the hospital or contact the LaLeche League, a certified lactation consultant, or a local breast-feeding agency as soon as you arrive home to ensure you get off to the right start! (See Box 9.1, "Is Your Baby Getting Enough to Eat?")

BOX 9.1   IS YOUR BABY GETTING ENOUGH TO EAT?

Nursing mothers often are concerned that their babies aren't eating enough. Unlike bottle-feeding, in which you can gauge how much your baby is getting, your only clue with breast-feeding is whether or not your breast feels "emptied" and your baby appears satisfied after a feeding. Nursing mothers also express concern that their milk looks diluted or "watery," and worry their baby isn't getting enough to eat.

One way to be assured your baby is eating well and thriving is to check the diapers. A newborn baby who nurses about ten times a day and wets six or more diapers every day is probably getting plenty to eat. Weight and height checks at your regular pediatrician visits also will give an indication of how well your baby is doing. Finally, how your baby acts often is an indicator of how well he or she is eating. A good indicator that a baby is healthy and eating well is whether he or she is happy and alert.

Benefits for Your Baby

Breast milk is the perfect food for your baby, providing all the nutrients in the right proportion and amount. It far outshines any other form of feeding a newborn because it supplies vital factors not found in formulas, including some trace minerals, such as chromium and selenium, and the essential omega-3 fatty acids (see below for information on DHA) for normal development of vision and the nervous system. Breast milk also contains unique forms of carbohydrates, called oligosaccharides, not found in commercial infant formulas. These special carbohydrates encourage the growth and establishment of healthy bacteria in the infant's gut, helping to boost natural defenses against disease and infection.

Breast milk also fluctuates to meet the changing nutritional needs of your baby. The thick, yellowish fluid called colostrum that is available first to your newborn is especially high in protein to help stabilize the newborn's fluctuating blood sugar levels. Colostrum is high in vitamins and minerals, which help clear the newborn's system of meconium—the first sticky, black stool—and prepare the baby's digestive system to handle the transitional milk and the mature milk to follow. Some of these unique components of breast milk are so essential to baby's growth that they are produced regardless of what the mother eats.

Breast milk also contains a host of health-enhancing compounds that are not supplied in formulas, such as IgA, an immunoglobulin that helps to kick start baby's immune system; lysozyme, an enzyme that gobbles up disease-carrying bacteria in the newborn's digestive tract; prolactin, a hormone that activates the baby's immune system; sialated mucins, a combination of carbohydrates and protein that help prevent infant diarrhea; and bifidobacterium, a healthy bacteria that destroy parasites. And, that's only a sample—there are many, many more benefits in breast milk!

Reduced Health Risks: Breast milk stimulates the growth of "friendly" bacteria in the infant's digestive tract and reduces the incidence of stomach upsets, diarrhea, or colic. The effect is dose-dependent. That is, the more breast milk a baby receives in the first six months and the longer a baby nurses, the greater the benefits. Limited evidence also shows that breast milk protects against the growth of a bacteria in the stomach called *H. pylori* that otherwise contributes to ulcers, gastritis, and even stomach cancer later in life.

Fewer Infections: Breast milk does something else that formulas cannot; it provides the newborn with a natural defense against colds, infections, allergies, and disease during the early months before the baby's own immune system is fully developed. This explains why breast-fed infants are much less likely to develop otitis media, or inner ear infections, not only while breast-feeding but for months after they have switched to solid foods and/or bottles. With more than 60 percent of children suffering from at least one inner ear infection during the early years of life, and since this infection can cause permanent hearing defects and subsequent problems with language development, the potential benefits of breast-feeding cannot be overemphasized. Infants also are at much lower risk of developing coughs and respiratory infections if they are breast-fed exclusively for at least fifteen weeks.

Smarter Babies: Breast milk makes smarter babies. In eight out of every ten studies, children who were breast-fed in the early months of life scored higher on IQ tests compared to children who had been formula-fed. For example, children who are breast-fed produce significantly higher scores on cognitive development compared to children who were bottle-fed, according to a study from the University of Kentucky in Lexington. The effect appears to be dose-dependent. A study from Christchurch School of Medicine in New Zealand found that the longer babies were breast-fed, the better they scored on verbal and performance IQ tests later in life. Children who had been breast-fed for eight months or longer averaged six points higher on verbal IQ tests than children who had not been breast-fed.

Reduced Risk for Obesity: Bottle-fed infants grow faster than breast-fed babies, but this could predispose them to a greater risk for being over-weight later in life. Numerous studies, including one from Harvard Medical School, have found that breast-fed infants are much less likely to battle weight problems in childhood, during the teen years, and into adulthood compared to formula-fed babies. In addition, the slower growth rates observed with breast-feeding might be beneficial for optimal nerve development.

Reduced Risk for Later Disease: Breast milk protects your child long after you've stopped nursing. Babies who are breast-fed are at lower risk of sudden infant death syndrome (SIDS). Later in life they are at much lower risk for developing heart disease, certain forms of cancer such as lymphoma and leukemia, asthma, celiac disease, and diabetes.

Better Eaters: Interestingly, breast-fed infants grow up to be more accepting of new foods. According to a study from the University of Illinois, breast-fed infants learned to enjoy a greater variety of vegetables than formula-fed infants, possibly because they were used to the varying tastes of breast milk, which changes from feeding to feeding depending on the mother's diet.

Benefits for the Mother

Breast-feeding benefits the mother just as much as the baby. She is more likely to regain her prepregnancy weight than is a woman who chooses not to breast-feed, although the last five pounds might not drop off until after she stops nursing. Breast-feeding might lower future risk of developing breast, endometrial, and ovarian cancers. It also blocks calcium loss from bones, reducing the risk for osteoporosis later in life. Breast-feeding helps the uterus contract, reducing blood loss after delivery and helping the uterus return to its prepregnancy state; delays the return to menstruation, which means you lose less iron and have a chance to restock iron stores after pregnancy; and reduces the risk for bladder infections.

While breast-feeding is a natural form of birth control, it is not a reli-able one; as many as 57 percent of women become fertile again while nursing and almost 80 percent of women begin menstruating within four weeks after they stop nursing. (See Box 9.2, "Overcoming Obstacles to Breast-Feeding.")

BOX 9.2

Overcoming Obstacles to Breast-Feeding

Many women have the best intentions about breast-feeding, but stop soon after starting. In one study, half of the women who had chosen to breast-feed had switched to formula after the twelfth week. Another study concluded that most women breast-feed for only one month. In some cases, early termination of nursing is associated with younger, working mothers or mothers suffering from postpartum depression. While you are most likely to continue nursing if you are older, well educated, relatively affluent, or live in the western United States, there is every reason to believe that any woman can nurse. Since many of the obstacles to nursing can be overcome, including a lack of support at the hospital, home, or the workplace, breast-feeding is a possibility for every woman.

Hospital practices are oriented toward bottle-feeding, as are the public displays of infant formula advertising in hospitals, public health programs, and doctors' offices. At the workplace, a lack of flexibility, role models, and privacy (to express milk) further complicates the nursing process. Coupled with self-doubts and lack of motivation or support from friends and family, these challenges can become obstacles to continuing nursing. Choosing a physician who supports your decision to breast-feed and selecting a hospital that allows "rooming in" (having the baby in the room with you) and provides breast-feeding guidance during your stay can greatly improve your chances of sticking with it after you get home.

By far the greatest factor influencing a woman's decision to breast- or bottle-feed is her motivation and support at home. Granted, it is difficult to combine a career with nursing; however, the overwhelming majority of women who successfully accomplish both report that it is worth the trouble, that they recommend it to other women, and that they feel they had done something special for their babies. In essence, they have adopted an attitude that nursing is important, they are proud of what they are doing, and they figure out a way to keep doing it. They get up a little earlier to express milk at home or express at the office. They develop a sense of humor to get them through the days when their milk leaks all over a new silk blouse. They surround themselves with the support of other women who have breast-fed. They overcome obstacles to nursing in public by draping a baby blanket over their shoulder to cover the nursing baby.

BOX 9.2 continued

Women who decide to breast-feed and continue for more than a few weeks usually have partners who are supportive of their decision. Fathers also can help their nursing partner by taking over some of the household work, making sure the mother has plenty of nutritious food to eat, helping care for the newborn, protecting her from people who don't understand breast-feeding, and being patient with her emotional ups and downs.

Whatever the cause, a woman should never feel guilty for deciding to stop nursing. Repeatedly, the research shows that women who stop nursing and those who nurse their babies for months are equally good parents, love their children, and do not differ in their perceptions of themselves as parents. They both report enjoying parenthood and view their babies as "easy" to manage.

What Should You Eat When Nursing?

Women who breast-feed continue to eat for two, just as they did when they were pregnant. The same concerns about what you eat and how it will affect your baby apply. Should you drink coffee? Is it safe to celebrate the new arrival with a glass of champagne? Could pesticides in foods find their way into breast milk and harm your baby? Can you breast-feed and still lose weight?

In most cases, your nutrient needs are even higher when breast-feeding than when you were pregnant. The plus side to this increased nutrient demand is that breast-feeding "burns" an additional 500 to 700 calories a day; that's the equivalent of running five or more miles without putting on your running shoes!

You need to be especially vigilant with your diet when nursing, since several studies have reported less-than-optimal nutrient intake in breast-feeding women, especially for critical nutrients, such as zinc, vitamins D and E, and iron. Other nutrients often found low in breast-feeding mothers' diets include calcium, magnesium, folic acid, vitamin B_2, and vitamin B_1.

A dietary slipup here and there, such as not drinking enough milk or falling short of your broccoli quota for a day, has little impact on the overall quality of your breast milk. On the other hand, frequently skipping meals, making poor food choices, or repeatedly consuming less than optimal amounts of one or more nutrients could have far-reaching effects on your health and your baby's.

Water, Water Everywhere

The most important determinant of how much milk is produced is your baby's demand for milk; in essence, the more you nurse, the more milk you will have. Your diet also has a significant effect on the quality and, in some cases, the quantity of that milk. First, drinking enough fluid is paramount. As a nursing mother, you lose considerably more fluid, up to twenty-three ounces or more daily. This fluid drain will automatically make you thirstier. However, thirst is not always a good indicator of fluid needs. If you are thirsty, you're already dehydrated. A general rule of thumb is to drink twice as much water or fluid as it takes to quench your thirst, or at least six glasses of water in addition to other drinks daily.

While you need more fluid, it is a myth that drinking large quantities of water will increase your milk supply. In one study, nursing women increased their fluid intake by 30 percent but produced no more milk than before the study. You may tax your kidneys to produce more concentrated urine or develop constipation when fluid intake is too low, and you are likely to feel fatigued and thirsty, but ignoring the need for water will not jeopardize your baby's nutrition.

The Calorie Nutrients: Fat, Protein, and Carbohydrate

The fat, protein, and carbohydrate content of milk varies little with the mother's intake; however, the type of fat in breast milk is a direct reflection of her diet now and while she was pregnant. Whether a woman is eighteen or eighty, active or inactive, healthy or ill, she should be following a low-fat diet that derives no more than 30 percent of its calories from fat. That recommendation also holds for the breast-feeding woman; however, there is more to the fat issue than just total fat. The type of fat in the nursing mother's diet also is important.

The composition of fats in milk is controlled primarily by the mother's diet during pregnancy (which established the type of fat buildup in her fat stores) and during lactation. If her diet is high in vegetable oils (polyunsaturated fats), her breast milk also will be high in these fats. If she is dieting, her breast milk will be higher in the saturated fats that have been stored in her fat tissue.

The Most Important Fat of All: A type of fat found in fish oils, called the omega-3 fatty acids and in particular docosahexaenoic acid or DHA, accumulates in the eye and brain of the infant during the last trimester of pregnancy. Breast milk also contains DHA, especially when the mother includes a few servings of fish in the weekly diet. Mother Nature wasn't fooling when she included these fats in breast milk. Your baby's visual development, intelligence, and even behavior depend, in part, on the omega-3s.

The link between DHA and vision first came to light in premature babies. These babies are at higher risk for vision problems when fed infant formulas, which do not contain DHA. Increasing the infant's intake of DHA improves visual acuity at four months and possibly beyond. The research now shows that even full-term infants need omega-3s, especially DHA. Babies fed breast milk from mothers who regularly eat fish concentrate more of these fats in their nerve tissues and are more alert and process information more quickly than babies who don't get enough of these fats.

The last trimester of pregnancy and the first year of a baby's life are critical periods for visual and nerve development. These processes require deposition of the omega-3 fats into cell membranes for normal cell structure and function. If these fats are in short supply, which is the case when a baby is formula-fed or a nursing mother consumes little or none of these fats, nerve tissue development might be jeopardized even though the baby is growing at a normal rate. Since the omega-3 content of breast milk reflects the mother's diet, it's easy to get enough of these fats just by including two servings of fish in your weekly diet. The best sources of the omega-3s are fatty fish, such as salmon.

How Much Protein? In contrast to fat, the amounts of protein and carbohydrate (that is, lactose) are relatively constant in all human milk, regardless of the mother's diet. But that does not mean you can take them lightly. Protein is your body's basic building block for muscles, organs, bones, cartilage, enzymes, skin, hormones, and numerous other body components. You need it, your baby needs it, and you lose quite a bit of it in breast milk. Consequently, your protein needs are higher during breast-feeding than at any other time in your life, or about twenty grams more than before you were pregnant. Fortunately, this requirement is easily met by increasing your intake of low-fat or nonfat milk. In addition, most diets already supply more than enough additional protein, so there is no reason to start ordering eight-ounce steaks or adding protein powders to your milkshakes. The chicken, fish, milk products, beans and peas, peanut butter, milk, and even whole grains in the Baby-wise Diet will more than meet your protein needs.

How Much Carbohydrates? Carbohydrates are the mainstay of your energy needs. If you are fatigued, look first at how much whole-grain breads and cereals, starchy vegetables, and fruit you are consuming and how often. The Baby-wise Diet supplies about 50 percent or more of its calories from high-quality carbohydrates, which is the perfect mix to help fuel your energy stores and your health.

Vitamins and Minerals for Breast-Feeding

When it comes to vitamins, what you eat is what your baby receives. The vitamin content of breast milk reflects the mother's diet. If your diet is rich in the B vitamins, vitamin A, or vitamin D, your milk will be high in these vitamins and your baby will receive ample amounts to sustain growth and health. In contrast, if your intake of vitamin-rich foods decreases, so does the vitamin content of your milk, and your baby's nutritional status suffers as well.

The Vitamins

While some is good, excessive dietary intake of the fat-soluble vitamins, such as vitamin A and vitamin D, can result in too high a concentration of these vitamins in breast milk. For example, women who supplement their diets with 20,000 IU of vitamin A produced a sevenfold increase of vitamin A in their milk. No harmful effects have ever been noted in these cases, but the potential for toxicity remains. Consequently, a nursing mother's goal is optimal, not excessive, when it comes to vitamins and minerals.

B Vitamins: The B vitamins provide a perfect example of how your diet affects your milk supply. In one study, women who consumed less than 2.5 mg of vitamin B_6 daily produced milk that also was significantly low in this B vitamin. A low intake of vitamin B_6, in turn, jeopardizes the infant's neurological development. As the mother's intake of B_6 increases, so does the B_6 concentration in her breast milk—up to two times the current Recommended Dietary Allowance of 1.9 mg. In another study conducted at the University of Maryland, women who supplemented with 4.0 mg of vitamin B_6 increased their blood levels of this vitamin, while their breast milk levels of vitamin B_6 also increased significantly. In contrast, the babies of women with low vitamin B intakes were more drowsy and less alert than babies nursing from well-nourished mothers. To compound the problem, the vitamin B–deficient mothers provided less stimulation and care to their less-alert babies, suggesting that low intake of this vitamin also affects the mother's mental or emotional health.

The intricate bond between the mother's and the infant's diet does not stop with vitamin B_6. The mother's dietary intake of other vitamins, such as vitamin B_1 and folic acid, directly influences the concentration of these nutrients in her milk. Breast-feeding women who follow strict vegetarian diets that exclude all foods of animal origin are likely to produce milk that is low in vitamin B_{12}, unless they take supplements or consume vitamin B_{12}–fortified foods, such as fortified soy milk. Babies fed vitamin B_{12}–deficient breast milk are at risk for developing nerve problems, anemia, and metabolic disorders associated with insufficient supply of this vitamin. A diet rich in water-soluble vitamins will produce breast milk that contains optimal levels of these nutrients.

The Baby-wise Diet supplies optimal amounts of all the B vitamins. However, if your diet frequently falls short of perfect when it comes to these guidelines, it would be wise to consider a moderate-dose multiple vitamin and mineral supplement that provides approximately 100 percent, and no more than 200 percent, of all the B vitamins, including vitamin B_1 (thiamin), vitamin B_2 (riboflavin), niacin, vitamin B_6 (pyridoxine), folic acid, vitamin B_{12} (cobalamin), biotin, and pantothenic acid. A study from Pennsylvania State University found that women who breast-feed might need more folic acid than the recommended amounts of 400 mcg. Following the Baby-wise Diet plus taking a multiple supplement that contains folic acid will meet these needs.

Vitamin C: Vitamin C is important to your baby throughout life. This water-soluble nutrient is essential in the formation of the body's most abundant tissue—connective tissue, which supports and strengthens all other tissues, from the gums to the blood vessels. The vitamin C content of breast milk varies somewhat depending on your dietary intake, so your baby will consume between 24 mg and 40 mg each day. The nursing mother should consume at least 95 mg of vitamin C daily during the first six months of nursing and 90 mg after that. This amount is easily obtained by including the recommended ten servings of fruits and vegetables in the Baby-wise Diet. Especially good sources of vitamin C include citrus fruit, dark green leafy vegetables, and green or red peppers.

Vitamin D: Vitamin D helps maintain your bones and build your baby's bones by enhancing calcium absorption and aiding in the transportation of calcium into the bones and teeth. Children who do not receive enough vitamin D develop bowed legs when they begin to walk, because the poorly calcified bones cannot withstand the weight of the body. Limited evidence suggests that vitamin D in breast milk is not affected by the mother's diet. Infant vitamin D status is more affected by sunlight exposure than by the mother's nutritional status.

Consequently, breast milk is a minor source of vitamin D during periods of adequate sunlight exposure, but during periods of reduced sunlight exposure, the vitamin D in milk becomes increasingly more important. The baby who is not in the sun and who is breast-fed by a mother who consumes a vitamin D–deficient diet is at highest risk for deficiency.

While there is no evidence that breast-feeding women need any more vitamin D than other women, in general, women often don't get enough of this vitamin. The only reliable dietary sources are vitamin D–fortified soy milk or milk (not yogurt, cheese, or other dairy products unless the label states they are made from vitamin D–fortified milk). As a nursing mom, you should consume at least three daily servings of nonfat or low-fat milk or fortified soy milk to ensure optimal intake of vitamin D, unless you are regularly out in the sun.

Vitamin K: Vitamin K is unusual as nutrients go, since most of a person's requirement is obtained from bacterial synthesis in the intestines rather than from the diet. Babies don't have a well-established bacterial colony in their intestines and are at risk for developing vitamin K deficiencies. In fact, newborn infants have low blood levels of this fat-soluble vitamin and are at elevated risk for developing hemorrhage, since vitamin K is essential in the normal blood-clotting mechanisms that stop a bruise or a cut from progressing into a hemorrhage. Consequently, the American Academy of Pediatrics recommends that all newborns get a onetime injection of vitamin K, which usually is administered at the hospital or soon after birth.

Typical dietary intakes or amounts found in supplements (i.e., 88 mcg/day) do not significantly affect milk concentrations. So, it is wise to consume a vitamin K–rich diet that contains several servings of dark green leafy vegetables, Brussels sprouts, nonfat milk, fruit, and whole-grain cereal, as outlined in the Baby-wise Diet, as well as a multiple supplement that contains a moderate dose of vitamin K.

The Minerals

Calcium: Calcium is the main mineral in bones and teeth and an important mineral in nerve transmission and muscle contraction. No one can do without it, especially a nursing mother who loses approximately 200 mg to 300 mg of calcium in breast milk every day. Consequently, optimal calcium intake remains a priority during breast-feeding to ensure that this calcium comes from your diet, not your bones. While your body adapts to the increased demand by increasing calcium absorption, you still need at least 1,200 mg of calcium—the equivalent of four glasses of nonfat or low-fat milk or fortified soy milk. A woman who consumes adequate amounts of calcium-rich foods can bear and breast-feed one or many children throughout her life with no harm to her bones. In fact, breast-feeding might have a protective effect against osteoporosis if calcium intake remains optimal.

Another reason to boost calcium intake is to prevent your baby from being exposed to lead. High-calcium diets during and following pregnancy help suppress lead mobilization from bone tissue, thus reducing both maternal and infant exposure to this toxic metal. Researchers at the U.S. Environmental Protection Agency in Cincinnati studied lead levels in women during gestation and for six months after pregnancy. Blood lead levels rose significantly after pregnancy (i.e., by 26 to 99 percent), primarily from lead leaching from bones into blood. Women who consumed adequate calcium had less bone loss, hence less lead was mobilized from bone, and blood levels of this metal remained lower. The researchers conclude that "calcium supplementation may be an important means of limiting [infant] exposure to lead."

Chromium: Chromium could be of particular concern for breast-feeding mothers. Insufficient intake of chromium is a problem for most adults, with only one in every ten people consuming enough of this essential mineral. However, chromium might be an even greater problem for breast-feeding women because of the increased demands for this mineral owing to milk production. Nursing women have lower levels of chromium in hair than do women who don't breast-feed. Hair chromium levels decrease after both pregnancy and lactation, and it takes four months or more between pregnancies to raise hair chromium levels back to prepregnancy levels.

While the baby can concentrate chromium from the mother and thus is protected to a certain extent from deficiency, research conducted by Richard Anderson, Ph.D., research chemist at USDA Vitamin and Mineral Nutrition Laboratory in Beltsville, Maryland, shows that breast-fed babies consume as little as 2 percent of their recommended levels of chromium. Insufficient intake of this trace mineral also can increase a woman's risk for developing high blood sugar and even heart disease.

To consume optimal amounts of chromium during breast-feeding, select several servings daily of chromium-rich foods, such as wheat germ, whole-grain breads and cereals, fish, cooked dried beans and peas, spinach, and orange juice.

Iron: Both you and your baby need iron to build hemoglobin, the protein in red blood cells that carries oxygen to all the body's tissues. Although the mother's iron intake has little effect on the iron concentration in breast milk, iron remains a primary concern for women after the baby is born. Even with iron supplementation, many women's iron reserves are depleted as a result of pregnancy. Breast-feeding delays the return of menstruation and so gives a woman a chance to replenish herself if she is eating an iron-rich diet. On the other hand, a nursing mother who also is menstruating has an even higher iron requirement because she is losing iron during her period and in her breast milk.

All women should continue eating iron-rich diets and possibly continue taking iron supplements for three months to one year after pregnancy to restock tissue iron stores. Also, don't drink coffee or tea at meals, since these beverages contain compounds called tannins that block iron absorption and possibly lower iron levels in breast milk. Consult your physician about iron supplements for your nursing baby, since some research shows that breast-fed infants are more prone to iron deficiency after the fourth month than are bottle-fed infants who are fed iron-fortified formulas.

Selenium: Selenium is another mineral of particular concern to breast-feeding women. The nursing baby's selenium status reflects the mother's intake, which is higher during lactation than at any other time in a woman's life. To add to the risk of developing a deficiency, the selenium content of most foods of plant origin—from fruits and vegetables to legumes and grains—is dependent on the selenium content of the soil in which the food is grown. Because of increased needs and suboptimal intakes, breast-feeding women often are low in selenium.

Poor selenium status is easily reversed by increasing consumption of selenium-rich foods, such as seafood (for example, salmon, shrimp, oysters, and trout), extra-lean meat, cooked dried beans and peas, and chicken. A moderate-dose supplement that contains 50 mcg to 200 mcg of selenium also raises blood selenium levels in breast-feeding women and improves the selenium content of breast milk.

Just because some is good does not mean more is better. Selenium is one nutrient that can be toxic if taken in large amounts, so limit intake from supplements to the above mentioned dose. In addition, the "organic" forms of selenium, such as selenium-rich yeast and selenomethionine, are particularly effective in raising selenium levels and may not be as potentially toxic as the inorganic forms, such as selenite.

Zinc: Several studies have reported that breast-fed infants don't get enough zinc, a trace mineral essential for growth and development. Granted, the zinc content of mother's milk is not high and babies often receive as little as 10 percent of their recommended intake when exclusively breast-fed. However, the zinc in breast milk is very well absorbed, while limited evidence shows that the mother's diet has little effect on the zinc concentration of breast milk. Unless a child shows delayed growth or a low resistance to colds and infections, there is little evidence that low zinc intake from breast milk is harmful.

While a woman should consume ample amounts of zinc from dietary sources to ensure her health and the health of her baby, there does not appear to be any reason to take extra zinc as supplements while breast-feeding. Infants who are breast-fed for more than four months and who show symptoms of delayed growth might be suffering from marginal zinc intake. Discuss with your physician the need to supplement your baby's diet with zinc under these conditions.

Other Minerals: All other minerals, from magnesium and manganese to iodine and copper, are important for the health of both the mother and her baby. Unfortunately, there is little or no research on how the mother's dietary intake of these minerals affects the baby's food supply. A diet of fewer than 2,200 calories daily is unlikely to supply all the minerals in optimal amounts, which is yet another reason why every bite counts when you are breast-feeding. The Baby-wise Diet supplies at least the recommended amounts of all the known minerals and, if followed closely, will guarantee optimal nutritional health for you and your baby.

Phytochemicals
A new field of nutrition has opened up in the past decade—the study of phytochemicals. More than 12,000 of these health-enhancing compounds have been identified in fruits, vegetables, whole grains, and other

unprocessed foods. Phytochemicals have a variety of functions from antioxidant capabilities to cancer-suppression and heart-disease prevention. While research clearly shows these compounds are essential to health in adults, little research has been done on their benefits during breast-feeding. What is known is encouraging. In one study from the Cancer Research Center of Hawaii, researchers found that breast-feeding women who consume ample amounts of daidzein and genistein, phytochemicals found in soy foods such as tofu and soy milk, pass along these health-enhancing compounds to their babies. While early exposure to these compounds reduces mammary cancer in animals, further research is needed to assess this effect in humans. Since our bodies evolved over hundreds of thousands of years on diets loaded with phytochemical-rich vegetables and other plants, it is likely that future research will show the benefits to both mother and baby of eating more phytochemical-rich produce, beans, and whole grains.

Garlic, Beer, Toxins, and Other Concerns

Wives' tales flourish when it comes to breast-feeding. One woman is told to drink more beer because it will boost her milk supply. Another is told to avoid eating onions and garlic because they cause colic. While some of these recommendations have some merit, many are more fiction than fact. For example, salt doesn't increase the sodium content of your breast milk and pepper won't make your milk "spicy." A bowl of beans can give you gas, but it won't affect your milk or your baby's health. Citrus fruits or tomatoes are thought to be acidic foods, but they have no effect on your blood or the acidity of your milk.

Garlic: Garlic is often avoided by breast-feeding mothers who fear it will cause colic in their newborns. However, research shows infants actually nurse longer and suck more overall, with no apparent discomfort, when there is a hint of garlic in the milk.

Cow's Milk: Infants who are sensitive to certain foods, such as cow's milk protein, might develop an allergic reaction or colic when these foods are included in the breast-feeding mother's diet. While cow's milk and soy products are commonly associated with colic, no one food can be attributed to colic in all children, so you must be your own sleuth and eliminate those foods in your diet that seem to be causing your baby discomfort. Be cautious when avoiding foods, since limiting variety in the diet can mean restricting essential nutrients. Always talk with your physician before eliminating a major food group, such as milk products or products made from wheat.

Beer and Alcohol: For centuries, women have been told that alcohol, in particular beer, would increase their milk supply and strengthen their nursing baby. In the early 1900s, beer companies advertised their products as "tonics" to stimulate appetite and enhance milk yield.

Beer consumption does increase blood levels of prolactin, a hormone necessary for milk production, in men and non-breast-feeding women. However, whether or not beer has a similar effect in breast-feeding women is unimportant, since regardless of the milk supply, babies prefer nonalcoholic breast milk and drink less milk (up to 23 percent less) after their mothers have consumed beer than they do after their mothers have consumed a nonalcoholic beverage.

Beer apparently flavors the milk and makes it less appetizing to the infant. In general, the Subcommittee on Nutrition during Lactation of the Food and Nutrition Board and the Institute of Medicine recommend that mothers who want to drink while breast-feeding should consume no more than two to two and a half ounces of liquor, eight ounces of wine, or two cans of beer a day.

Wine drinkers should be careful not to expose their babies to lead. Foil-wrapped wine bottles leave lead-salt deposits on the bottle's rim. Unless the drinker carefully wipes the rim and the exposed cork before pouring, these deposits can dissolve when the wine is poured and raise the lead content of the beverage. Better yet, choose wines that do not have this type of wrapper.

Caffeine: After the baby is born, some women mistakenly think they can resume their prepregnancy coffee intake. Caffeine does stimulate milk production; however, a nursing baby does an even better job of increasing the milk supply by suckling. Although one cup of coffee, tea, cola, or a small amount of chocolate or other caffeinated foods and beverages appear to be harmless, by the second serving the caffeine is accumulating in breast milk to levels that could affect the baby.

Babies eliminate caffeine from their systems more slowly than do adults, so accumulation can occur in the infant, prolonging the effects of this drug. Although caffeine is poorly researched, anecdotal reports include irritability, wakefulness, and poor eating habits following maternal consumption of caffeine. In addition, coffee and tea inhibit iron absorption, and anemia is common in countries where there is heavy coffee consumption. At a time when a woman needs to be stockpiling iron, coffee may undermine her efforts.

Pesticides: Pesticides are another concern for the breast-feeding mother. It is virtually impossible to avoid these environmental contaminants, and almost all women carry contaminants such as PCBs and dioxin in their bodies. Dioxin is a by-product of chemical manufacturing and is most commonly remembered as the contaminant in Agent Orange, the defoliant used in Vietnam. This chemical has accumulated in the soil and in our food since the 1940s and is stored in fat tissue of all animals from fish to humans. The best a woman can do is limit her intake of fatty meats and dairy products so as not to concentrate too much of these stored contaminants into her system. Also, lose weight slowly, so you don't dump large amounts of these stored toxins into your blood supply where they could enter your milk. To minimize exposure—yours and your baby's—to harmful chemicals:

- Eat a variety of wholesome, minimally processed foods to limit your intake of any one food.
- Avoid fatty cuts of meat, trim all meats, and skin poultry before cooking.
- Avoid fatty dairy products, such as cheese, whole milk, sour cream, cream cheese, whipping cream, and butter.
- Purchase foods in season and local produce (or at least produce grown in the United States) when possible.
- Wash produce, peel waxed foods such as cucumbers or apples, discard outer leaves on vegetables, and peel any suspect fruits or vegetables.
- If you purchase "organic" produce, verify that the food really is grown without the use of pesticides.

Drugs, Medications, and Tobacco: As with pregnancy, drugs of any kind, from the chemicals in cigarettes to prescription or street drugs, should be viewed with concern. Tobacco smoke could increase your child's risk for asthma, respiratory infections, and possibly even lung cancer. If you or someone in your household smokes, now is the time to quit. (See Chapter 1 for more on smoking.)

Many prescription and over-the-counter medications can be absorbed into breast milk, thus exposing the infant to unwanted and potentially harmful substances. A partial list of medications is found in Table 9.1,

"The Dos and Don'ts of Medications When Breast-Feeding." If you must take one of these drugs, always check with your physician and your pharmacist about safer alternatives. To relieve pain, for example, your physician might recommend acetaminophen rather than aspirin, since the former medication is not absorbed into breast milk. Another way to minimize your baby's exposure is to take a medication just after breast-feeding or just before your baby takes a long nap. This will allow time for the drug to be metabolized and reduce its accumulation in your milk.

TABLE 9.1

The Dos and Don'ts of Medications When Breast-Feeding

Even if a medication is listed as safe, always check first with your physician. According to the American Academy of Pediatrics, the following medications probably are safe:

Acetaminophen, codeine, ibuprofen (painkillers)
Amoxicillin, streptomycin (antibiotics)
Birth control pills
Lidocaine (anesthetic)
Loperamide (antidiarrhea medication)
Naproxen (anti-inflammatory)

The following medications are not recommended:

Aspirin
Clemastine (antihistamine)
Diazepam (antianxiety medication)
Ergotamine (antimigraine medication)
Caffeine
Sulfasalazine (antiulcer medications)

Can You Eat to Avoid Colic?

For no apparent reason, approximately 20 percent of healthy, happy babies develop colic. They start crying, usually in the evening and usually when they are between three weeks and three months of age. To express their discomfort, their fists clench, their faces turn red, their legs pull up to their chests, and they howl in pain for up to an hour or more. Then, as quickly as they started, those babies stop crying and start to smile again.

Although most babies have fussy periods, especially later in the day, they usually are comforted by the breast when they are tired, bored, lonely, or uncomfortable. The difference between normal fussiness and colic is that the colicky baby has periods of intense crying that are difficult to soothe.

There are as many folk remedies for colic as there are parents who have survived a colicky baby. Holding the baby in a sitting position on your lap and pulling the baby's knees up to his or her chest may help. Some parents find ingenious ways to soothe the troubled baby. They place the infant in a baby seat on top of the washer during the spin cycle. They go for a car ride. They pace up and down the hallway singing whatever song seems to work.

No one knows exactly what colic is, but more than likely it's an umbrella term for a variety of troubles. The most commonly held belief is that colic is related to the baby's immature digestive tract with the pain caused by spasms, cramps, or gas. Limited evidence shows that some cases of colic might be remedied by the mother avoiding cow's milk in her diet for the first few months of the baby's life; as many as one-third of colicky babies improve when the mothers adopt milk-free diets. One study showed that mothers of colicky babies have higher levels of cow antibodies in their breast milk than do other mothers, suggesting that some component of cow's milk actually passes into the mother's breast milk.

This does not mean all breast-feeding mothers should give up cow's milk, especially since this is one of the best dietary sources of calcium, vitamin D, and other essential nutrients. However, if you have a colicky baby, try avoiding cow's milk for a week to see if your baby's symptoms improve. If so, avoid cow's milk for the baby's first few months and look to other dietary sources of calcium, such as fortified soy milk, spinach, turnip greens, broccoli, canned salmon with bones, tofu, and collard greens, or calcium supplements. If not, there is no reason to avoid this nutritious food.

While you might hear that a baby will develop diarrhea or eczema if you eat chocolate, there is no scientific evidence that this is true. On the other hand, a study from the University of Minnesota found that chocolate (as well as cruciferous vegetables and onions) in the mother's diet was associated with an increased risk for colic in babies that were exclusively breast-fed. You might try temporarily eliminating these foods for a week from your diet and watch for improvements in colic symptoms.

The "Weighting" Game

Breast-feeding is a natural way to lose weight after the baby is born. You have stored added fat during pregnancy in preparation for breast-feeding. Studies on animals show that if the mother nurses her pups, all this stored fat is "burned" by the end of the nursing period. In contrast, the fat remains if the mother is not allowed to breast-feed. Even more fat is likely to be stored if the animal becomes pregnant shortly after the first baby. In studies on humans, women who nurse their babies are more likely to lose excess pounds and return to their prepregnancy weights than are women who bottle-feed their infants. In short, women who do not breast-feed are more likely to stay "fatter" for a longer period of time than those who breast-feed.

What Not to Do: After the baby is born, you probably will be eager to lose some pounds. You've watched your figure change and your tummy grow; now you want to fit back into those jeans. Many women jump on the diet bandwagon immediately upon returning home from the hospital. But if you cut calories too far, you deprive your body and your baby of essential energy and nutrients, thus placing yourself and your baby at nutritional risk. Big mistake. This is no time to diet. You need about 2,700 calories daily when nursing. You can't afford to drop much below this.

Cutting calories while breast-feeding can result in fatigue, poor milk supply, and a reduction in the immune factors in breast milk that provide your newborn with a resistance to colds and infections. Women who try to lose too much weight too fast by severely restricting calories jeopardize the health and well-being of their babies. Strict dieting also is an underlying reason why some women are unable to produce enough milk.

A hidden concern about losing too much weight while breast-feeding is the potential for chemical contaminants to migrate into the baby's milk supply. The breakdown of fat tissue could release fat-soluble contaminants, such as PCBs, that are stored in this tissue. The risk of unacceptable pesticide levels in breast milk is especially high for women who have consumed high-fat diets (pesticides accumulate in the fatty portions of foods, such as meat). This concern is theoretical, since there has not been research to test the contaminant levels in the breast milk of women who are dieting. However, since severe weight loss is not recommended, this adds one more argument against strict dieting while breast-feeding.

How to Lose Weight Safely: You can lose weight and breast-feed safely. However, as a new mom, you shouldn't worry about losing weight for the first six weeks after delivery. Use those first few weeks to focus solely on the care of yourself and your baby.

After the first six weeks and when breast-feeding is established, you can begin a weight-loss program based on a mild calorie restriction that allows gradual weight loss. The key word here is *gradual*. Prior to pregnancy the weight-loss goal could have climbed as high as two pounds a week. Now it is only two pounds lost per month for most women and no more than one pound a week for overweight nursing mothers who use a combination of diet and exercise to shed pounds. Keep in mind it took nine months to gain the weight and it could take as long or longer to reach a desirable weight after the baby is born.

Whatever your weight goal, add five pounds for the extra tissue your body retains while breast-feeding. So, if you ultimately want to lose twenty pounds, aim for fifteen pounds for now. The final five pounds usually drop off when you stop nursing. According to Lindsay Allen, Ph.D., professor of nutrition at the University of Connecticut, "breast-feeding stimulates a woman's appetite, but once she stops producing milk, her weight drops off." Consequently, whatever your weight is at six months postpartum, minus five pounds if you are breast-feeding, is approximately where you need to start in your weight-management goals.

Another key to weight loss while breast-feeding is timing. The first four to six months is the most calorie-intensive period for breast-feeding, since during these early months the baby is exclusively drinking breast milk. Milk production gradually decreases as solid foods are added to the diet in later months. Consequently, the nursing mother must decrease her food intake after six months, or she is likely to gain weight. The best indicator of your varying calorie needs is the scale. If you are gaining weight, your calorie intake is too high (or your exercise is too low).

While 2,700 calories or more is optimal, an average calorie intake of 2,200 to 2,500 calories is associated with adequate milk production and appropriate infant growth and allows most women to lose about one to two pounds a month. The extra 36,000 or more calories stored in fat reserves during pregnancy can help make up the energy difference. In fact, most women will gradually lose weight (on average about one to one and a half pounds monthly for the first four to six months) without even trying. How do you know if you are getting enough to eat? The most obvious signs are your hunger and the scale. If you are hungry all of the time or if you are losing more than one pound a week, you're not eating enough.

A breast-feeding mom has an additional 500 calories above the 2,200 quota from pregnancy. That means she can eat an additional three slices of bread, three ounces of lean chicken, a serving of a fruit or vegetable, and a cup of nonfat yogurt for a total of 500 calories. It doesn't mean she can order an extra cheeseburger, French fries, and a soda pop, which would add more than 1,000 calories and far fewer vitamins and minerals. In short, breast-feeding gives you some extra calories to work with, but you need to use them wisely.

Some Women Gain Weight: About one in every five women doesn't automatically lose weight and might even gain a little weight after pregnancy. One study found that stubborn weight gain is more than just retaining your pregnancy weight. For some women, staying home with the children and being around food all day encourages them to eat more and gain more weight. First-time moms and women who have closely spaced pregnancies (less than two years between one pregnancy and the next) are at highest risk for putting on a few pounds after the baby is born. If you find that this applies to you, turn to pages 243–45 for tips on how to handle the nibbling syndrome.

Reasons Not to Lose: No woman, especially one who is nursing, should lose weight to please anyone else or should even consider trying to achieve unrealistic, and potentially harmful, fashion-model thinness. A new mother's greatest and most important task is to love and nourish both her baby and herself. She should be proud of herself and her accomplishment and should never feel apologetic or guilty about a few extra pounds.

Exercise and Breast-Feeding

Daily exercise is an excellent alternative to dieting. Moderate physical activity helps mobilize fat from the mother's fat stores and burns calories, creating a calorie deficit, which is what you need to lose weight. You also lose the right kind of weight—body fat—whereas relying solely on diet for weight loss results in the loss of both body fat and muscle. Staying fit also helps avoid the postpartum blues that many women experience in the first few weeks after delivery. It helps you feel livelier and boosts your confidence. In fact, women who exercise during pregnancy and resume a modified exercise plan after delivery report they get their "life back in order" in half the time—that is, in approximately two weeks, compared to women who haven't exercised postpartum.

TABLE 9.2

No Time to Snack? Get a Life!

The following snacks take less time to prepare than grabbing a soda pop. Just remember to bring them along! For each snack, pick at least two items from Group A and one or more items from Group B.

Group A:

Fresh fruit (the easiest to carry and eat include apples, oranges, bananas, grapes, peaches, nectarines, or tangerines)

Applesauce or fruit cocktail packaged in individual containers

Single-serving packages of dried fruit, such as boxed raisins or minibags of dried cranberries

A mixture of raisins (or other dried fruit), almonds, and your favorite cereal

Raw vegetables (buy the precut versions or the baby carrots and save even more time!)

A tomato

100 percent juice in a box (orange juice is the most nutritious)

Mini-cans of tomato, V8, or carrot juice

Salsa, preferably fresh

Group B:

Fat-free cottage cheese or ricotta cheese

Low-fat or nonfat yogurt, plain or fruited

8-ounce carton of low-fat milk (regular or chocolate)

1 ounce extra-lean sandwich meat

⅓ cup hummus

1 tablespoon peanut or almond butter

Fat-free whole-wheat crackers

Microwave fat-free popcorn

Minibagels

Graham crackers

Oven-baked tortilla chips

Low-fat bran muffins (from bakery)

Whole-wheat bread sticks

Premade crepes (some grocery stores carry these in the produce section)

Fat-free dips, such as salad dressings or fat-free sour cream dips

Limited research has been done on exercise during breast-feeding; however, the information that is available supports the benefits to both the mother and the baby. Women who exercise are leaner, have a higher fitness level, and produce more milk than do couch potatoes. They burn more calories, so they can eat more food while still losing weight; consequently, they are more likely to eat an optimal diet. Breast-feeding women who exercise have the best of all worlds. "Research shows that these women consume more calories, lose weight more consistently, and their milk production is better than sedentary women," says Bonnie Worthington-Roberts, Ph.D., former professor of nutrition at the University of Washington in Seattle. So, get moving!

Women who have exercised throughout their pregnancies often resume physical activity sooner and will be capable of doing more than women who remained sedentary during those nine months. If you plan to exercise during lactation, the same guidelines apply as during pregnancy, which includes obtaining medical clearance, exercising at least three times a week, beginning and ending the session with a warm-up and cooldown period, and gradually increasing the frequency and intensity. Avoid intense exercise, since this can raise lactic acid levels in breast milk, which changes the taste of the milk and might cause your baby to drink less. In addition, avoid any jarring or bouncing movements and maximal exertion until your pelvic area is completely healed, which usually takes at least six weeks postpartum. Always consult your physician before beginning any exercise program.

Probably the biggest challenge to exercise after the baby is born is time. You will need to set aside a half hour or hour and arrange child care ahead of time. Gyms and health clubs often have baby-sitting services, or you can purchase a baby jogger or a backpack and bring the baby on your walks. Some mothers get together and share child care or take turns watching the kids so they can exercise. You will need to decide how you will take time for yourself, while staying realistic about how much you can take on while caring for a new baby. Keep in mind your exercise program will be in transition during the first few months after the baby is born. Some days you will find time to exercise for an hour, other days you will be lucky if you fit in a walk around the block. Don't let a slip progress to a relapse; just do it—exercise, that is—when and where you can!

Postpartum Blues

Eight out of ten women experience "the blues" after the baby is born. For some, the transient weepiness, mood swings, hopelessness, anxiety, and irritability are only minor nuisances that last a few days. For 10 to 15 percent of new mothers, the depression is more serious or lasts for weeks or months.

Defining the problem is difficult and the causes are unknown. Some researchers theorize that fluctuations in hormones or other brain chemicals called endorphins might underlie postpartum depression (PPD). Just as women vary in their experience with premenstrual syndrome, so do women vary in how they react to hormonal changes after pregnancy. Other experts believe that feelings of anxiety or depression are a normal phase everyone experiences during major life changes. Women with a family history of depression, alcoholism, or psychological problems could be at higher risk for PPD, but many women with PPD have no known risk factors. (See Table 9.3, "Postpartum Depression: What's Normal and What's Not.")

TABLE 9.3

Postpartum Depression: What's Normal and What's Not

Eight out of ten women experience a little moodiness after pregnancy. However, up to 15 percent of women suffer symptoms serious enough to need professional help. If you recognize any of the symptoms in the right-hand column as pertaining to yourself, you might want to discuss these with your physician.

What's Normal	What's Not
Feeling a little overwhelmed.	Thoughts of hurting yourself or your baby.
Feeling tired all the time.	Feeling so exhausted you don't get out of bed for days.
Not falling madly in love with your new baby right off the bat.	Feeling increasingly detached from your baby.
Feeling disappointed in how your labor and delivery turned out.	Feeling like a total failure.

Mild depression or mood swings are normal and temporary. As with many other adjustments during the early weeks of parenthood, ride the storms and revel in the tender moments. Ask for help from loved ones or even seek a few therapy sessions to help you cope in the first few weeks. Your moods should start stabilizing within a few months. However, you should consult with your physician if you experience severe depression. You might need more aggressive treatments, such as antidepression medications, to help stabilize your moods.

Postpartum depression can take several forms. The most common is ordinary depression, characterized by sadness, overwhelming fatigue, crying, and inability to sleep. A small percentage of women (3 to 5 percent) experience depression accompanied by anxiety attacks that can include frequent thoughts of hurting themself or the baby. Some women experience a rare form of postpartum depression accompanied by psychosis, including delusions and paranoia.

Finally, forget the rules when it comes to adjusting to parenthood. The recommendation that you should be back to normal in six weeks is now recognized to be outdated and downright sexist. The ovaries might have recovered, but your body and emotions still might need some tender loving care. Some women take from three months up to one year to start feeling like their old selves again. Many suffer from colds, sinus trouble, earaches, bronchitis, hair loss, acne, poor appetite, memory loss, and loss of sexual drive for months, without feeling tired or depressed. Pregnancy and delivery might not be categorized as a sickness, but they are major stresses to the body, so give yourself plenty of time to heal, physically and emotionally.

Nursing Meals and Snacks

A new mother has a difficult time trying to feed herself and keep up with the new commitment of caring for a baby. Women with small children and a new baby have even more trouble taking time to eat well. At the same time, there is almost nothing more important than to make sure you follow the Baby-wise Diet for at least a year after the baby is born.

Eating well doesn't need to take time; it does mean planning ahead and listening to your body's needs. A bowl of cereal and a glass of orange juice for breakfast; a turkey sandwich, baby carrots, apple, and milk for lunch; cold chicken, a salad, and lots of steamed vegetables for dinner; and several nutritious snacks in between is all it takes. Each of these meals takes less than ten minutes to prepare. Keep track of your food intake by using Worksheet 9.1, "My Postpregnancy Daily Checklist (for the Breast-Feeding Mother)."

Worksheet 9.1 My Postpregnancy Daily Checklist
(for the Breast-Feeding Mother)

Food Groups	Minimum Servings	Actual Intake
Calcium-rich foods	3–4	_____
Vegetables (at least 2 folic acid–rich choices)	6	_____
Fruits (at least 2 vitamin C–rich choices)	4	_____
Grains (at least 4 whole-grain choices)	9	_____
Extra-lean meats and legumes	3	_____
Quenchers	8	_____

Did I reach my goals? _____

What needs improvement? _____

What will I do differently next week? _____

Chapter 10

❧

The Postpregnancy Diet: Regaining Your Figure and Eating for the Next Baby

If you choose to formula-feed your baby, if you have stopped breast-feeding, or if you are are planning another baby:

1. **Nutrition:** Follow the guidelines outlined in the Baby-wise Diet. One out of every two pregnancies is unplanned, so restock your nutritional stores in the likelihood of another pregnancy.
2. **Weight:** Lose weight gradually by cutting fat and increasing fruits, vegetables, whole grains, and low-fat milk and lean meat products.
3. **Supplement:** Continue to take a multiple vitamin and mineral that contains 100 to 200 percent of the Daily Value for all vitamins and minerals plus at least 18 mg of iron each day.
4. **Exercise:** Exercise daily, but only when your body is ready and even then, adjust the routine, intensity, or duration as needed.
5. **Medical Checkups:** Regularly check your iron levels (serum ferritin levels should be 20 mcg/L or above).

After delivering a baby, the challenge for the woman who does not breast-feed is to nourish her body to restock depleted nutrient stores while slowly regaining a desirable figure. Sacrificing either optimal nutrition or a desirable weight can affect your physical and emotional health later on.

As always, eating right is not an instinctive process, so you must take time to plan a healthful eating style that will suit your new, busy lifestyle while nourishing you and your baby. As with pregnancy, your goal for the first year after pregnancy, whether you choose to breast-feed or not, is to eat enough nutrient-packed foods to stay healthy, feel satisfied, and rebuild your nutritional stores.

In addition, it's never too late to start nourishing the next baby. Since one in every two babies are unplanned and some are complete surprises, maintaining optimal nutritional status during the childbearing years is an essential part of being a woman. So, if you plan to have a second baby, resume competition sports, or even survive the additional stress of juggling family, work, and home, then restocking nutrient stores should begin immediately after the baby is born.

Having a baby is a nutritionally draining experience. Breast-feeding that baby for six months or more adds to the nutritional stress. Ideally, a woman should wait a year or two between babies and follow the Baby-wise Diet during that time to gear up for the next pregnancy. However, some women either intentionally or unintentionally have babies in quick succession. To reduce the nutritional risk that comes from having a large or closely spaced family, there are a few dietary guidelines worth following.

When and What to Eat and Drink

Once your baby is on formula, the goal is to consume optimal amounts of all the essential nutrients in order to maintain health and restock dwindling nutrient stores, while gradually attaining a desirable weight. Your diet should resemble the one you followed for the months prior to pregnancy, including:

   2 servings from the Calcium-Rich Group
   5 servings from the Vegetable Group (at least 2 of these should be folic acid–rich selections)
   3 servings from the Fruit Group (2 of these should be vitamin C–rich selections)
   6 servings from the Grains Group (at least 4 of these should be whole-grain or mineral-rich selections)
   2 servings from the Extra-Lean Meats and Legumes Group, with at least 1 serving being fish or legumes
   5 servings from the Quenchers Group

(See Worksheet 10.1, "My Postpregnancy Daily Checklist [for the Non-Breast-Feeding Mother]," at the end of this chapter.)

Eating on the Run

Whether you are a working mother or a full-time mom, other matters often interfere with the best eating plans. However, with a little planning, there is no excuse for not eating well.

It takes as little as five minutes to fix a nutritious meal or snack. A container of yogurt, a piece of fruit, a handful of fat-free whole-wheat crackers, and a few slices of low-fat luncheon meats can make a nutritious, easy, and fast lunch. Or prepare a big pot of homemade vegetable soup on Sunday and serve it with bread and cheese for several meals throughout the week. Even a ready-to-eat turkey sandwich (hold the mayonnaise), an apple, and a carton of nonfat milk fit well into the Baby-wise Diet. Don't forget to bring snacks with you. Pack your purse, briefcase, glove compartment, baby bag, or desk drawer with nuts, dried fruit, crackers and a jar of peanut butter, individual packs of applesauce, or cartons of 100 percent orange juice. Might as well make it a habit now, because once your baby is eating solid foods you will be carrying snacks with you for many years to come.

Stockpiling Nutrients

If you followed the Baby-wise Diet prior to and during your pregnancy, it should take only a few months of eating well after the baby is born to return your body to optimal nutritional health. Even if you are only now beginning to eat better, following these dietary guidelines will help you restock the nutrient stores in your tissues and energize you for parenthood. If you entered pregnancy only marginally nourished or if morning sickness and other pregnancy-related problems were roadblocks to eating well during your pregnancy, don't be surprised if it takes a year or more of eating well to restock your nutrient stores and regain a high level of wellness.

The Skinny on Fat

The foremost dietary guideline to remember is to cut the fat. By reducing your fat intake you automatically consume fewer fatty meats, dairy products, oils, convenience and snack foods and more nutrient-packed foods, such as fruits, vegetables, whole grains, and legumes. A low-fat diet also helps you regain and maintain your figure while reducing your risk for diseases later in life. Also, remember to eat as many minimally processed foods as possible. That means choosing whole-wheat bread instead of white bread, baked potatoes instead of potato chips, and fresh broccoli instead of frozen broccoli in cream sauce.

While fat is the most important consideration in our diets, we may not have been given the whole scoop. For one thing, the "30 percent fat calories" rule was recommended because researchers didn't think Americans could handle going any lower (we've cut fat by only a few percentage points in the past two decades and currently hover between 34 and 37 percent). According to William Connor, M.D., professor of medicine and clinical nutrition at Oregon Health Sciences University in Portland, we would be a lot better off if we aimed for about 25 percent of our calories as fat. "That recommendation fits the epidemiological evidence and allows us to eat some fat, but not much," says Dr. Connor. This goal can be met only if the diet is planned around whole grains, vegetables, fruits, and legumes. There is little room for fatty foods, from hamburgers and French fries to ice cream.

When fat does creep into your food, be sure it's the "good" fat from fish, nuts, or canola or olive oil. These fats lower, rather than raise, the risk of heart disease. But, this doesn't give us a blank check to overdose on oil. "Olive oil is an acceptable fat, but the idea that pouring it on food is all right is as absurd as the belief years ago that it was good to douse everything in corn oil," says Dr. Connor. In order to reach the 25 percent fat goal, you must cut fat everywhere.

Grains and Veggies

When it comes to advice on carbohydrates, do you feel like a Ping-Pong ball? First, grains are good for you. Then they're bad. Let's set the record straight once and for all. Grains *are* good for you. The trick is choosing the right ones, in the right amounts.

Grains: The claims made in fad diet books that carbohydrates make you fat are partly right. In the past few decades, our appetites have dramatically increased for thousands of highly refined, calorie-dense grain-based foods, including doughnuts, cookies, white pasta, sweetened cereals, white bread and bagels, sports bars, and snack foods. Along with our increasingly sedentary lives, these carbs have packed on the weight, especially with the super-sized portions to which we've grown so accustomed. Along with the pounds has come an escalating risk for disease.

The main paradox in the controversy over grains is that excessive intake of refined grains *causes* the same diseases that whole grains help to *prevent*. Fiber-rich whole grains lower our risks for everything from heart disease and cancer to diabetes, and they fill us up without filling us out, so they help with weight loss. Unlike processed refined grains, whole grains are low-fat, high-fiber, and packed with vitamins, minerals, and antioxidant phytochemicals. In short, making sure at least half the grains you eat every day are whole grains, along with loading the plate with tons of vegetables and fruit, is the smartest thing a woman can do for her health and waistline after the baby is born.

Ideally you should be eating at least six to nine servings daily of grains. At least four servings should be whole grains, such as whole-wheat bread, brown rice, oatmeal, or stoneground cornmeal. It is easy to meet this quota by including a bowl of oatmeal and a piece of whole-wheat toast for breakfast and a sandwich made from whole-grain bread for lunch; the other servings can come from additional whole-grain selections or from a few refined grain sources, such as white rice or white bread. However, the whole-grain varieties are higher in fiber and almost all vitamins and minerals compared to their enriched or refined counterparts. For example, a slice of white bread has only

- 22 percent of the magnesium,
- 38 percent of the zinc,
- 28 percent of the chromium,
- 12 percent of the manganese,
- 4 percent of the vitamin E,
- 18 percent of the vitamin B_6, and
- 63 percent of the folic acid of whole-wheat bread.

Veggies: One thing is for sure—most women need to include a lot more fresh fruits and vegetables in their daily routines. It is impossible to reach the nutritional goals without them. Take for example, the dark green leafies, which are nature's closest thing to the "perfect" food. They provide ample amounts of the antioxidants (vitamin C and beta carotene), folic acid, iron, calcium, and numerous other minerals essential to a woman during the childbearing years—all with virtually no fat and minimal calories.

A woman preparing for her next pregnancy should eat eight to ten servings daily of these nutritional powerhouses. But nine out of ten women don't eat even half this recommended amount, and when they do, more often than not the vegetable is fatty French fries, nutrient-poor iceberg lettuce, or sugary apple juice. To ensure you get your fair share, include at least two fruits and/or vegetables at each meal and at least one at every snack.

Losing Those Extra Pounds

The average woman has about eight to ten pounds of extra fat tissue that is her energy bank account for breast-feeding. Whereas most women who breast-feed will lose the weight because of the added energy drain of producing milk, the woman who chooses not to breast-feed must cut her calories or increase activity to achieve the same results. Keep in mind, however, that while most women can lose weight after pregnancy and many can attain a weight close to their prepregnancy weight, pregnancy can change your body shape somewhat and may even cause some weight gain that persists despite the best of weight-management efforts.

If you struggle with five or more pounds after the baby is born, avoid quick weight-loss diets, which actually work against your intentions to maintain a healthy eating plan. Researchers at the Karolinska Institute in Stockholm found that women who lost the excess postpartum weight were more likely to have gained an appropriate amount of weight during pregnancy, to have exercised and eaten regularly, and to have avoided skipping meals compared to women who retained excess postpartum weight. In essence, a woman's weight is more a reflection of her lifestyle during pregnancy and after the baby is born than of what she ate or how much she exercised before pregnancy. If you follow the Baby- wise Diet and exercise regularly, you should reach your weight goals within the first year.

For the non-breast-feeding woman, a prepregnancy calorie allotment of approximately 2,000 calories from nutrient-packed foods, such as those recommended in the Baby-wise Diet, will guarantee optimal intake of nutrients, while helping to lose weight. It is impossible to guarantee optimal intake of all the vitamins and minerals on a low-calorie intake. You have just completed one of life's most strenuous feats, and you have to do a lot of nutritional rebuilding and restocking. You cannot afford to cut yourself short when it comes to even one nutrient. Consequently, if you can't lose weight on 2,000 calories a day, then increase your exercise! (See Box 10.1, "Debunking Those Diet Myths.")

BOX 10.1   DEBUNKING THOSE DIET MYTHS

Diet dogma has a life of its own. Even when science reveals the truth behind a diet fad, the myth lingers. Here's the skinny on a few diet myths.

1. **Your weight is just a matter of calories in versus calories out.**
    There is more to weight management than the first law of thermodynamics (the amount of stored energy equals the difference between energy intake and work). Some people gain weight easier and faster than others, probably because of what scientists call "thrifty genes," or a genetically based ability to get and store calories with exceptional efficiency. "The very genes that helped humans survive and evolve in a world that demanded high energy expenditures and frequent food shortages are now a liability in a world with ample food and little reason to move," says John Foreyt, Ph.D., obesity expert at Baylor College of Medicine.

2. **Don't eat between meals.** The nibbler's diet has replaced the "three squares" diet as a better way to manage weight, cut heart-disease and diabetes risk, and curb cravings. A study from the University of Michigan School of Public Health found that women who divided their food intakes into several little meals and snacks throughout the day were leaner with less body fat than were women who ate the same calories, but packed them into two or three big meals. Why nibbling helps weight management is poorly understood; however, one theory is that dividing the same amount of calories into five or more little meals and snacks encourages the body to "burn" the food for immediate energy rather than store it in the hips and thighs.

3. **Fatty foods curb hunger better and keep you full longer than starchy foods.**Fat might take longer to clear the stomach than other foods, but it is the least filling of any food. Protein is the most satiating, followed by carbohydrate, and then by fat. So fatty foods are the easiest to overeat and are likely to encourage overeating at the next meal.

4. **Skipping meals is one surefire way to cut back on calories.** People who skip meals, especially breakfast, are more likely to overeat later in the day. "The body regulates itself by diurnal rhythms, including cycles of light and dark, sleep and wakefulness, and hunger. A person who skips meals upsets one of these cycles; the system tries to right itself by overcompensating and the person eats from midafternoon until bedtime," says Wayne C. Callaway, M.D., associate clinical professor of medicine at George Washington University in Washington, D.C.

5. **Giving in to cravings is sure to put on the pounds** Humans don't take well to being told no. The more you try to willpower away a craving,

the stronger becomes the urge; eventually you give in, often with a vengeance. Instead, enjoy the foods you crave in moderation.

6. Big evening meals cause weight gain. It's not the time of day, but the amount of food that impacts your waistline. If dinner contributes to a weight problem, it's because people tend to de-stress by overeating in the evening.

7. Women gain weight after menopause. Menopause is not the inevitable ticket to middle-age spread; age and loss of muscle mass is. Maintain muscle mass by strength training, and boost your body's natural fat burning with endurance activity to offset the drop in estrogen that aggravates weight gain in the second fifty years.

8. Nuts are a no-no on any weight-loss diet. Don't stop eating nuts just because you're worried about your weight. In a study from Loma Linda University, people did not gain weight when they added two ounces of nuts to their normal diets every day for six months. It's likely the body compensates by cutting back elsewhere on calories. Nuts also help lower heart-disease risk and are good sources of folic acid, vitamin E, fiber, and healthy monounsaturated fats.

The Nibbling Syndrome: A few new challenges to good nutrition develop after the baby is born. For women who have worked outside the home, staying home with a baby can mean battling more than just diapers. These women are more likely to gain weight or retain the extra pounds of pregnancy, possibly because they have easy access to the refrigerator. Food can become the entertainment or stimulation that was once supplied by work.

In addition, after the baby is born a woman might spend increasing time feeding other family members, and the increased time spent tasting and preparing food can put on the pounds. Finally, the changed self-image a woman can experience as she makes the transitions from seeing herself as a young woman to seeing herself as someone's mother can shift her priorities from herself to the needs of others. Along with this change in self-image can come a more relaxed attitude toward weight.

Any of these factors might result in the "nibbling syndrome," whereby small bites, snacks, or tastes while cooking; frequent high-calorie snacks; or "grazing" from the refrigerator result in weight gain. Keep in mind that an extra 100 calories above what you need to maintain a desirable weight will result in a one-pound weight gain per month. That calorie allotment can be reached easily by finishing the buttered toast your husband left at breakfast, eating the leftover creamed tuna while cleaning up after dinner, or nibbling on two oatmeal cookies.

On the other hand, eating frequently can help you control hunger and overeating that can lead to weight gain, but it must be done wisely and with some planning. While skipping meals in an effort to lose weight is more likely to send you to the refrigerator during the afternoon or evening with a license to eat anything in sight, planned nutritious snacks can maintain a steady blood sugar and energy level, curb hunger, and prevent impulse eating, which almost always is high in sugar, fat, salt, and other unhealthful choices. What can you do?

First, forget the supersimplified promises of all those fad diet books. Carbs don't make you fat, just as food combining and cabbage soup aren't the cures for permanent weight loss. According to John Foreyt, Ph.D., obesity expert at Baylor College of Medicine in Houston, the only way to lose weight and keep it off is to focus on balance, variety, and moderation, which in a nutshell means following these four food tips:
Food must be:

1. tasty,
2. satisfying,
3. good for you, and
4. varied.

The Yum Factor: If a truckload of salad isn't your idea of the perfect dinner, you're not likely to eat it for very long. All the obesity experts agree that whatever eating plan you choose after the baby is born must be one you can stick with for life. "Your diet must fit your taste buds and lifestyle. You'll feel deprived when forced to give up favorite foods, which will ricochet you back to the very eating habits that caused the weight gain in the first place," says Barbara Rolls, Ph.D., at Pennsylvania State University in University Park.

Portions play a role here, since you still need to pay attention to serving size depending on what you want to eat. That means moderate portions of the processed, low-fiber, high-fat stuff like fast, convenience, and processed foods, and platters of unprocessed goodies.

Savor the Satisfaction: "A big factor in successful weight management is making sure your meals are filling and satisfying," warns Dr. Foreyt. A snack of five cantaloupes might be filling (for about five minutes), but it's likely to leave you hankering for pizza. According to Dr. Rolls, protein-rich foods, such as grilled salmon or baked chicken breast, have a high satiety effect, so you feel both full and satisfied longer if you add a little extra-lean meat to vegetable-based dishes. Fiber-rich and water-packed foods—say carrot-raisin salad, black bean burritos, or vegetable soup— also are satisfying because their high volume and weight signals the stomach that it is full on fewer calories.

The trick is to find foods you love that also fill you up without filling you out. That means focusing on tummy-filling stuff from the Baby-wise Diet, like chicken breast, extra-lean meats, and seafood; fresh fruits and vegetables; whole-grain breads and cereals; legumes; nonfat milk products such as plain yogurt; and nuts and seeds. Calorie-packed foods, like a small double-fudge brownie or a ladle of gravy on roast beef, are tasty trimmings added to an otherwise waist-slimming food plan.

Focus on Health: Why did you choose the foods you did today? If you're like most people, you probably grabbed that energy bar because it was handy and quick. You had a slice of pizza for lunch because it was tasty or because your friends were having pizza. Or you nibbled on those baked tortilla chips because they were lower in calories than the regular ones. Seldom does someone say, "because it was nutritious."

The quality and length of our lives depends on our health; we thrive only when our bodies are nourished with optimal amounts of the 40-plus nutrients and the 12,000-plus phytochemicals in minimally processed foods. "The irony is, if we just focused more on our health and less on our waistlines, we'd automatically eat more nutrient-packed, low-calorie foods, such as fruits, vegetables, whole grains, nonfat milk products, and legumes, that help us manage our weights," says Dr. Foreyt.

The good news is that many of the food cravings and aversions you lived with during pregnancy are likely to subside after the baby is born. A random sample of new mothers who had experienced one or more food cravings during pregnancy found that food cravings did not continue into the post-partum period. In addition, there was no evidence to support the theory that cravings are caused by dietary deficiencies. Without the weird food cravings and aversions, you can settle into a healthful diet based on preferences and good nutrition. (See Box 10.2, "What If You're a Vegetarian?")

Keep Exercising!

A little exercise can go a long way in helping you adjust to motherhood. The key is to start at the right time and at the right intensity. Your uterus needs time to heal and an episiotomy can be sore for days or even a few

---

BOX 10.2   WHAT IF YOU'RE A VEGETARIAN?

Planning a successful weight-loss diet remains the same for the vegetarian as it does for the meat eater, with the exception that the two to three daily servings from the meat group must come from cooked dried beans and peas, nuts and seeds, and/or eggs. Base the diet on whole grains, fruits, legumes, and vegetables, with three to four servings of low-fat milk products or fortified soy milk and limited intake of sugars, oils, and alcohol. As with any diet, avoid or limit fried foods; instead, bake, broil, and steam foods. To boost the nutritional value of your vegetarian diet:

- add tofu and beans for protein, iron, and zinc.
- drink soy milk fortified with calcium, vitamin D, and vitamins B_2 and B_{12}.
- include at least one whole grain and two fruits and/or vegetables at every meal and snack.
- replace iceberg lettuce with leaf lettuce or spinach in salads and add toppings such as nuts, low-fat cheese, kidney beans, and winter pears.
- avoid drinking tea or coffee with meals, since compounds called tannins in these beverages inhibit iron absorption by up to 75 percent.
- take a daily moderate-dose multiple supplement that supplies 100 percent of the Daily Value for a broad range of vitamins and minerals.

---

weeks postpartum. You can start a gentle walking schedule as soon as you feel up to it if you've had an uncomplicated vaginal delivery. Gradually work up to brisk walking with your baby in a stroller. You'll need more time to heal if you've had a cesarean, so discuss the best exercise schedule with your physician.

Six weeks is usually the earliest most doctors recommend returning to a more vigorous exercise routine after an uncomplicated birth. But in reality, it can take up to a year before some women feel enough like themselves to even think about vigorous exercise. One study of mothers who had given birth to healthy, full-term babies found that one in every four of them did not feel physically recovered even six months after delivery. They were battling fatigue, hemorrhoids, constipation, low sex drive, frequent colds, and . . . well, you name it. The message here is to be patient with yourself, but at the same time start including some form of exercise as soon as you are ready.

Start back slowly. Your abdominal muscles are stretched so they won't give your back much support right now. Your center of gravity also has shifted, so you can't strap on those in-line or ice skates right away without feeling a bit wobbly. One good option is to join a postpartum fitness class at the local gym or YMCA where you can bring your baby and share advice with new moms.

Time can be a new mom's greatest barrier to exercise. So get creative.

- Take a daily walk with your baby in the stroller.
- Put your newborn in a front pack and ride a stationary bike.
- Rent exercise videos that you can follow at home with your baby next to you.
- Have your partner watch the baby while you exercise.
- Join a gym that has a baby-care facility.

Fatigue: A New Mother's Biggest Challenge

Fatigue tops the list when it comes to postpregnancy problems. You're home all day but seldom have a chance to put your feet up, and then you're up half the night with a hungry or tearful baby. New mothers have less time to spend on themselves and often dream of the days when they had an uninterrupted night's sleep.

Iron Up: To help prevent exhaustion you must eat well, which means eating plenty of the right foods without overeating and gaining weight. The first concern is to eat enough iron-rich foods to help restock drained iron stores. So be sure to include at least four or five iron-rich foods, such as extra-lean meat, dark green leafy vegetables, whole-grain breads and cereals, and cooked dried beans and peas, in the daily diet. In addition, cook in cast-iron pots, combine a vitamin C–rich food such as orange juice with all iron-rich foods, and take a moderate-dose iron supplement for at least the first year after the baby is born. Monitor your iron status closely by requesting a serum ferritin test from your physician at least every six months. Once your serum ferritin value rises above 20 mcg/L, you can stop taking the iron supplement unless you are planning another pregnancy, in which case you should continue the iron-rich regimen indefinitely.

Eat Regularly: Another fatigue-fighting tactic is to eat regularly or at least every four hours. Always combine a carbohydrate-rich food such as whole grains, vegetables, or fruit with a protein-rich food such as nonfat milk products, cooked dried beans and peas, or chicken to help regulate energy and blood sugar levels. Always eat breakfast, even if it is only a piece of whole-wheat toast and a glass of nonfat milk, and include at least two or three small snacks between meals to keep yourself energized. Finally, drink water! Often fatigue is caused by mild dehydration. (See Table 10.1, "Just Say No to Temptation.")

Rest and Relaxation: Other tactics for warding off fatigue are to take a nap when the baby is sleeping, limit social commitments for the first few months after the baby is born, concentrate on you and your baby and cut

---

TABLE 10.1

Just Say No to Temptation

At no other time in your life are you more ready to make dietary changes for your health and the health of your baby. However, even when you are your most motivated self, you may find yourself faced with the temptation to overeat, choose the wrong foods, or give in to cravings. Here are a few tips for resisting the impulse to slip from your best intentions.

1. Schedule snack times and come prepared. When you skip meals or forget to bring nutritious foods with you, you are setting yourself up for temptation.
2. At the first sign of an urge to splurge, drink two glasses of water and wait fifteen minutes. Often a drink can provide instant relief from a craving.
3. The "out-of-sight-out-of-mind" motto holds true for cravings. The sight, aroma, and taste of a food can undermine the best of intentions, especially during your high-risk times of day such as midafternoon or after work. So keep the cookies and cake out of the house, avoid driving by the bakery, or bypass the kitchen when you arrive home from work.
4. Switch to a mood-elevating activity. A doughnut or candy bar may give you a mental lift, but so can a brisk walk, listening to your favorite music, or spending time with people who make you laugh.
5. Work with, not against your cravings. You are likely to swing from abstinence to bingeing if you try using willpower against your chocolate cravings. So, plan a small "treat" into the day. Have a chocolate Kiss or a small peanut butter cup, or dip fresh strawberries in low-fat chocolate sauce, rather than turn to a large candy bar or pint of ice cream.
6. Reprogram your taste buds. Often a craving for sweets is a craving for carbohydrate. Identify when you are most prone to these crave attacks, then plan to eat a carbohydrate-rich bagel with all-fruit jam, toasted English muffin with marmalade, or other nutritious, starchy snack.
7. Remember that nothing is forbidden, but everything counts.

back on other tasks such as housework, and remind yourself that life will regain a normal pace in time.

Your Hair

If your hair starts falling out a few weeks after your baby arrives, don't despair. Some women lose up to 40 percent of their normal hair, but in most cases the hair grows back. Although the phenomenon is poorly understood, one theory for postpartum hair loss is that the hormones that stimulate the growth of the baby also affected your hair by stimulating growth. When the hormone storms of pregnancy subside during the weeks following birth, hair completes its natural cycle and begins falling out.

Another theory states that it is the physical and emotional trauma or shock of giving birth that causes the hair loss. A third theory is that marginal nutrient deficiencies of zinc, folic acid, or other B vitamins might contribute to the shedding. In the latter case, try increasing your intake of foods rich in these nutrients, such as extra-lean meats, whole grains, dark green vegetables, and cooked dried beans and peas. Or take a moderate-dose multiple vitamin and mineral supplement.

Spacing Pregnancies

A woman should wait at least eighteen months, and ideally two and a half years, between babies to restock her nutrient stores and allow her body time to mend and prepare for the next pregnancy. For example, it takes approximately three months to one year to replenish iron stores after pregnancy. The stress of pregnancy and delivery also increases the body's need for other vitamins and minerals, from vitamin A to zinc. It can take months to restock these depleted tissue stores and allow the body time to heal. Reentering pregnancy before you've given your body a chance to recuperate increases the risk for premature or undersized babies.

Back-to-back pregnancies also can interfere with your first baby's nutrition if you are breast-feeding. Frequent cycles of reproduction increase the risk that nursing will overlap with pregnancy and shorten the duration of the recuperative time.

Women who do find themselves pregnant within a few months of giving birth can give birth to a healthy baby, but they must take extra precautions.

They must eat for the growing baby, for the first child who is nursing, and for their own health. They also will battle the physical and emotional stresses of juggling family, work, and pregnancy. That means taking extra care to eat even more fresh fruits and vegetables, nonfat dairy foods, whole grains, and cooked dried beans and peas. There is little or no room for high-fat or high-sugar items.

Eating for the Next Baby

Most women are very concerned about their health and diet during their first pregnancy. They want the very best for the babies growing inside them, and they take the time to revel in the baby-making process. By the time the second or third baby comes along, those same women have their hands full with toddlers, work, and other responsibilities. The baby-making process is not as special as it was the first time around and less time is devoted to taking care of themselves. The mother who religiously took her prenatal supplements during her first pregnancy might let weeks lapse before beginning supplementation the second time around. Another woman who steamed dark green vegetables every night for dinner during her first pregnancy now skips these vegetables because her toddler won't eat them.

According to Andrew Czeizel, M.D., director of the Department of Human Genetics and Teratology at the National Institute of Hygiene in Budapest, nutrition is likely to slip in these experienced mothers unless they make a concerted effort to stick with the guidelines outlined in the Baby-wise Diet as they prepare for their next pregnancy. The research supports this finding and shows that women having their first babies gain more weight than women having their second and third babies, which suggests that women are not as nutritionally conscientious the second and third time around.

Babies, unlike birthdays and Christmas, often arrive unexpectedly. While you may not have saved your nest egg, reached the pinnacle of your career, or finished remodeling the spare bedroom before your next baby arrives, you should make sure your body is well nourished in preparation for the coming addition (planned or unplanned) to your family. It is never too late—nor too early—to begin giving your next baby the best chances for a healthy life. The second or third baby also needs the same nutrients as your first baby, or even more, especially since your body may be entering pregnancy not fully recovered from the last pregnancy.

If you conceive while nursing, you will have an increased demand for all nutrients, from protein and carbohydrate to vitamins and minerals. You will need to consume optimal amounts of all the nutrients essential to pregnancy, including folic acid and iron, plus all the nutrients needed for nursing, including calcium, zinc, and protein. In all cases, the Baby-wise Diet is the mainstay of your eating plan, with added servings from each of the food groupings to make up the difference in calories.

The abundance of nutrients in the Baby-wise Diet allows you to stockpile all of the essential vitamins and minerals that you and your baby will need. And by starting early you can build your nutritional defenses before the onset of morning sickness, heartburn, and other pregnancy-related stumbling blocks to eating perfectly.

Other lifestyle habits, including your level of exercise and alcohol consumption, and maintaining a positive mental state continue to be important contributors to your next baby's health. During the childbearing years, and especially as you get ready for your next pregnancy, avoid tobacco and ask that other people not smoke around you. Exposure to tobacco smoke could affect the future health of your baby before you even know you are pregnant, so why take the risk?

Dad's Diet
Dad's diet may have little to do with your baby's health while you are pregnant, but how your partner eats prior to pregnancy might affect whether or not you conceive and even the future health of your next baby. As discussed in Chapter 1, if your partner drinks heavily, eats poorly, takes drugs, or smokes cigarettes, those habits could jeopardize the number and viability of his sperm, which would make the sperm less capable of fertilizing an egg or producing a healthy baby. On the other hand, a dad-to-be who eats well and takes good care of himself is optimizing his health and potentially the health of his offspring. Even if all he does is choose better foods when he snacks, he'll be helping to ensure a healthy next baby! (See Table 10.2, "Twenty-five Super Snacks.")

Tell your mate also to avoid workplace radiation and chemicals that can damage sperm, which in turn lowers the sperm count or causes genetic defects in children. Researchers at McGill University in Montreal report that more than fifty industrial, medical, and other chemicals can harm sperm. (Call the National Institute for Occupational Safety and Health, or NIOSH, at 800-356-4674 for more information.)

The period when you are looking foward to pregnancy is an ideal time

TABLE 10.2

Twenty-five Super Snacks

Each of the following twenty-five snacks is packed with vitamins and minerals, yet tallies one hundred calories or less.

1 large orange
1 cup nonfat milk (plain or steamed with flavorings)
1 medium apple (raw or baked with cinnamon)
50 pretzel sticks
3 servings of Cucumber Toss*
2½ cups fresh strawberries
1 papaya (tastes especially good if flavored with lemon or lime juice)
6 ounces nonfat plain yogurt (sweeten with fresh fruit)
1 small sweet potato
3 cups air-popped popcorn
5 tablespoons dried fruit (raisins, cranberries, apricots, etc.)
½ cup sorbet (mango, lemon, or passion fruit)
2 cups cubed cantaloupe
1½ servings of Spicy Carrots*
1 ounce low-fat cheese
1 slice whole-wheat toast with 1 tablespoon jam
¾ cup canned pineapple chunks, drained
2 kiwi
1 pear
1 cup grapes
5 vanilla wafers
2 fat-free fig bars
1 small banana
1 small serving of Naughty Nachos*
3½-ounce fat-free pudding

*See Recipes section.

to improve the eating habits of the entire family. What is good for mom also is good for everyone else. So while you are following the guidelines of the Baby-wise Diet, everyone else will benefit as well. Encourage everyone to support and join you in eating healthfully in preparation for the next member of your family.

Dad also can be a big help as you recuperate from one pregnancy and build yourself up for the next. Your mate can get involved in the process by:

- Encouraging your good eating habits.
- Making sure there are always good foods, plenty of milk, and iron-rich snacks on hand.
- Reminding you to take your supplements, eat regularly, or limit the intake of not-so-nutritious foods.
- Avoiding bringing home tempting foods, such as cookies, cakes, candy, or doughnuts. (If he wants these foods, ask him to eat them outside the home and away from you!)
- Helping with household chores, cooking nutrient-packed meals, or grocery shopping.
- Bringing home fresh fruits and vegetables (and an occasional bouquet of flowers).
- Encouraging you to stick with your nutrition plan even when dining out.

Light Meals

Good nutrition does not have to be time-consuming and, in fact, can be simple and elegant. For example, little, light meals—simple, elegant meals that are bigger than a first course, but smaller than a main course—are one way to nourish your body while feeling satisfied, not stuffed. They also can be a way to manage your weight and even spice up your marriage.

Little, light meals can be gourmet minimeals that emphasize nutritious foods—that is, grains, vegetables, fruits, and legumes—but they do it with flair. You can blend unusual ingredients to tantalize the taste buds and accent the sensuous side to food—its color, texture, and aromas. A little, light meal can be anything from a tabbouleh salad to lemon chicken with minted rice.

Little, light meals may be just the ticket for adding a little romance to your marriage. For example, you can share a bowl of frozen blueberries and grapes on the floor in front of the TV, some fresh strawberries and a glass of sparkling apple cider at your own private backyard picnic, or several small, tasty dishes for a cozy candlelight dinner.

In fact, good nutrition can be a family affair if your partner or other family members help with food preparation. You may find that you have wonderful talks or laughs while preparing dinner or a snack. Try working out shared roles, so that everyone does something he or she enjoys. One person may take over the barbecuing, while the other experiments with one-dish meals. Toddlers can help set the table and older children can help with the shopping, food preparation, or cleanup. In this way everyone is part of the process of planning and making ready for the next pregnancy.

Worksheet 10.1   My Postpregnancy Daily Checklist (for the Non-Breast-Feeding Mother)

Copy this master sheet to complete daily.

Food Groups	Minimum Servings	Actual Intake
Calcium-rich foods	2	_____
Vegetables (at least 2 folic acid–rich choices)	5	_____
Fruits (at least 2 vitamin C–rich choices)	3	_____
Grains (at least 4 whole-grain choices)	6	_____
Extra-lean meats and legumes	2	_____
Quenchers	5	_____

Did I reach my goals? _____

What needs improvement? _____

What will I do differently next week? _____

Appendix:

❧

Twenty-Eight Days' Worth of Menus Based on the Baby-wise Diet

The following four weeks of menus are based on the guidelines outlined in the Baby-wise Diet. Each basic menu is designed for women gearing up for pregnancy, in the first trimester, and recovering from pregnancy. Additional suggestions to meet the calorie and nutrient needs of women in their second and third trimesters or when breast-feeding are listed on page 284. Items marked with an * are found in the Recipes section, starting on page 287.

Day 1

Breakfast:

1 cup whole-wheat raisin bran
1 cup nonfat milk (drink the remaining milk after the cereal is gone!)
1 banana

Lunch:

1 serving Spinach and Red Pepper Quiche*
Confetti Salad: Mix 2 tablespoons thinly sliced red onion, 2 tablespoons corn kernels, 1 diced tomato, and 2 tablespoons low-calorie ranch dressing. Place on top of 2 cups baby lettuce greens.
1 slice French bread
Water

Dinner:

Herb-Roasted Chicken: Combine 1 minced clove garlic, a pinch each of finely chopped rosemary and thyme, and salt. Rinse 1 four-ounce skinned chicken breast, pat dry, and rub with herb mixture. Spray baking pan with vegetable spray and place chicken in pan. Bake at 400° for about 15 minutes. Turn and bake another 15 minutes, or until no longer pink in the center. Drizzle with 1 teaspoon balsamic vinegar while still in hot pan.

1 cup asparagus, sauteed in 3 tablespoons chicken broth over high heat until heated through (about 7 minutes). Salt to taste.

1 small sweet potato, baked

½ cup cooked instant brown rice mixed with 2 tablespoons caramelized onion (spray small skillet with vegetable spray, cook onions over medium-low heat with a pinch of brown sugar until golden brown).

Tomato Salad with Mozzarella: Slice a medium tomato, top with a thin slice of fresh mozzarella cheese, fresh basil leaves, and 1 teaspoon non-fat vinaigrette dressing.

Snacks:

Snack #1: Open-Face Creamy Peach Sandwich: Blend 2 tablespoons fat-free cream cheese, 1 teaspoon honey, and 1 peach, peeled and chopped. Spread on a slice of seven-grain bread and sprinkle with ½ teaspoon of chopped walnuts. Water.

Snack #2: 1 cup chocolate low-fat soy milk and ½ whole-wheat bagel with 1 tablespoon almond butter. Water.

Snack #3: 1 serving Spinach Hummus* with ½ whole-wheat pita bread. Water.

Nutrition Score: 2,237 calories, 20 percent fat, 59 percent carbohydrates, 21 percent protein, 1,227 mg calcium, 1,224 mcg folic acid, 28.7 mg iron, 40 g fiber.

Day 2

Breakfast:

2 toaster whole-wheat waffles topped with 2 tablespoons maple syrup and 1 teaspoon chopped pecans

1 cup fortified vanilla soy milk

½ honeydew melon or cantaloupe

Lunch:

Pacific Northwest Salmon Sandwich: Blend ½ teaspoon dry dill with 1 tablespoon fat-free cream cheese and spread inside one whole-wheat pita bread cut in half. Fill sandwich with 3 ounces smoked salmon, 4 thick slices cucumber, and lettuce.

1 cup fresh-squeezed orange juice

Coleslaw: 1 cup preshredded cabbage mixed with 1 tablespoon low-calorie coleslaw dressing.

Water

Dinner:

1 3-ounce pork loin chop, trimmed and broiled

Mashed green potatoes: Whip together 1 large baker or Russet potato, peeled and boiled, ½ cup chard steamed and chopped, ¼ cup nonfat milk, 1 tablespoon Parmesan cheese, and salt and pepper to taste.

2 carrots, peeled, sliced into diagonals and steamed until heated through, but still crunchy. Sprinkle with ½ teaspoon chopped chives, salt, and pepper.

1 serving Red Beet Salad with Vinaigrette Dressing*

Water

Snacks:

Snack #1: 1 12-ounce nonfat decaffeinated café latte (optional: sweeten with aspartame) with 1 almond biscotti. Water.

Snack #2: 1 cup fresh fruit with 4 ounces low-fat fruit yogurt and topped with 1 tablespoon light whipped cream. Water.

Snack #3: 1 serving Naughty Nachos*. Water.

Nutrition Score: 2,232 calories, 29 percent fat, 51 percent carbohydrates, 20 percent protein, 1,704 mg calcium, 608 mcg folic acid, 19.1 mg iron, 32 g fiber.

Day 3

Breakfast:

Veggie Omelet: Spray a medium skillet with vegetable spray and saute ½ carrot peeled and thinly sliced, ¼ cup broccoli pieces, 2 tablespoons sliced yellow onion over medium heat until heated through but still firm. Whip together two medium whole eggs, salt, and pepper to taste. Pour over vegetable mixture, top with 1 ounce shredded cheddar cheese, cover, reduce heat to medium-low, and cook until firm (about 15 minutes).

1 piece seven-grain toast

½ broiled grapefruit (cut grapefruit in half, top with pinch of sugar, cinnamon and nutmeg and broil until bubbly).

Decaffeinated tea

Lunch:

Crunchy Tuna Sandwich: Blend 3 ounces water-packed tuna with 1 tablespoon fat-free mayonnaise and 1 tablespoon chopped green onion. Spread on whole-wheat bread with ½ cup grated carrot, lettuce, and ½ teaspoon sunflower seeds.

1 serving Cucumber Toss*

Sparkling water

Dinner:

Spaghetti: 2 cups cooked spaghetti topped with 1 cup Chunky Spaghetti Sauce* and 2 tablespoons low-fat grated Parmesan cheese.

1 cup Italian vegetables, steamed

Tossed salad: 2 cups chopped romaine lettuce, 2 tablespoons thinly sliced red onion, 1 chopped medium tomato with oil and vinegar dressing (2 teaspoons olive oil and 2 teaspoons balsamic or red wine vinegar).

Snacks:

Snack #1: 5 lemon-flavored pitted dried plums each stuffed with 1 almond. Serve with 1 cup warmed nonfat milk flavored with 1 tablespoon almond syrup. Water.

Snack #2: Blend 1 tablespoon chutney with 2 tablespoons fat-free cream cheese. Spread on 5 fat-free whole-wheat crackers. Serve with 1 sliced pear. Water.

Snack #3: 1 slice raisin-cinnamon toast with 1 cup nonfat milk.

Nutrition Score: 2,250 calories, 21 percent fat, 59 percent carbohydrates, 20 percent protein, 1,324 mg calcium, 465 mcg folic acid, 21.5 mg iron, 45.5 g fiber.

Day 4

Breakfast:

1 cup shredded wheat cereal
⅔ cup low-fat fortified soy milk
1 banana, sliced
1 cup orange juice

Lunch:

Spinach-Chicken Wrap: Fill one whole-wheat tortilla with 3 ounces grilled or roasted chicken breast, ¼ cup baby spinach leaves, ¼ cup roasted red peppers (from jar), and 2 tablespoons low-fat cream cheese. Heat in microwave. Top with 2 teaspoons salsa.
1 cup mandarin oranges drained and topped with 1 teaspoon candied ginger
1 cup 1 percent low-fat milk

Dinner:

4 ounces salmon brushed with lemon juice and dill. Bake, broil, or barbecue.
½ cup cooked instant brown rice
2 cups steamed broccoli
Tomato-Corn Salad: Mix two chopped tomatoes, ⅓ cup corn kernels, 2 tablespoons diced red onion, and 2 teaspoons chopped cilantro with salt and rice wine vinegar to taste.
Water

Snacks:

Snack #1: 4 cups air-popped popcorn and 1 cup tomato juice.
Snack #2: 1 cup hot cocoa made with 1 percent low-fat milk and 5 graham crackers.
Snack #3: 1 serving Berry-Banana Salad* and 1 Currant-Date Muffin.* Water.

Nutrition Score: 2,225 calories, 18 percent fat, 62 percent carbohydrates, 20 percent protein, 1,454 mg calcium, 570 mcg folic acid, 17.5 mg iron, 43 g fiber.

Day 5

Breakfast:

1 cup regular oatmeal cooked in 1 cup 1 percent low-fat milk and topped
    with 2 tablespoons toasted wheat germ, 1 tablespoon chopped wal-
    nuts, and 1 tablespoon brown sugar.
1 cup orange juice

Lunch:

Shrimp Salad Sandwich: 3 ounces precooked salad shrimp mixed with
    2 teaspoons minced celery, 1 teaspoon chopped green onions, and
    2 tablespoons low-calorie mayonnaise. Layer shrimp mixture, 3 slices
    tomato, and lettuce on two slices whole-wheat bread.
1 serving Savory Potato Salad*
20 baby carrots
Water

Dinner:

1 slice homemade meat loaf (made with extra-lean ground round)
1 small sweet potato, baked or microwaved
1 cup steamed green peas
Tossed Salad: 2 cups mixed leaf lettuce, 1 tablespoon thinly sliced red
    onion, ½ winter pear sliced, and 1 tablespoon oil-free vinaigrette
    dressing.
Water

Snacks:

Snack #1: 1 cup 1 percent low-fat milk, warmed and flavored with almond
    syrup/flavoring.
Snack #2: 5 dates each stuffed with one pecan and a 6-ounce custard-style
    lemon yogurt. Water.
Snack #3: 2 cups slightly steamed vegetables, such as broccoli, cauliflower,
    carrots, and/or Chinese pea pods, dunked in 1 tablespoon low-calorie
    ranch dressing. Water.

Nutrition Score: 2,230 calories, 25 percent fat, 56 percent carbohydrates,
19 percent protein, 1,280 mg calcium, 712 mcg folic acid, 19.3 mg iron,
44 g fiber.

Day 6

Breakfast:

2 six-inch whole-grain pancakes topped with¼ cup fat-free sour cream
 and 1 serving Raspberry Sauce*
1 cup orange juice
Water

Lunch:

Portobello Mushroom Burger: Saute in a nonstick frying pan one large
 Portobello mushroom cap in 1 teaspoon olive oil. Top with 1 ounce
 Gruyère cheese (or cheese of your choice), 1 medium tomato sliced,
 1 slice red onion, and 2 teaspoons Dijon mustard. Place on whole-
 wheat bun.
1 cup celery sticks
Water

Dinner:

4 ounces halibut steak, grilled and topped with Corn Salsa: Mix 3 tablespoons corn kernels, 1 medium tomato chopped, 1 tablespoon chopped
 cilantro, 1 tablespoon chopped red onion, 1 teaspoon finely chopped
 canned chilies.
1 cup Wehani Rice with Dried Cherries: Cook ¼ cup wehani rice in ½-
 plus cup chicken broth until done (about 55 minutes). While rice is
 cooking, saute ¼ sliced onion in 1 teaspoon butter and a pinch of
 brown sugar over low heat until caramelized. Mix 3 tablespoons dried
 cherries (dried cranberries also are good) into cooked rice. Let stand
 for 5 minutes then add and stir onions, 1 teaspoon chopped walnuts,
 and pinch of orange zest.
Spinach Salad: 2 cups baby spinach leaves, ¼ cup canned and drained
 kidney beans, 2 ounces water-packed artichoke hearts, 2 tablespoons
 diced red onion, and 1 tablespoon light Dijon vinaigrette dressing.
Water

Snacks:

Snack #1: 2 cups frozen blueberries and 1 cup 1 percent low-fat milk,
 warmed and sprinkled with nutmeg. Water.

Snack #2: 1 cup fresh fruit mixed with 4 ounces low-fat fruit yogurt and topped with 2 tablespoons light whipped cream. Water.

Snack #3: 1 cup 1 percent low-fat milk and 2 chocolate-chip cookies. Water.

Nutrition Score: 2,216 calories, 23 percent fat, 59 percent carbohydrates, 18 percent protein, 1,569 mg calcium, 687 mcg folic acid, 19.2 mg iron, 44 g fiber.

Day 7

Breakfast:

2 eggs scrambled using vegetable spray, salt and pepper to taste, and/or a dash of tabasco sauce

2 slices whole-wheat toast topped with 2 teaspoons jam

1 tomato, sliced

1 cup fresh-squeezed orange juice

Lunch:

1 Spicy Black Beans* burrito: Prepare beans according to recipe, fill a 10" flour tortilla with ½ cup of beans, top with 1 ounce sliced low-fat cheddar cheese, and heat in microwave for one minute.

1 serving Spicy Carrots*

1 orange

Herb iced tea

Dinner:

Spicy Ginger Salmon: Blend 2 tablespoons chopped cilantro, 2 table-spoons hoisin sauce, 2 teaspoons minced fresh ginger, 1 teaspoon chopped canned chipotle peppers, and a dash of lemon juice. Rub a 5-ounce salmon fillet. Broil or grill until done (approximately 6 minutes per side, depending on thickness of fillet).

1 cup steamed asparagus, drizzled with lemon juice

½ cup couscous (made according to package directions)

Tossed salad: 2 cups chopped romaine lettuce, 1 tablespoon sliced red onion, 4 cucumber slices, and 3 tablespoons low-calorie creamy dressing.

Water

Snacks:

Snack #1: 1 cup nonfat plain yogurt mixed with 1 tablespoon apricot jam and 3 canned apricot halves, chopped. Water.

Snack #2: 4 orange-essence-flavored pitted prunes, 2 chocolate kisses, and 1 cup warmed milk flavored with almond extract and sugar substitute, sprinkled with nutmeg. Water.

Snack #3: 1 serving Apple Bread Pudding* with ¼ cup low-fat frozen yogurt.

Nutrition Score: 2,227 calories, 28 percent fat, 54 percent carbohydrates, 18 percent protein, 1,566 mg calcium, 760 mcg folic acid, 16 mg iron, 30g fiber.

Day 8

Breakfast:

Decadent Pancakes: 1 eight-inch pancake made with low-fat pancake mix, 1 egg, 1 tablespoon wheat germ, and nonfat milk. Place 1 sliced banana along middle of pancake and roll into a "burrito." Top with 4 tablespoons apricot sauce and 2 tablespoons light whipped cream.

1 cup hot cocoa made with nonfat milk

Lunch:

Peanut Butter Candy Sandwich: Mix 2 tablespoons peanut butter, 1 tablespoon honey, and 2 tablespoons toasted wheat germ. Spread between 2 slices whole-wheat bread.

½ papaya drizzled with lime juice

15 baby carrots

Dinner:

3 ounces roasted chicken with 3 roasted red potatoes and 1 cup roasted carrots (all cooked in a roasting pan together)

2 cups steamed broccoli

Romaine Leaf Caesar Salad: 10 inner romaine leaves sprinkled with 1 ounce grated Parmesan cheese, 2 tablespoons low-calorie Caesar dressing, and ground black pepper.

Snacks:

Snack #1: 1 cup frozen blueberries and 1 cup nonfat milk.

Snack #2: 1 6-ounce container of strawberry-kiwi, custard-style low-fat yogurt, mixed with 1 chopped kiwi, and a diet soda.

Snack #3: Root beer float, made with 8 ounces root beer and ½ cup vanilla ice cream.

Nutrition Score: 2,196 calories, 27 percent fat, 55 percent carbohydrates, 18 percent protein, 36 g fiber, 1,740 mg calcium, 608 mcg folic acid, 13.1 mg iron.

Day 9

Breakfast:

1 cup low-fat granola
1 cup nonfat milk
½ cup cantaloupe, cubed and drizzled with lemon juice
1 cup Fruity Spritzer*

Lunch:

Cajun Chicken Salad: 4 ounces chicken breast rubbed with Cajun seasonings and broiled, 2½ cups chopped romaine lettuce, 1 tablespoon chopped red onion, and 2 tablespoons honey mustard dressing.
1 slice French bread
1 cup nonfat milk
2 soft chocolate-chip cookies

Dinner:

Linguini with clams: 9 ounces fresh linguini cooked until barely tender (about 5 minutes). Sauce: Saute 4 minced cloves of garlic in 2 tablespoons butter. Add two 6½-ounce cans minced clams and 1 bottle clam juice, and cook until heated through. Add ¼ cup chopped parsley, 2 tablespoons dry vermouth,† and white pepper to taste. Heat through. Top drained pasta with sauce and sprinkle with ½ cup low-fat Parmesan cheese. (Makes 4 servings. Use extra servings for leftovers later in week.)

†The alcohol cooks off with heating.

1 cup steamed peas and carrots

2 cups coleslaw made with 2 cups preshredded cabbage and 2 tablespoons coleslaw dressing

Snacks:

Snack #1: 1 cup strawberries dunked in 1 tablespoon fat-free dark
chocolate syrup. Sparkling water.

Snack #2: 2 cups air-popped popcorn and a diet soda.

Snack #3: ¼ cup trail mix (nuts, dried fruit, chocolate bits). Water.

Nutrition Score: 2,238 calories, 24 percent fat, 56 percent carbohydrates,
20 percent protein, 1,217 mg calcium, 809 mcg folic acid, 42 mg iron,
27 g fiber (clams are a particularly rich source of iron!).

Day 10

Breakfast:

1 slice French toast with fresh Raspberry Sauce*

¾ cup cubed honeydew melon

1 cup steamed nonfat milk flavored with nutmeg and ½ teaspoon vanilla
extract (aspartame optional)

Water

Lunch:

Egg Salad Sandwich: 1 large egg boiled and chopped, mixed with 1 tablespoon fat-free mayonnaise, 1 tablespoon diced celery, ½ teaspoon
Dijon mustard (optional), salt and pepper to taste; 2 lettuce leaves;
and 2 slices whole-wheat bread.

1 ounce potato chips

1 apple sliced and sprinkled with ½ teaspoon cinnamon sugar

Water

Dinner:

Juicy, Thick Cheeseburger: 3 ounces extra-lean grilled or broiled ground
beef, 1 ounce low-fat cheddar cheese, 1 medium sliced tomato, 2 lettuce leaves, 1 slice red onion, catsup and mustard to taste, and
1 whole-grain hamburger bun.

Sweet Potato Fries: 1 sweet potato, cut into wedges, sprinkled with salt, and placed on a vegetable-sprayed cookie sheet and baked at 425° until slightly crispy (about 25 minutes).

Spinach Salad: 2 cups chopped or baby spinach leaves, 1 tablespoon sliced red onion, ½ cup raspberries, and 2 tablespoons fat-free raspberry vinaigrette dressing.

1 cup chocolate milkshake

Snacks:

Snack #1: 1 ounce peanut brittle, and herbal iced tea.

Snack #2: ½ cup grapes and 1 cup nonfat milk.

Snack #3: 1 cup slightly steamed and cooled broccoli florets and 2 carrots peeled and sliced. Sparkling water flavored with lemon juice.

Nutrition Score: 2,212 calories, 24 percent fat, 59 percent carbohydrates, 17 percent protein, 1,636 mg calcium, 617mcg folic acid, 18 mg iron, 34 g fiber.

Day 11

Breakfast:

Sunrise Smoothie: In a blender, whip ½ cup nonfat plain yogurt, 2 table-spoons orange juice concentrate, 1 banana, 4 canned apricot halves, 2 tablespoons toasted wheat germ, ½ teaspoon lemon peel.

Lunch:

BLT Deluxe: 3 slices cooked bacon, 1 medium sliced tomato, 2 lettuce leaves, 1 tablespoon low-calorie mayonnaise, and 2 slices whole-wheat toast.

Fruit Salad: 1 peeled and sectioned orange, 1 peeled and sliced kiwi, ½ cup strawberries, ¼ cup papaya slices, 1 teaspoon lemon juice, and ½ teaspoon grated lemon peel.

Sparkling water

Dinner:

2 cups tomato soup made with 1 percent low-fat milk (per directions on can)

Grilled Cheese Sandwich: Spray a griddle or frying pan with vegetable spray and grill until cheese is melted and bread is toasted: 1 ounce cheddar cheese slices, ½ medium tomato sliced, 1 canned chili (optional), 2 slices whole-wheat bread.

Raw Vegetable Platter, such as ½ cup broccoli florets, ⅓ cup cauliflower florets, 10 baby carrots, and ½ cup fresh green beans steamed slightly, but still crisp. Dip in ⅓ cup of any fat-free sour cream–based dip.

Sparkling water flavored with lemon

Snacks:

Snack #1: 1 peanut granola bar and 2 ½ tablespoons craisins. Water.

Snack #2: ½ cup berry sorbet topped with ¼ cup raspberries. Water.

Snack #3: 1 brownie and 1 cup Mexican Hot Chocolate: 1 cup nonfat milk heated in a saucepan with 4 teaspoons unsweetened cocoa, 4 teaspoons granulated sugar, ¼ teaspoon ground cinnamon, and 1 small vanilla bean split (or ½ teaspoon vanilla extract; add extract after removing pan from burner).

Nutrition Score: 2,198 calories, 22 percent fat, 64 percent carbohydrates, 14 percent protein, 1,420 mg calcium, 506 mcg folic acid, 18.5 mg iron, 39 g fiber.

Day 12

Breakfast:

1 cup whole-wheat flaked ready-to-eat cereal (i.e., Post Whole Wheat Raisin Bran)

1 tablespoon raisins

1 cup 1 percent low-fat milk

1 banana

1 cup grapefruit juice

Lunch:

Fast-Food Restaurant lunch: Grilled chicken sandwich on hamburger bun with 1 tablespoon mayonnaise, tomato, and lettuce, 1 tossed salad with 1 tablespoon ranch dressing, 1 eight-ounce carton 1 percent low-fat milk.

1 orange (brought from home)
1 small bag baby carrots (brought from home)

Dinner:

Frozen entree: Healthy Choice Grilled Glazed Pork dinner
1 cup frozen asparagus, steamed
Coleslaw made with 1 cup shredded cabbage (purchase preshredded),
   2 tablespoons low-fat bottled coleslaw dressing, 2 tablespoons canned
   pineapple chunks, and salt and pepper to taste.
Water

Snacks:

Snack #1: 2 cups microwave air-popped popcorn and 1 cup 1 percent
   low-fat milk.
Snack #2: 1 cup whole strawberries dunked in 2 tablespoons fat-free
   chocolate syrup.
Water.
Snack #3: 1 Oat Bran and Fig Muffin* with 1 teaspoon all-fruit jam.
   Water.

Nutrition Score: 2,202 calories, 26 percent fat, 57 percent carbohydrates,
17 percent protein, 1,359 mg calcium, 839 mcg folic acid, 25 mg iron,
42 g fiber.

Day 13

Breakfast:

2 packets instant oatmeal cooked and topped with 1 cup 1 percent low-
   fat milk, 2 tablespoons toasted wheat germ, 1 packet non-calorie
   sweetener (optional)
1 cup calcium-fortified orange juice

Lunch:

Chicken Salad Sandwich: Mix together 3 ounces diced chicken, 1 tablespoon finely chopped celery, 1 teaspoon finely chopped green onion,
   2 tablespoons mayonnaise, salt and pepper to taste. Spread on 2 slices
   whole-wheat bread with 1 leaf lettuce.

Tomato-Corn Salad: Toss together 2 chopped tomatoes, ¼ cup corn kernels, 1 tablespoon chopped fresh cilantro, 1 tablespoon chopped red onion, 1 tablespoon rice vinegar, and salt and pepper to taste.

1 peach, orange, or nectarine

10 baby carrots

Water or diet soda

Dinner:

At-the-Restaurant Dinner: 2 cups tossed salad with 1 teaspoon oil and vinegar dressing, served on the side. Share an entree (ask for extra vegetables, steamed, and for a potato served without butter): ½ 6-ounce sirloin steak, ½ baked potato, and 1 cup vegetables. Water with lemon or iced tea.

Snacks:

Snack: #1: ⅔ cup grapes and 5 graham crackers. Water.

Snack #2: 1 half-pint carton 1 percent low-fat chocolate milk.

Snack #3: ½ cup vanilla ice cream topped with 1 tablespoon chocolate syrup or maple syrup. Water.

Nutrition Score: 2,222 calories, 27 percent fat, 55 percent carbohydrates, 18 percent protein, 1,279 mg calcium, 733 mcg folic acid, 29 mg iron, 40 g fiber.

Day 14

Breakfast:

Breakfast Burrito: ⅓ cup scrambled egg substitute, ½ ounce grated cheddar cheese, ¼ cup grated zucchini, 1 tablespoon salsa, 1 8-inch heated flour tortilla.

1 cup grapefruit juice (from carton)

Lunch at the Deli:

Roast beef sandwich made with 2 ounces extra-lean roast beef, mustard, lettuce, tomato, and 2 slices whole-wheat bread

1 cup carrot-raisin salad

Bottled orange juice

Dinner:

Linguini with Pesto: 2 cups fresh linguini, prepared according to package instructions and topped with 2 tablespoons pesto sauce (in refrigerator section of grocery store), and 1 tablespoon grated Parmesan cheese.

1 cup frozen mixed vegetables, steamed

Tossed salad: 2 cups bagged salad greens, ½ cup drained canned kidney beans, 2 tablespoons drained canned plain (not marinated!) artichoke hearts, 1 tablespoon low-fat bottled salad dressing.

Water

Snacks:

Snack #1: 1 piece cinnamon-raisin bread dunked in a 6-ounce container of low-fat cinnamon-apple yogurt. Water.

Snack #2: 1 cup chocolate fortified soy milk.

Snack #3: Ginger Smoothie: In a blender, whip: ½ cup nonfat milk, 1 tablespoon orange juice concentrate, 1½ teaspoons candied ginger.

Nutrition Score: 2,208 calories, 23 percent fat, 59 percent carbohydrates, 18 percent protein, 1,425 mg calcium, 488 mcg folic acid, 20 mg iron, 38 g fiber.

Day 15

Breakfast:

2 frozen whole-wheat waffles, topped with 2 tablespoons fat-free sour cream and ½ cup fresh or thawed blueberries

6 ounces fresh orange juice

1 tall decaffeinated café latte, made with nonfat milk (optional: sweeten with sugar substitute)

Lunch:

Spicy Grilled Chicken Sandwich: 3 ounces roasted chicken breast, 1 drained canned fire-roasted green chili, 2 teaspoons honey mustard, 1 tablespoon mayonnaise, 1 lettuce leaf, and 2 slices whole-wheat bread.

10 baby carrots

1 cup 1 percent low-fat milk

Sparkling water, flavored with lime and fresh mint

Dinner:

1 serving Polenta and Black Bean Casserole*
2 cups lightly steamed broccoli sprinkled with red pepper flakes
Tossed Salad: 1 cup chopped romaine lettuce, 4 cucumber slices, 1 table-
    spoon thinly sliced red onion, and 2 tablespoons ranch dressing
Water

Snacks:

Snack #1: 6-ounce container of low-fat fruit yogurt with 2 chopped kiwi.
    Water.
Snack #2: 1 cup drained canned mandarin oranges sprinkled with candied
    ginger. 1 cup 1 percent low-fat milk. Water.
Snack #3: 1 serving Chocolate Mousse Parfait*. Water.

Nutrition Score: 2,214 calories, 27 percent fat, 54 percent carbohydrates,
19 percent protein, 1,897 mg calcium, 597 mcg folic acid, 16.3 mg iron,
41 g fiber.

Day 16

Breakfast:

1 whole-grain bagel, toasted and topped with 2 thin slices of cheddar
    cheese
1 cup fresh orange juice

Lunch:

1 serving Wild Mushroom Tart*
2 cups mixed raw vegetables, cut into large pieces (i.e., carrot and jicama
    sticks, broccoli or cauliflower florets, zucchini strips), dunked in
    4 tablespoons fat-free sour cream, seasoned with fresh herbs, garlic,
    salt, and pepper
Sparkling water flavored with fresh lemon slices

Dinner:

5 ounces salmon fillet, seasoned with dill and lemon juice, baked or grilled
1 cup wild rice, cooked
1 serving Fresh Green Beans with Shallots and Feta Cheese*

1 cup crookneck squash, steamed
Water

Snacks:

Snack #1: 1 cup frozen blueberries with Frothy Freeze: In a blender, mix 1 cup nonfat milk, 1 teaspoon vanilla extract, ¼ teaspoon nutmeg, 1 packet sugar substitute, and 1 ice cube. Water.
Snack #2: 1 cup pineapple chunks and 1 cup nonfat milk. Water.
Snack #3: 1 Razz 'n' Blues Muffin,* 1 banana, and 1 cup low-fat chocolate soy milk. Water.

Nutrition Score: 2,235 calories, 26 percent fat, 53 percent carbohydrates, 21 percent protein, 1,647 mg calcium, 416 mcg folic acid, 14.9 mg iron, 41 g fiber.

Day 17:

Breakfast:

Sunrise Smoothie: In a blender combine 1 cup nonfat milk, 1 banana, ⅓ cup drained canned apricot halves, 2 tablespoons orange juice concentrate, 2 tablespoons toasted wheat germ, 1 teaspoon vanilla extract.

Lunch:

1 serving Shrimp Quesadillas with Peach Chutney*
Tossed Salad: 2 cups butter lettuce, 1 winter pear sliced, 2 tablespoons sliced red onion, and 2 tablespoons raspberry vinaigrette dressing.
Iced herb tea with lemon

Dinner:

Pork-Vegetable Stir-Fry: Over high heat in chicken broth and soy sauce, cook 4 ounces extra-lean pork cut into thin slices, 1 sliced celery stalk, ½ sliced onion, 1 thinly sliced carrot, 5 halved mushrooms, and ½ cup pea pods. Sprinkle ¼ cup mung bean sprouts and ¼ teaspoon sesame seeds over top before serving over 1½ cups cooked chow mein noodles.
Herb tea

Snacks:

Snack #1: 1 slice whole-wheat toast topped with 1 tablespoon almond butter, 1 sliced banana, and 3 pitted dried plums. Water.

Snack #2: 1 cup low-fat hot cocoa and 2 chocolate-covered graham crackers. Water.

Snack #3: 1 mango, sliced and drizzled with lime juice. Water.

Nutrition Score: 2,233 calories, 29 percent fat, 54 percent carbohydrates, 17 percent protein, 1,132 mg calcium, 498 mcg folic acid, 18.5 mg iron, 36 g fiber.

Day 18

Breakfast:

Breakfast Wrap: 1 whole-wheat or spinach tortilla filled with: ½ cup egg substitute scrambled with 2 tablespoons diced green pepper, 1 tablespoon diced onion, 1 ounce grated or sliced cheddar cheese. Top with 1 tablespoon salsa.

1 cup pink grapefruit juice

Tea or coffee (sweetened with sugar substitute, optional)

Lunch:

1 serving Spinach and Red Pepper Quiche*

1 whole-wheat roll

1 papaya, sliced and topped with 1 teaspoon lime juice and a sprig of fresh mint

Dinner:

Beef and Vegetable Shish Kebabs:

Marinate the following in low-calorie teriyaki sauce, skewer, and barbecue: 3 ounces extra-lean beef cut into ¾" pieces, ½ green bell pepper cut into 1" pieces, ½ onion cut into 1" pieces, 6 whole or halved mushrooms, 2 carrots cut into ½" slices and slightly steamed before skewering, and 1 small zucchini cut into ¾" slices.

⅔ cup brown rice, cooked

1 artichoke, steamed with garlic cloves. Dip leaves in 1 tablespoon mayonnaise seasoned with fresh herbs, fresh ground pepper, and salt.

Snacks:

Snack #1: 1 cup nonfat milk, steamed and flavored with almond extract, and 1 cup grapes. Water.

Snack #2: ⅓ cup black bean dip, 1 ounce baked tortilla chips, and 2 table-spoons salsa. Water.

Snack #3: 4 cups air-popped popcorn and 1 cup 1 percent low-fat milk with 1 tablespoon flavored syrup.

Nutrition Score: 2,194 calories, 22 percent fat, 57 percent carbohydrates, 21 percent protein, 1,484 mg calcium, 693 mcg folic acid, 20 mg iron, 45 g fiber.

Day 19

Breakfast:

1 cup oatmeal cooked in 1 cup 1 percent low-fat milk and topped with 2 tablespoons toasted wheat germ, 2 tablespoons dried cranberries, 2 tablespoons chopped walnuts, and 2 teaspoons maple syrup

1 cup orange juice

1 banana

Herb or green tea

Lunch:

Thai Tofu Salad (serve hot or cold): 3 ounces firm tofu, cut into cubes and heated in a nonstick pan for 5 minutes. Add 2 cups preshredded cabbage mix, 1 tablespoon peanut sauce, and 1 tablespoon sunflower seeds. Heat over medium heat for 2 minutes (or until heated through, but still crunchy). Top with ¼ cup chopped fresh cilantro and serve.

2 medium tomatoes, sliced and topped with 2 cloves minced garlic, 2 tablespoons chopped fresh basil, 1 teaspoon balsamic vinegar

Sparkling water with lemon or herb tea

Dinner:

1 serving Salt-Rubbed Roasted Chicken with Herbs*

1 serving Oven-Roasted Vegetables*

Orange-Spinach Salad: 2 cups fresh spinach leaves, ½ can drained mandarin oranges, and 1 tablespoon chopped walnuts. Dressing: 1 tablespoon orange juice, 1 tablespoon olive oil, salt and fresh ground pepper.

Sparkling water with lime juice

Snacks:

Snack #1: 1 cup nonfat, plain yogurt mixed with 2 tablespoons chopped dates, 1 tablespoon chopped almonds, and 1 tablespoon all-fruit jam. Water.

Snack #2: 1 cup nonfat milk blended with 1 teaspoon nutmeg, 1 teaspoon honey, and 1 ice cube. ½ whole-wheat bagel toasted and topped with 1 tablespoon peanut butter. Water.

Snack #3: 2 cups frozen grapes. Water.

Nutrition Score: 2,190 calories, 31 percent fat, 49 percent carbohydrates, 20 percent protein, 1,658 mg calcium, 685 mcg folic acid, 21 mg iron, 37 g fiber.

Day 20

Breakfast:

Veggie Omelet: Whip 2 whole eggs and pour into nonstick 10" frying pan coated with vegetable spray. Cover and cook over medium heat until cooked through and firm. Remove in one piece, place on plate, fill with ½ cup steamed vegetables (onions, garlic, zucchini, mushrooms, red peppers, etc.) and fresh herbs. Fold egg mixture over vegetables and herbs to form an omelet. Salt and pepper to taste.

1 slice whole-wheat bread, toasted, topped with 1 tablespoon apricot preserves

1 cup pink grapefruit juice

Herb or green tea

Lunch:

Black Bean Burrito: 1 whole-wheat tortilla, warmed and filled with ½ cup Spicy Black Beans,* 1 ounce grated fat-free cheddar cheese, 3 tablespoons canned chopped green chilies, 3 tablespoons chopped fresh cilantro, and 2 tablespoons enchilada sauce. Top with 2 tablespoons fat-free sour cream and 3 tablespoons salsa.

½ cup instant brown rice, cooked

1 medium orange, cut into wedges
½ papaya, peeled and cut into slices
Iced tea

Dinner:

1 serving Oven-Roasted Halibut with Lemon, Basil, and Capers*
1 serving Curried Couscous with Cranberries*
15 mushrooms, sauteed in ¼ cup chicken broth with 3 cloves garlic, minced
1 serving Fresh Green Beans with Shallots and Feta Cheese*
Sparkling water, herb tea, or water

Snacks:

Snack #1: 1 cup 1 percent low-fat milk and 1 banana. Water.
Snack #2: ⅓ cup Spinach Hummus,* 1 whole-wheat pita, 1 carrot, peeled and cut into sticks, and ⅓ cup jicama, peeled and cut into strips. Water.
Snack #3: 1 cup 1 percent low-fat milk, warmed and flavored with almond extract and nutmeg, 1 banana, and 1 cup blueberries.

Nutrition Score: 2,207 calories, 19 percent fat, 61 percent carbohydrates, 20 percent protein, 1,310 mg calcium, 897 mcg folic acid, 19 mg iron, 58 g fiber.

Day 21

Breakfast:

2 whole-wheat waffles topped with 1 tablespoon fat-free cream cheese, 1 tablespoon marmalade, and 1 tangerine, peeled, sectioned, and seeded
1 cup 1 percent low-fat milk

Lunch:

1 serving Southwest Tuscany Soup*
1 slice whole-wheat bread
1 ounce cheddar cheese
½ cup coleslaw
Sparkling water or herb or green tea

Dinner:

1 4-ounce extra-lean steak, grilled

1 baked potato with 1 tablespoon butter

Spinach with a Zing: In a medium skillet, add 2 tablespoons chicken broth, 2 teaspoons balsamic vinegar, 1 teaspoon olive oil, 1 tablespoon dried cranberries, 2 minced cloves garlic, and a dash of red pepper flakes and nutmeg. Bring to a simmer. Add ⅓ pound fresh spinach, washed and stemmed. Toss and cook until spinach is wilted, or about 1 to 3 minutes.

Water

Snacks:

Snack #1: 1 serving Frozen Frappaccino* and 1 Oat Bran and Fig Muffin.*

Snack #2: 1 cup tomato juice, and celery sticks.

Snack #3: 1 sliced banana and 3 canned apricot halves. Water.

Nutrition Score: 2,191 calories, 30 percent fat, 51 percent carbohydrates, 18 percent protein, 1,603 mg calcium, 747 mcg folic acid, 23 mg iron, 33 g fiber.

Day 22

Breakfast:

1 six-inch pancake made from reduced-fat pancake mix according to directions on box with 1 tablespoon toasted wheat germ added per pancake. Top with 2 tablespoons maple syrup.

½ cantaloupe with lemon juice and a sprig of fresh mint

Herb or green tea

Lunch:

Turkey Sandwich: 4 ounces turkey breast, 2 lettuce leaves, 2 slices of tomato, 1 teaspoon honey mustard, 1 tablespoon mayonnaise, 2 slices whole-wheat bread.

Tossed Salad: 2 cups chopped leaf lettuce, ½ sliced winter pear, 2 tablespoons fat-free vinaigrette dressing.

Water

Dinner:

Prawn Kebabs: Brush with 2 tablespoons teriyaki sauce, skewer, and barbecue, grill, or broil the following: 6 jumbo shrimp (peeled and deveined), 2 bell peppers cut into strips or 1" pieces, ½ cup thickly sliced red onions, and 6 large mushrooms.

½ acorn squash, baked

Sparkling water with lime or herb or green tea

Snacks:

Snack #1: 1 cup nonfat, plain yogurt mixed with 2 tablespoons dried fruit, 2 tablespoons slivered almonds, 2 tablespoons sunflower seeds, and 1 tablespoon all-fruit jam.

Snack #2: 4 large celery stalks filled with 2 tablespoons peanut (or almond) butter.

Sparkling water with lemon.

Snack #3: Tropical Fruit Salad: ½ peeled and sliced papaya, ½ cup pineapple chunks, 3 tablespoons mandarin orange slices, ⅓ cup sliced avocado, 1 tablespoon orange zest, and 2 tablespoons low-fat bottled lime salad dressing.

Nutrition Score: 2,210 calories, 30 percent fat, 51 percent carbohydrates, 19 percent protein, 1,415 mg calcium, 719 mcg folic acid, 20 mg iron, 41 g fiber.

Day 23

Breakfast:

1 whole-wheat English muffin toasted and topped with 2 tablespoons peanut butter

1 cup hot cocoa made with nonfat milk

½ cup stewed prunes

Tea

Lunch:

2 cups canned chunky split-pea soup

1 slice whole-wheat bread

1 ounce cheddar cheese

1 cup mixed fruit salad
Water

Dinner:

1 four-ounce barbecued chicken breast
1 large corn-on-the-cob
Spinach Salad: 3 cups baby spinach leaves, 2 tablespoons sliced red onion, and 2 tablespoons low-fat creamy dressing.
Water

Snacks:

Snack #1: ½ cup pineapple chunks and ½ cup fat-free cottage cheese. Water.

Snack #2: 1 cup tomato juice with a dash of tabasco, and celery sticks. Water.

Snack #3: Warm Sweet Potato Salad: Mix together 1 warm medium sweet potato cooked and cubed, ½ cup cooked corn, ¼ cup diced red onion, 1 tablespoon olive oil, 1 tablespoon red wine vinegar, 2 teaspoons chopped cilantro, and salt/pepper to taste. Sparkling water.

Nutrition Score: 2,226 calories, 30 percent fat, 49 percent carbohydrates, 21 percent protein, 1,150 mg calcium, 624 mcg folic acid, 19 mg iron, 46 g fiber.

Day 24

Breakfast:

2 cups shredded wheat topped with 1 cup 1 percent low-fat milk
1 cup orange juice
Tea

Lunch:

Grilled Vegetable Sandwich: 2 slices eggplant and ⅓ sweet red pepper cut into slices, brushed with 1 teaspoon olive oil and grilled. Place on 2 slices of French bread with 1 slice of fresh, low-fat mozzarella cheese and 3 teaspoons fresh basil chopped. Drizzle vegetables and cheese with balsamic vinegar (¼ teaspoon or less).

1 cup nonfat plain yogurt mixed with 1 tablespoon orange juice concentrate and topped with ½ cup apricots canned in juice

Dinner:

Fettuccine with Scallops and Vegetables: 1 cup cooked fettuccine topped with a sauce made with 2 minced cloves of garlic, 3 chopped green onions, and ½ cup fresh scallops sauteed in 1 teaspoon olive oil, mixed and heated with 2 tablespoons dry white wine,[†] 3 tablespoons chicken broth, salt, pepper, ⅔ cup cooked broccoli florets, and ⅔ cup cooked carrot rounds.
1 serving Red Beet Salad with Vinaigrette*
Water

Snacks:

Snack #1: 1 mango, sliced and drizzled with lemon juice. Water.
Snack #2: 2 cups slightly steamed asparagus dipped in ranch-style dressing. Water.
Snack #3: 2 cups jicama slices. Water.

Nutrition Score: 2,194 calories, 25 percent fat, 61 percent carbohydrates, 15 percent protein, 1,514 mg calcium, 788 mcg folic acid, 16 mg iron, 36 g fiber.

Day 25

Breakfast:

Tomato-Based Poached Eggs: In a small, nonstick skillet sprayed with vegetable spray, place 2 tablespoons diced onion and heat until softened. Add two chopped tomatoes, ½ teaspoon thyme, and salt/pepper to taste and cook until well heated. Make a hole in center of tomato and gently break two eggs into center. Cover pan, reduce to low heat, and cook until poached, approximately 4 minutes. Serve over 1 slice whole-wheat toast.
1 cup orange juice
Water

[†]The alcohol cooks off with heating.

Lunch:

Tuna Sandwich: Mix 3 ounces drained water-packed tuna with 2 table-spoons diced celery and 1 tablespoon low-fat mayonnaise. Place on two slices whole-wheat bread.
1 cup vegetable soup with ½ cup extra mixed vegetables
1 cup 1 percent low-fat milk

Dinner:

1½ cups chili made with extra-lean meat
1 corn bread muffin
Spinach Salad: 2 cups spinach leaves, 1 sliced tomato, and 2 tablespoons oil and vinegar dressing.
Water

Snacks:

Snack #1: ½ cup fat-free frozen yogurt and 2 vanilla wafers.
Snack #2: 1 Oat Bran and Fig Muffin* and 1 cup nonfat milk.
Snack #3: Fruit Plate: 1 winter pear sliced and 1 orange sliced. Alternate slices on plate and drizzle with lemon juice.

Nutrition Score: 2,182 calories, 25 percent fat, 55 percent carbohydrates, 20 percent protein, 1,408 mg calcium, 666 mcg folic acid, 21 mg iron, 42 g fiber.

Day 26

Breakfast:

1 whole-wheat bagel toasted and topped with 2 tablespoons fat-free cream cheese and ½ cup crushed pineapple
1 cup strawberries
Tea or water

Lunch:

Hamburger made with 3 ounces extra-lean meat, 1 medium sliced tomato, 2 lettuce leaves, 2 tablespoons catsup, and 1 whole-wheat hamburger bun
20 baby carrots

Chocolate Milkshake: 1 cup nonfat milk, ½ cup fat-free chocolate frozen yogurt, and 1 tablespoon chocolate syrup.
Water

Dinner:

1 low-calorie cheese lasagna frozen meal
Sauteed Spinach: 2 minced cloves garlic sauteed over medium heat in 1 teaspoon olive oil until softened. Add 3 cups fresh spinach and toss. Cover, reduce heat, and cook until spinach wilts down, approximately 4 minutes. Salt and pepper to taste.
1 cup cubed butternut squash, baked and drizzled with 1 teaspoon maple syrup
Water

Snacks:

Snack #1: 6 ounces low-fat fruit yogurt, ½ sliced banana, 2 teaspoons semisweet chocolate chips. Sparkling water flavored with lemon juice.
Snack #2: 1 cup sparkling apple juice, ½ whole-wheat pita bread dunked in ¼ cup Spinach Hummus.*
Snack #3: 1 papaya, sliced and drizzled with lime juice. Water.

Nutrition Score: 2,215 calories, 19 percent fat, 62 percent carbohydrates, 19 percent protein, 1,551 mg calcium, 850 mcg folic acid, 23 mg iron, 49 g fiber.

Day 27

Breakfast:

1 slice French toast topped with 2 tablespoons maple syrup
1 cup 1 percent low-fat milk
½ grapefruit, broiled and sprinkled with 1 teaspoon sugar
Tea or water

Lunch:

Ham Sandwich: 4 ounces extra-lean ham, 2 teaspoons mustard, 2 lettuce leaves, 2 slices rye bread.

2 cups grapes
1 cup 8th Continent chocolate soy milk
Water

Dinner:

1 serving Polenta and Black Bean Casserole*
Tossed Salad: 2 cups red-leaf lettuce, 2 tablespoons diced red onion, 1 chopped tomato, and 2 tablespoons creamy Italian dressing.
Water or herb tea

Snacks:

Snack #1: 1 cup orange juice and 5 pitted dried plums each stuffed with an almond. Water.
Snack #2: 1 cup slightly steamed broccoli, cooled and dipped in low-calorie ranch-style dressing. Water.
Snack #3: 1 slice angel food cake topped with 1 cup thawed frozen raspberries. Water.

Nutrition Score: 2,203 calories, 22 percent fat, 62 percent carbohydrates, 16 percent protein, 1,492 mg calcium, 563 mcg folic acid, 16 mg iron, 42 g fiber.

Day 28

Breakfast:

Scrambled Egg Sandwich: Place one scrambled egg topped with 1 slice cheddar cheese on a toasted whole-wheat English muffin. Optional: 1 teaspoon salsa.
1 cup orange juice
Tea or water

Lunch:

Salmon Wrap: Warm a 10" spinach tortilla and fill with 3 ounces broiled salmon, ¼ cup instant brown rice, 1 tablespoon gari or Oriental pickled ginger, 1 tablespoon chopped green onions, 2 avocado slices, and 1 tablespoon wasabi vinaigrette dressing.

1 cup pink grapefruit juice
Water

Dinner:

1 serving Glazed Chicken with Orange and Ginger*
1 serving Curried Couscous with Cranberries*
1 serving Fresh Green Beans with Shallots and Feta Cheese*
1 serving Spinach, Pear, and Pecan Salad*
Water

Snacks:

Snack #1: 1 cup nonfat milk, warmed and flavored with almond extract.
Snack #2: 1 cup cocoa made with nonfat milk, and 1 oatmeal-raisin cookie.
Snack #3: 1 soft granola bar.

Nutrition Score: 2,214 calories, 32 percent fat, 46 percent carbohydrates, 22 percent protein, 1,490 mg calcium, 454 mcg folic acid, 14 mg iron, 21 g fiber.

Mix and Match Choices:

Additions for the Second and Third Trimesters and When Breast-Feeding

The preceding menus are your basic plan when gearing up for pregnancy, during the first trimester, and when you are not breast-feeding. You'll need an additional 300 calories during the second and third trimesters and 500 or more calories if you breast-feed.

The following additions each supply about one hundred calories. Select three to five each day to meet your calorie and nutrient needs. See Table 10.2, "Twenty-five Super Snacks," on page 252, for more one-hundred-calorie additions to your diet. Items marked with an * are found in the Recipes section.

Fruit Additions:

1 cup unsweetened applesauce sprinkled with cinnamon
2 cups cubed casaba melon

1 grapefruit sweetened with 2 teaspoons sugar
⅓ cup guacamole

Vegetable Additions:
1 small baked potato
½ cup Southwest Tuscany Soup*
2 celery stalks filled with 1 tablespoon peanut butter
2 cups broccoli with 1 tablespoon ranch dressing
1 thin slice Wild Mushroom Tart*
1 thin slice Spinach and Red Pepper Quiche*
2 sliced carrots and 1 tablespoon sour cream dip
3 cups chopped leaf lettuce with 1½ tablespoons French dressing

Dairy Additions:
1 cup nonfat milk with almond extract and sugar substitute
6 ounces nonfat plain yogurt and ¼ cup blueberries
½ cup fat-free cottage cheese

Grain Additions:
½ whole-wheat bagel (1.2 ounces)
10 thin twist pretzels
1 thin slice Glazed Blueberry-Lemon Bread*
1 slice cinnamon-raisin toast with 1 tablespoon jam
8 tortilla chips with 2 tablespoons salsa
8 saltine crackers
1 rice cake topped with 1 tablespoon fat-free cream cheese and 2 teaspoons jam
4 graham crackers
1 whole-wheat freezer waffle
6 long, thin breadsticks dipped in 4 tablespoons low-fat spaghetti sauce
14 Ritz Bits peanut butter sandwiches

Protein/Iron Additions:
1 tablespoon peanut butter
2 small eggs
8 large shrimp, peeled, deveined, and boiled. Dip in 4 teaspoons tomato-based cocktail sauce.
½ serving Spinach Hummus*
4 slices fat-free bologna

Dessert Additions:

½ cup Kiwi Ice*

½ cup Banana Ice*

4 Hershey's Kisses

½ cup fat-free chocolate frozen yogurt

1 small brownie with nuts

Major Splurge: 4 cups sugar-free gelatin topped with 4 tablespoons light non-dairy topping

10 animal crackers

32 Gummi Bears

20 plain M&M's

Fat / Sugar / Convenience Food Additions:

1 tablespoon butter

2 tablespoons ranch dressing

1 ounce fat-free potato chips, either baked or made with Olestra

Recipes

STARTERS AND SIDES

✄ Shrimp Quesadillas with Peach Chutney

This simple dish makes a great appetizer, snack, or accompaniment to lunch. The chutney gives it a sweet, exotic taste. Best of all, it takes only five minutes to make!

Ingredients:
6 whole-wheat tortillas
½ pound small cooked shrimp, rinsed and drained
¼ cup thinly sliced green onions
¼ cup spreadable brie cheese (or remove skin from regular brie and heat in microwave for 15 seconds)
⅓ cup chutney (peach or Major Grey's is especially good)

Directions:
1. Spray large skillet with nonstick spray and heat over medium heat.
2. Add one tortilla, sprinkle with 2 heaping tablespoons of shrimp and a teaspoon or two of green onions. On another tortilla spread 1 tablespoon brie cheese and 1 tablespoon chutney, and place on top of shrimp and green onion (sandwich style). Cook until golden brown and a bit crunchy, then flip and toast other side. Remove from skillet.
3. Cool slightly, slice into wedges, and serve warm. Repeat twice more.

Yield: Makes 6 servings, ½ quesadilla each.

Nutrition Score per serving: 145 calories, 14 percent fat, 57 percent carbohydrates, 29 percent protein, 42 mg calcium, 17 mcg folic acid, 2.1 mg iron, 2.2 g fiber.

✂ Spinach Hummus

This twist on traditional hummus is a great dip for whole-wheat pita bread or vegetables or makes a good sandwich spread. It keeps for a week in the refrigerator.

Ingredients:
1 16-ounce can garbanzo beans (chickpeas), rinsed and drained
¼ cup raw sesame tahini
3 to 4 tablespoons fresh lemon juice
2 garlic cloves
½ teaspoon light soy sauce
Dash of ground cumin
1 cup fresh spinach leaves, washed and patted dry

Directions:
1. Combine all ingredients in a food processor and process until smooth. Add water, if needed, a tablespoon at a time until desired consistency is reached.
2. Serve with toasted pita bread wedges, whole-grain crackers, or as a dip for fresh vegetables.

Yield: Makes 5 servings, ⅓ cup each.

Nutrition Score per serving, without bread: 209 calories, 36 percent fat, 46 percent carbohydrates, 18 percent protein, 70 mg calcium, 171 mcg folic acid, 3.4 mg iron, 6.5 g fiber.

✂ Naughty Nachos

While typical nachos are more than 40 percent fat calories, this revised, yet just as tasty, version is only 11 percent fat calories.

Ingredients:
1 14-ounce bag oven-baked tortilla chips
½ cup fat-free refried beans
¼ cup grated, low-fat cheddar cheese
¼ cup bottled salsa

Directions:
Preheat oven to 400°.
Place chips on a large oven-proof platter. Top with beans and cheese and bake until heated through and cheese melts, about 10 minutes. Serve with salsa.

Yield: Makes 4 servings.

Nutrition Score per serving: 110 calories, 11 percent fat, 70 percent carbohydrates, 19 percent protein, 110 mg calcium, 36 mcg folic acid, 1.2 mg iron, 3.6 g fiber.

✂ Spicy Black Beans

These beans are great as a burrito filling, as a dip topped with salsa, or as a side dish.

Ingredients:
½ cup finely chopped onion
1 teaspoon olive oil
2 16-ounce cans black beans, drained (do not rinse)
1 garlic clove, minced
¼ teaspoon black pepper
Dash of cayenne pepper
½ teaspoon sugar
¼ teaspoon ground cumin
¼ teaspoon ground ginger

Directions:

In a saucepan, saute onion in olive oil for 3 to 4 minutes, or until soft. Add the remaining ingredients. Bring to a boil, reduce heat, and simmer 5 minutes to heat through and blend flavors.

Yield: Makes 8 servings, ½ cup each.

Nutrition Score per serving: 141 calories, 7 percent fat, 68 percent carbohydrates, 25 percent protein, 29 mg calcium, 149 mcg folic acid, 2 mg iron, 6 g fiber.

✌ Curried Couscous with Cranberries

Couscous is a simple grain to serve. It takes only five minutes to prepare, but is a great base for any meat or vegetable dish, or stew. This couscous is especially good with the Glazed Chicken with Orange and Ginger and the Fresh Green Beans with Shallots and Feta Cheese.

Ingredients:

1 box curry couscous (Near East brand is very good)
¼ cup orange juice
½ cup dried cranberries (more if you like)

Directions:

Prepare couscous according to package directions, with the exception of replacing ¼ cup water with orange juice, not adding olive oil, and adding the dried cranberries in with the spice sack. Follow all other directions.

Yield: Makes 4 servings, a generous ½ cup each.

Nutrition Score per serving: 194 calories, 1 percent fat, 88 percent carbohydrates, 10 percent protein, 21 mg calcium, 22 mcg folic acid, 1 mg iron, 4 g fiber.

SALADS

✂ Red Beet Salad with Vinaigrette Dressing

The blend of flavors in this salad is a great accompaniment to any dinner dish, including meat, chicken, or fish, as well as a side dish to a light lunch.

Ingredients:

Salad:
1 head red leaf lettuce, washed, dried, and chopped
1 cup cooked beets, julienned
¼ cup red onion, slivered
¼ cup toasted chopped walnuts*

Vinaigrette Dressing:
3 tablespoons olive oil
2 tablespoons balsamic vinegar
1 teaspoon Dijon mustard
½ teaspoon sugar

Directions:
1. Place lettuce in a large salad bowl. Place beets in center of lettuce, place red onion along edges of salad, and sprinkle salad with toasted walnuts.
2. Mix vinaigrette ingredients together in a small bowl; drizzle over salad just before serving.

Yield: Serves 4.

Nutrition Score per serving: 178 calories, 71 percent fat, 21 percent carbohydrates, 8 percent protein, 73 mg calcium, 83 mcg folic acid, 2 mg iron, 2.8 g fiber.

*To toast walnuts: Preheat oven to 350°, place chopped walnuts on a small double piece of aluminum foil, and bake for 5 to 7 minutes until lightly brown. Remove from oven and cool.

Recipes

✂ Spinach, Pear, and Pecan Salad

An elegant salad with unusual flavors in a delightful blend. Goes well with any meat, chicken, or fish dish. This salad is surprisingly high in calcium, folic acid, and iron, as well as magnesium, vitamin A, and vitamin C.

Ingredients:

Dressing:
2 tablespoons green onion, chopped fine
2 tablespoons sherry vinegar
1 tablespoon balsamic vinegar
2 teaspoons Dijon mustard
3 tablespoons olive oil
Salt and freshly ground pepper to taste

Salad:
2 10-ounce bags baby spinach leaves
1 large Belgian endive, cut into thin slices
1 large red winter pear, seeded and sliced into thin strips
1 ounce blue cheese
⅓ cup pecans toasted in maple syrup (roll pecans in 1 teaspoon maple syrup, place on cookie sheet sprayed with vegetable spray, and bake at 350° until golden, about 15 minutes)

Directions:
1. Dressing: Place all ingredients in a jar. Tighten the lid and shake well. Let stand while you prepare the salad.
2. In a large bowl, place spinach, endive, and pear. Toss. Divide into four salad bowls and sprinkle blue cheese and pecans on top of each. Drizzle dressing over each salad.

Nutrition Score per serving: 245 calories, 66 percent fat, 23 percent carbohydrates, 11 percent protein, 208 mg calcium, 335 mcg folic acid, 5 mg iron, 6 g fiber.

✣ Berry-Banana Salad

This quick-fix fruit salad goes well with sandwiches at lunch or as a mid-morning snack.

Ingredients:
1 pound blueberries, raspberries, and blackberries, washed
1 cup nonfat custard-style vanilla yogurt
1 medium banana
¼ cup orange juice

Directions:
1. Gently mix berries in a large bowl and divide evenly into 3 serving bowls.
2. Combine the yogurt, banana, and orange juice in a blender. Puree until smooth and pour over berries. Chill and serve.

Yield: Makes 4 servings.

Nutrition Score per serving: 148 calories, 8 percent fat, 82 percent carbohydrates, 10 percent protein, 115 mg calcium, 24 mcg folic acid, less than 0.5 mg iron, 3.2 g fiber.

✣ Cucumber Toss

If you need a crunchy snack that has almost no calories, this dish is for you! The vinegar soothes a troubled stomach during the first trimester, too.

Ingredients:
2 medium cucumbers, peeled and thinly sliced
1 medium Walla Walla or other sweet onion, thinly sliced
1 teaspoon Mrs. Dash or other herb seasoning mix
1 teaspoon sugar
1½ teaspoons dill weed
¾ cup rice wine vinegar

Directions:

Mix the cucumber and onion slices in a medium bowl. Blend other ingredients, then pour over cucumbers and onion. Chill and serve.

Yield: Makes 6 servings.

Nutrition Score per serving: 30 calories, 4 percent fat, 84 percent carbohydrates, 12 percent protein, 21 mg calcium, 18 mcg folic acid, 0.5 mg iron, 1.3 g fiber.

✄ Savory Potato Salad

This simple potato salad is a great side dish to a lunch sandwich or makes a tasty carbohydrate-rich midafternoon snack.

Ingredients:
1½ pounds small red potatoes (approximately 12)
1½ tablespoons fresh chives, minced
1½ tablespoons fresh basil or dill, chopped
1 tablespoon fresh parsley, minced
½ cup carrots, grated
½ cup diced celery
1 tablespoon wine vinegar
1 tablespoon olive oil
Salt and pepper to taste

Directions:
1. Scrub potatoes, cover with water in a medium saucepan, and gently boil until soft but firm, approximately 20 minutes. Drain the potatoes, then cool and cut into quarters.
2. Blend the remaining ingredients in a large bowl, then add the potatoes and toss well. Serve chilled or at room temperature.

Yield: Makes 6 servings, approximately ⅔ cup each.

Nutrition Score per serving: 142 calories, 15 percent fat, 78 percent carbohydrates, 7 percent protein, 20 mg calcium, 18 mcg folic acid, 0.6 mg iron, 2.6 g fiber.

SOUP

✣ Southwest Tuscany Soup

Who says eating healthy has to take more time! This tasty soup is ready in thirty minutes and preparation time depends on how quickly you can open a can! Rich in flavor, B vitamins, folic acid, iron, magnesium, fiber, protein, and a host of other nutrients, yet low in fat, this soup makes a great dinner, lunch, and snack. The recipe makes enough to last a few days and is even better if you add leftover chicken breast! Serve with corn tortillas or cornbread and cheese for a full meal.

Ingredients:
2 15½-ounce cans great northern beans, undrained
1 15½-ounce can hominy (white or yellow), undrained
2 14½-ounce cans stewed tomatoes, undrained and chopped
1 10-ounce can diced tomatoes and green chilies (Hunt's or other brand), undrained
1 4-ounce can diced green chilies
2 cups chicken broth
1 cup cilantro, chopped
1 teaspoon cumin
1 teaspoon chili powder
1 teaspoon coriander
1 10-ounce package frozen whole kernel corn
2 cups leftover chicken breast, chopped (optional)

Directions:
Combine all ingredients in a large Dutch oven, bring to a boil, then simmer for 30 minutes.

Yield: Serves 10 (1-cup serving without chicken, a generous cup with chicken).

Nutrition Score per 1-cup serving without chicken: 193 calories, 6 percent fat, 75 percent carbohydrates, 19 percent protein, 94 mg calcium, 107 mcg folic acid, 3.3 mg iron, 11 g fiber.

Nutrition Score per 1-cup serving with chicken: 221 calories, 8 percent fat, 67 percent carbohydrates, 25 percent protein, 97 mg calcium, 107 mcg folic acid, 3.5 mg iron, 11 g fiber.

MAIN DISHES AND LIGHT LUNCHES

✺ Wild Mushroom Tart

The rich, earthy taste of this tart is a meal in itself, accompanied by a tossed salad and French bread. Or, serve as a light lunch or for breakfast. It reheats well.

Ingredients:

1 nine-inch frozen unbaked pie crust
2 tablespoons tub margarine
4 cups fresh brown mushrooms, sliced
2 cups fresh oyster mushrooms, sliced
1 teaspoon minced fresh marjoram, or ½ teaspoon dried
1 teaspoon minced fresh thyme, or ½ teaspoon dried
1 cup reduced-fat Swiss cheese, shredded
2 well-beaten eggs
½ cup low-fat milk
1 tablespoon chives, chopped

Directions:

Preheat oven to 450°.

1. Leave pastry in original pie tin, prick crust, line with foil, and bake for 7 minutes. Remove foil and continue baking for 5 minutes or until golden brown. Remove from oven. Reduce heat to 375°.
2. In a large skillet over medium-high heat, melt margarine. Add mushrooms, marjoram, and thyme. Saute for 4 to 5 minutes, or until mushrooms are tender and liquid has evaporated. Remove from heat.
3. In a large bowl, combine mushroom mixture, Swiss cheese, eggs, milk, and chives. Stir well to mix thoroughly.
4. Pour mushroom-egg mixture into partially baked pastry shell. Bake at 375° for approximately 30 minutes or until set and top is golden.
5. Cool in pan for 15 minutes. Cut into wedges and serve warm or at room temperature.

Yield: Serves 8.

Nutrition Score per serving: 202 calories, 54 percent fat, 28 percent carbo-hydrates, 17 percent protein, 192 mg calcium, 21 mcg folic acid, 1.4 mg iron, 1.1 g fiber.

℀ Polenta and Black Bean Casserole

This Mexican-style lasagna is just the right amount of spicy to satisfy your taste buds, and makes a good dinner meal and a great leftover for lunches. It's surprisingly rich in vitamin C, calcium, and folic acid and takes only minutes of preparation time.

Ingredients:
2 15-ounce cans black beans, rinsed and drained
1 15-ounce can Mexican tomatoes, chopped
1 4-ounce can diced green chilies
1 teaspoon cumin
1 teaspoon coriander
½ teaspoon chili powder
1 cup of your favorite salsa
1 cup cilantro, chopped
1 18-ounce package precooked, ready-to-eat rolled polenta (plain or basil flavored)
1 cup low-fat Monterey Jack cheese, shredded

Directions:
Preheat oven to 350°.
1. In large Dutch oven, combine all ingredients except polenta and cheese. Cover and simmer over medium heat for 15 minutes, to enhance flavors.
2. While bean mixture is simmering, slice polenta into ¼-inch-thick rounds. Spray a 9 x 5 x 3-inch loaf pan or a 1-quart casserole with non-stick spray.
3. Layer bottom of pan with ⅓ of bean mixture, then add one layer of polenta rounds (½ of the polenta). Sprinkle with ⅓ cup of cheese. Add another layer of beans, polenta, cheese, then beans, and finish with cheese. Bake for 50 to 55 minutes, or until bubbly hot.
4. Drain any liquid from the pan, cool for 5 minutes, then slice and serve.

Yield: Serves 4.

Nutrition Score per serving: 365 calories, 23 percent fat, 53 percent carbohydrates, 24 percent protein, 415 mg calcium, 152 mcg folic acid, 4.5 mg iron, 9 g fiber.

✂ Oven-Roasted Halibut with Lemon, Basil, and Capers

Halibut is a firm, flavorful fish, and topped with fresh herbs, lemon, and capers, this dish is great for any season. Serve with the Fresh Green Beans with Shallots and Feta Cheese and/or the Red Beet Salad with Vinaigrette Dressing. Makes a great leftover for lunch; for example, debone and use for a fish burrito along with salsa and fat-free sour cream.

Ingredients:
¼ cup fresh basil leaves, chopped
2 tablespoons olive oil
2 tablespoons fresh-squeezed lemon juice
2 tablespoons capers, rinsed
2 firm Italian tomatoes, diced
1 teaspoon garlic, minced
1 pound halibut or 2 8-ounce halibut steaks

Directions:
Preheat oven to 450°.
1. In a small bowl, whisk first 6 ingredients.
2. Brush bottoms of halibut steaks with sauce and arrange on baking sheet. Brush tops of halibut steaks with half of the sauce.
3. Roast in oven for approximately 15 to 25 minutes (depending on thickness of steaks), or until opaque. Remove from oven, transfer to fish platter or plate, drizzle with remaining basil mixture and serve.

Yield: Makes 4 servings of approximately 4 ounces each.

Nutrition Score per serving: 196 calories, 44 percent fat, 6 percent carbohydrates, 50 percent protein, 58 mg calcium, 20 mcg folic acid, 1 mg iron, 0.5 g fiber.

Beef Fajitas

These spicy fajitas are a great snack, lunch, or dinner meal. They're high in iron, too!

Ingredients:
½ cup onion, sliced
½ medium green bell pepper, seeded, cored, and slivered
½ cup fresh mushrooms, sliced
½ cup zucchini, slivered
6 ounces flank steak, cut into ½-inch strips
3 tablespoons bottled fajita seasoning
4 8-inch flour tortillas
1 medium tomato, chopped
1 ounce low-fat cheddar cheese, grated
½ cup bottled salsa

Directions:
1. Coat a large nonstick skillet with cooking spray. Stir-fry the onion, green pepper, and mushrooms on medium heat until tender, but still crisp, about 3 minutes.
2. Remove vegetables and stir-fry flank steak until browned and cooked through, about 2 minutes.
3. Stir the vegetables back into the pan and stir in fajita seasoning.
4. Wrap the tortillas in a paper towel and heat in microwave on high for 10 seconds.
5. Fill each tortilla with one-fourth of the beef-vegetable mixture, then sprinkle on some chopped tomato and grated cheese. Fold the tortillas over and top with salsa.

Yield: Makes 4 fajitas.

Nutrition Score per serving: 244 calories, 25 percent fat, 48 percent carbohydrates, 27 percent protein, 114 mg calcium, 35 mcg folic acid, 3 mg iron, 3 g fiber.

✿ Spinach and Red Pepper Quiche

This light and flavorful crustless quiche is creamy and rich, yet surprisingly low-calorie. It's easy to make and high in vitamin C, calcium, B vitamins, and vitamin A. Serve for dinner or lunch with a tossed salad and bread. You even could serve this for breakfast! It also reheats well.

Ingredients:
1 10-ounce package fresh spinach (ready to eat), chopped
¾ cup bottled roasted red peppers (rinse, chop, and pat dry)
1 cup fat-free cottage cheese
½ cup fat-free sour cream
½ teaspoon salt
3 eggs, beaten well
½ cup 1 percent low-fat milk
½ teaspoon thyme
¼ cup reduced-fat Parmesan cheese

Directions:
Preheat oven to 350°.
1. In a medium saucepan, sauté chopped spinach quickly to wilt; drain well.
2. Combine all ingredients in a large bowl; mix well.
3. Spray a 10 x 6 x 2-inch baking dish or a deep-dish pie pan with non-stick vegetable spray. Pour mixture into pan. Bake 50 to 55 minutes, or until set in center.
4. Let stand for 10 minutes, slice into wedges.

Yield: Serves 6.

Nutrition Score per serving: 192 calories, 26 percent fat, 33 percent carbohydrates, 41 percent protein, 182 mg calcium, 160 mcg folic acid, 2.6 mg iron, 2.2 g fiber.

✿ Chicken Parmesan

A quick, low-fat version of a traditional recipe. Use leftovers for salads and sandwiches later in the week.

Ingredients:
3 tablespoons plain bread crumbs
3 tablespoons reduced-fat Parmesan cheese
¼ teaspoon ground pepper
1 teaspoon fine herbs*
4 skinless and boneless chicken breasts, about 4 ounces each
2 egg whites, lightly beaten

Directions:
Preheat the oven to 350°.
1. Combine and blend bread crumbs, cheese, pepper, and herbs in a shallow bowl.
2. Dip the chicken breasts in egg white and roll in bread-crumb mixture.
3. Place chicken on a baking pan coated with cooking spray and bake for 20 minutes, or until cooked through.

Yield: Makes 4 servings.

Nutrition Score per serving: 173 calories, 15 percent fat, 14 percent carbohydrates, 71 percent protein, 47 mg calcium, 6 mcg folic acid, 1 mg iron, 1 g fiber.

*Fine herbs is a mixture of dried herbs, especially parsley, chervil, and tarragon. It is available in most supermarkets.

✂ Salt-Rubbed Roasted Chicken with Herbs

The salt seals in moisture and flavor, while the herbs and lemon give the meat extra flavor. Serve with Oven-Roasted Vegetables, mashed potatoes, or any vegetable. For best results, refrigerate salt-rubbed chicken overnight before cooking to seal in juices.

Ingredients:
2 tablespoons coarse salt (canning salt will do)
2 teaspoons dried thyme
3 tablespoons fresh marjoram, chopped fine (save stems for stuffing bird)
¼ teaspoon freshly ground pepper
1 5½-pound roasting chicken, rinsed and patted dry
1 lemon, cut into pieces
6 cloves garlic, peeled

Directions:
Preheat oven to 350°.
1. Combine salt, thyme, chopped marjoram leaves, and pepper.
2. Stuff cavity of chicken with lemon, marjoram stems, and garlic. Pat outside with salt mixture. If possible, refrigerate overnight.
3. Place chicken in covered roasting pan and roast for 3 hours, or until thigh meat is cooked to 170° and juices run clear. Periodically baste with juices from pan.
4. Let stand 10 minutes before carving and serving. Do not use juices for gravy, since they will be too salty.

Yield: Serves 5 to 6.

Nutrition Score per 4-ounce serving of breast meat: 186 calories, 21 percent fat, 0 percent carbohydrates, 79 percent protein, 17 mg calcium, 4.5 mcg folic acid, 1.2 mg iron, 0 g fiber.

Nutrition Score per 4-ounce serving of dark meat: 195 calories, 31 percent fat, 0 percent carbohydrates, 69 percent protein, 14 mg calcium, 10 mcg folic acid, 1.5 mg iron, 0 g fiber.

✌ Glazed Chicken with Orange and Ginger

This chicken is easy to fix and great with the Curried Couscous with Cranberries. Leftovers can be used for sandwiches and salads later in the week.

Ingredients:
⅓ cup orange marmalade
1 tablespoon orange juice
1 tablespoon fresh ginger, minced
1 teaspoon dried thyme
1 tablespoon balsamic vinegar
Salt and freshly ground pepper to taste
4 boneless, skinless chicken breasts halves, 4 ounces each

Directions:
Preheat oven to 375°.
1. In a small saucepan, combine all glaze ingredients (everything but the chicken) and warm over low heat for 3 minutes.
2. Place chicken in ungreased baking pan and brush with half of glaze/sauce mixture. Bake in oven for 15 minutes. Remove from oven, brush again with remaining glaze, and continue to bake for 20 to 25 minutes, or until chicken juices run clear.
3. Place chicken on plate and drizzle with any remaining sauce from pan.

Yield: Serves 4.

Nutrition Score per serving: 321 calories, 38 percent fat, 24 percent carbohydrates, 38 percent protein, 28 mg calcium, 19 mcg folic acid, 1.2 mg iron, 0 g fiber.

✒ Chunky Spaghetti Sauce with Pasta

This spaghetti is chock-full of vegetables with old-country flavor. Cook the sauce in a cast-iron kettle and you'll boost the iron content severalfold! Serve over spaghetti or use the sauce for manicotti or lasagna.

Ingredients:
1 tablespoon olive oil
1½ large yellow onions, peeled and chopped
5 cloves garlic, peeled and diced
1 green bell pepper, seeded and chopped
15 brown mushrooms, washed and sliced
1 pound extra-lean ground beef (7 percent fat by weight or less)
1 26-ounce bottle spaghetti sauce (I prefer Classico Tomato & Basil)
1 14½-ounce can diced tomatoes
1 14½-ounce can tomato sauce
3 bay leaves
2 tablespoons Italian seasoning
Salt and freshly ground pepper
1 20-ounce bag spaghetti

Directions:
1. In a large kettle or Dutch oven, heat oil over medium heat. Add onions, garlic, pepper, and mushrooms and saute, stirring occasionally, until onion is transparent, about 10 minutes.
2. Add beef. Break into small bits, and continue to saute until beef is cooked through, about 7 minutes.
3. Add spaghetti sauce, tomatoes, tomato sauce, and bay leaves. Stir well, cover, and reduce heat to low. Let simmer for 1 to 2 hours. Add Italian seasoning about 30 minutes before serving. Salt and pepper to taste.
4. Cook spaghetti according to directions on package.

Yield: Makes 8 one-cup servings.

Nutrition Score per serving without pasta: 243 calories, 41 percent fat, 28 percent carbohydrates, 31 percent protein, 55 mg calcium, 31 mcg folic acid, 3.5 mg iron, 4 g fiber.

Nutrition Score per serving with pasta: 507 calories, 22 percent fat, 55 percent carbohydrates, 23 percent protein, 96 mg calcium, 65 mcg folic acid, 5 mg iron, 9 g fiber.

✄ Spinach-Cheese Manicotti

Another great way to use Chunky Spaghetti Sauce is in this yummy, low-fat manicotti. With just a hint of garlic, this dish makes a great dinner served with a tossed salad. It also makes leftover lunches, freezes well, and is loaded with calcium, iron, magnesium, and zinc.

Ingredients:
2 15-ounce containers fat-free ricotta cheese
2 cups shredded low-fat mozzarella cheese
½ cup grated low-fat or fat-free Parmesan cheese
2 large eggs, beaten
2 cloves garlic, minced
1 10-ounce package frozen spinach, thawed and drained thoroughly
¼ cup green onions, chopped fine
⅛ teaspoon nutmeg
Salt and freshly ground pepper to taste
1 8-ounce box manicotti shells (14 shells), cooked according to directions on box
2 cups Chunky Spaghetti Sauce (see page 304)

Directions:
Preheat oven to 350°.
1. In a large bowl, mix thoroughly ricotta, 1½ cups mozzarella, half the Parmesan, eggs, garlic, spinach, onions, nutmeg, and salt and pepper.
2. Spoon mixture into shells, about ⅓ to ½ cup per shell. Place shells in 14 x 10-inch baking pan.
3. Spread spaghetti sauce over top and sprinkle with remaining mozzarella and Parmesan cheeses. Cover with foil and bake for 1 hour, or until hot and bubbly.

Yield: Serves 8.

Nutrition Score per serving: 382 calories, 26 percent fat, 39 percent carbohydrates, 35 percent protein, 538 mg calcium, 75 mcg folic acid, 3 mg iron, 4 g fiber.

VEGETABLES

℀ Oven-Roasted Vegetables

These hearty roasted vegetables go well with roasted chicken. The roasting brings out the natural sweetness and the sliced fennel adds a delicate flavor.

Ingredients:
1 large red onion, sliced thickly*
1 head garlic (about 16 cloves), peeled
2 fennel bulbs, sliced thin
1 small eggplant, cut into 2-inch cubes (leave skin on)
½ pound baby carrots
½ pound green beans (blanch in hot water to preserve color, if desired)
½ pound baby red potatoes, cut in half
¼ cup olive oil
2 tablespoons balsamic vinegar
¼ cup fresh chives, chopped
1 teaspoon fresh chopped marjoram, or ½ teaspoon dried
1 teaspoon fresh chopped rosemary, or ½ teaspoon dried
Salt and freshly ground pepper to taste

Directions:
Preheat oven to 500°.
1. Combine all vegetables, except eggplant, in a large 13 x 9 x 2-inch baking dish or pan.
2. Blend olive oil, vinegar, salt, pepper, and fresh herbs, and pour mixture over vegetables. Toss to cover vegetables thoroughly.
3. Roast for 25 minutes, stirring every 15 minutes. Add eggplant, toss thoroughly, and continue to roast for an additional 20 minutes, stirring after 10 minutes.

Yield: Serves 8.

Nutrition Score per serving: 151 calories, 40 percent fat, 52 percent carbohydrates, 8 percent protein, 76 mg calcium, 48 mcg folic acid, 2 mg iron, 6.2 g fiber.

*May use any combination of vegetables to roast. Keep in mind some vegetables cook more quickly than others.

✌ Fresh Green Beans with Shallots and Feta Cheese

These flavorful green beans are a refreshing alternative to steaming, yet they are easy to make and take no more than ten minutes to prepare. They go well with any meat, chicken, or fish entree. One serving meets a third of your day's need for vitamin C, with ample amounts of calcium, vitamin A, magnesium, and potassium.

Ingredients:
1½ pounds fresh green beans, stemmed and rinsed
2 tablespoons olive oil
2 large shallots, minced
2 garlic cloves, minced
¼ cup feta cheese, crumbled
Salt and freshly ground pepper to taste

Directions:
1. Place beans in a large pot of boiling water. Cook for 5 minutes or until tender, yet still bright green. Drain beans, rinse under cold water, pat dry.
2. In a large skillet, on medium heat, saute shallots in oil for 5 minutes, then add garlic for 1 minute. Add cool beans to skillet, toss to coat with olive oil/shallot mixture; this will reheat the green beans.
3. Spoon onto a platter, sprinkle with feta cheese.

Yield: Serves 4.

Nutrition Score per serving: 131 calories, 43 percent fat, 41 percent carbohydrates, 16 percent protein, 144 mg calcium, 70 mcg folic acid, 2 mg iron, 5.4 g fiber.

✌ Spicy Carrots

The jalapeño peppers in these carrots give them a zing, making them a great accompaniment to burritos or fajitas.

Ingredients:
1 pound carrots, washed, peeled, and cut into ⅛-inch slices
⅙ cup vinegar
1 cup water
½ teaspoon black peppercorns
⅓ cup onion, chopped
Pinch of dried oregano
1 small bay leaf
1 teaspoon safflower oil
1½ teaspoons salt
2 garlic cloves, minced
¼ cup canned whole jalapeño peppers with juice (remove seeds and cut into ⅛-inch slices)

Directions:
1. Place carrots in a saucepan, cover with water, and bring to a low boil. Cook until tender but still crisp, about 10 minutes. Drain and let cool.
2. In medium bowl, combine the next 9 ingredients.
3. Place carrots and jalapeños in a medium bowl and pour marinade over the top. Cover and place in refrigerator for 12 to 24 hours (the longer the better to bring out the flavor).

Yield: Makes three servings, ½ cup each.

Nutrition Score per serving: 60 calories, 22 percent fat, 70 percent carbohydrates, 8 percent protein, 29 mg calcium, 15 mcg folic acid, 0.6 mg iron, 5 g fiber.

SWEETS

✱ Chocolate Mousse Parfait

It doesn't get any easier than this, or any more chocolaty either! Indulge your chocolate cravings with this low-calorie pudding and avoid the guilt! The soy even boosts your intake of phytoestrogens, which lower heart-disease risk.

Ingredients:
1 package European-style mousse mix by Nestlé (usually found next to
    powdered pudding mixes)
⅔ cup 8th Continent chocolate soy milk
¼ cup light nondairy dessert topping
4 teaspoons nonfat dark chocolate syrup

Directions:
1. Make mousse according to package using soy milk.
2. Fill 2 parfait glasses with a dollop of soft topping, followed with a
   dollop of mousse; continue until filled. Drizzle the top of each parfait
   with 2 teaspoons chocolate syrup. Keep chilled in refrigerator, for 1 to
   2 hours before serving.

Yield: Serves 2.

Nutrition Score per serving: 278 calories, 25 percent fat, 63 percent carbohydrates, 12 percent protein, 135 mg calcium, 4.5 mcg folic acid, 2 mg
iron, 7 g fiber.

✱ Currant-Date Muffins

Muffins are a great quick-fix, nutritious snack. This recipe makes twenty-four, so you can freeze some for later.

Ingredients:
1 cup unsweetened applesauce
½ cup granulated sugar
¼ cup brown sugar
¼ cup canola oil

3 egg whites
3 tablespoons 1 percent low-fat milk
1 cup all-purpose flour
1 cup whole-wheat flour
1 teaspoon baking soda
1 teaspoon baking powder
½ teaspoon ground cinnamon
¼ teaspoon ground nutmeg
½ cup dried currants or raisins
½ cup pitted dates, chopped
¼ cup walnuts, chopped

Directions:
Preheat oven to 350°.
Coat two 12-muffin tins with vegetable spray and set aside.

1. In a large bowl, combine the applesauce, sugars, oil, egg whites, and milk. Mix thoroughly. Set aside.
2. In a medium bowl, blend flours, baking soda, baking powder, cinnamon, and nutmeg. Stir in currants, dates, and walnuts until thoroughly coated.
3. Add flour mixture to applesauce mixture and blend only until dry ingredients are wet.
4. Spoon batter into tins and bake for 15 minutes or until springy and lightly brown on top. Do not overbake.

Yield: Makes 24 muffins.

Nutrition Score per serving: 112 calories, 24 percent fat, 68 percent carbohydrates, 8 percent protein, 19 mg calcium, 5.5 mcg folic acid, 0.7 mg iron, 1.5 g fiber.

✿ Razz 'n' Blues Muffins

One way to meet your fruit and vegetable needs is to sneak them into other foods. This muffin recipe contains loads of antioxidant-packed berries!

Ingredients:
1½ cups all-purpose flour
¾ cup rolled oats

⅓ cup sugar
1 tablespoon baking powder
1 teaspoon ground cinnamon
1 cup buttermilk
3 egg whites
2½ tablespoons safflower oil
1 cup fresh blueberries and raspberries, washed and drained

Directions:
Preheat oven to 350°.
Coat one 12-muffin tin with vegetable spray and set aside.
1. In a large bowl, combine flour, oats, sugar, baking powder, and cinnamon.
2. In a small bowl, combine the buttermilk, egg whites, and oil.
3. Add the liquid mixture to dry mixture and stir until just blended. (Do not overstir!) Fold in berries and spoon batter into muffin cups.
4. Bake for 20 to 25 minutes or until springy and golden brown on top.

Yield: Makes 12 muffins.

Nutrition Score per serving: 143 calories, 22 percent fat, 67 percent carbohydrates, 11 percent protein, 76 mg calcium, 7.7 mcg folic acid, 1 mg iron, 1.2 g fiber.

✼ Oat Bran and Fig Muffins

These muffins are packed with fiber, vitamins, and minerals. Oat bran is especially high in soluble fiber, the type of fiber that lowers heart-disease and diabetes risk, and keeps you regular, too! Top these muffins with peanut butter or jam, or serve as an accompaniment to applesauce or a fruit salad for a snack.

Ingredients:
2 cups oat bran
¼ cup wheat germ
2 teaspoons baking powder
2 teaspoons orange peel, grated
1 teaspoon cinnamon
¼ teaspoon nutmeg
¼ teaspoon salt

¾ cup dried figs, dates, or prunes, chopped
½ cup maple syrup
½ cup nonfat, sugar-free orange yogurt
¼ cup canola oil
2 eggs, well beaten

Directions:
Preheat oven to 400°.
Spray one 12-muffin tin with nonstick vegetable spray.

1. Combine first 7 ingredients in medium bowl.
2. Add figs, dates, or prunes and toss to coat.
3. Blend liquid ingredients (syrup, yogurt, oil, and eggs) in large bowl. Pour liquid ingredients into dry ingredients and mix gently, only until dry ingredients are wet.
4. Spoon batter into muffin cups. Bake until golden brown, approximately 20 minutes.

Yield: Makes 12 muffins.

Nutrition Score per serving: 178 calories, 30 percent fat, 60 percent carbohydrates, 10 percent protein, 79 mg calcium, 22 mcg folic acid, 2 mg iron, 4.1 g fiber.

Apple Bread Pudding

The perfect comfort food for breakfast, lunch, or snacks, this spiced pudding is loaded with B vitamins, fiber, and selenium.

Ingredients:
2½ cups vanilla-flavored soy milk
1½ cups apples, peeled and chopped into ½-inch cubes
½ cup raisins or dried cranberries
½ cup fat-free sweetened condensed milk
2 teaspoons vanilla extract
1 teaspoon cinnamon
¼ teaspoon nutmeg
⅛ teaspoon cardamom
¼ teaspoon salt
3 eggs, well beaten

8 cups 1-inch bread cubes (whole-wheat, sourdough, egg bread, or a combination)

Directions:
Preheat oven to 325°.
Spray a 9 x 9-inch baking dish with vegetable spray.
1. Combine first 10 ingredients in large bowl and blend well.
2. Add bread cubes to soy milk mixture, tossing to coat. Let stand for 15 minutes, then stir again.
3. Spoon bread mixture into baking dish, bake for 1½ hours or until firm in the center. Serve warm with nonfat frozen vanilla yogurt, or at room temperature.

Yield: Serves 8.

Nutrition Score per serving (without frozen yogurt): 245 calories, 20 percent fat, 65 percent carbohydrates, 15 percent protein, 189 mg calcium, 26 mcg folic acid, 1.4 mg iron, 1.6 g fiber.

✙ Glazed Blueberry-Lemon Bread

This yummy bread is easy to make, tastes delicious, and is loaded with vitamins, minerals, and health-enhancing phytochemicals from the blueberries and soy milk. It makes a great snack, breakfast bread, or dessert.

Ingredients:
1¾ cups unbleached, all-purpose flour
⅔ cup sugar
1 tablespoon baking powder
¼ teaspoon salt
1 cup 8th Continent vanilla soy milk
3 tablespoons canola oil
1 tablespoon lemon peel, grated
2 large eggs
2 cups frozen blueberries, partially thawed
¼ cup unbleached, all-purpose flour
¼ cup ready-to-spread vanilla or cream cheese frosting
2 teaspoons 8th Continent vanilla soy milk
1 teaspoon grated lemon peel

Directions:

Preheat oven to 350°. Spray loaf pan, 9 x 5 x 3 inches, with vegetable cooking spray.

1. In large bowl, stir together 1¾ cups flour, sugar, baking powder, and salt.
2. In small bowl, whip until thoroughly blended 1 cup soy milk, oil, 1 tablespoon lemon peel, and eggs. Gently stir soy milk mixture into flour mixture, just until moistened.
3. Toss slightly thawed blueberries (no longer icy, but still firm) with ¼ cup flour until thoroughly coated. Place in sieve to remove excess flour, then fold gently into batter.
4. Pour batter into pan and bake for 55 minutes or until toothpick inserted into center comes out clean. Cool for 10 minutes in pan on wire rack, then remove from pan and cool completely for about 1 hour.
5. While bread is baking or cooling, stir together frosting, 2 teaspoons soy milk, and 1 teaspoon lemon peel. Let sit to blend lemon flavor. Drizzle or spread over top of cooled bread.

Yield: Makes 1 loaf, 12 slices.

Nutrition Score per serving: 204 calories, 24 percent fat, 68 percent carbohydrates, 8 percent protein, 82 mg calcium, 12 mcg folic acid, 1.2 mg iron, 1 g fiber.

Glazed Blueberry-Lemon Bread is reprinted and amended by Elizabeth Somer with permission of 8th Continent LLC.

Frozen Frappaccino

Just because you're pregnant doesn't mean you can't have a life! This decaf icy coffee drink is a perfect treat. While it tastes great, it also supplies lots of calcium, vitamin D, and B vitamins.

Ingredients:

1 cup vanilla soy milk
1½ cups frozen low-fat yogurt, chocolate or vanilla flavored
½ cup cold, strong decaffeinated coffee
2 cups crushed ice

1 scant teaspoon almond extract
4 tablespoons fat-free, dark chocolate syrup

Directions:
1. In a blender, whirl all ingredients except the chocolate syrup. Blend until thick and creamy. Pour into four glasses.
2. Add 1 tablespoon chocolate syrup to each prepared glass. Stir to mix.

Yield: Makes 4 one-cup servings.

Nutrition Score per serving: 152 calories, 22 percent fat, 67 percent carbohydrates, 11 percent protein, 155 mg calcium, 7 mcg folic acid, 0.6 mg iron, less than 1 g fiber.

FRUIT ICES

For each of the four recipes, blend all ingredients in a blender until smooth. Pour into glasses and freeze. Serve frozen for a healthy alternative to ice cream.

✂ Blueberry Ice

Yield: Makes 2 generous one-cup servings

2 cups frozen blueberries
1 cup nonfat milk
2 tablespoons sugar

Nutrition Score per serving: 172 calories, 4 percent fat, 85 percent carbohydrates, 11 percent protein, 159 mg calcium, 16 mcg folic acid, less than 0.5 mg iron, 3.3 g fiber.

✂ Banana Ice

Yield: Makes 3 one-cup servings

4 frozen bananas, sliced
1 cup nonfat plain yogurt

1 tablespoon vanilla extract
⅛ teaspoon ground nutmeg
2 tablespoons sugar

Nutrition Score per serving: 216 calories, 3 percent fat, 86 percent carbohydrates, 11 percent protein, 172 mg calcium, 39 mcg folic acid, 0.5 mg iron, 3 g fiber.

✿ Kiwi Ice

Yield: Makes 2 generous one-cup servings

4 frozen kiwis, peeled and sliced
¾ cup evaporated nonfat milk
2 tablespoons sugar

Nutrition Score per serving: 216 calories, 3 percent fat, 81 percent carbohydrates, 15 percent protein, 316 mg calcium, 42 mcg folic acid, 1 mg iron, 5.2 g fiber.

✿ Orange, Pineapple, Apricot Ice

Yield: Makes 4 one-cup servings

1 20-ounce can crushed or cubed pineapple, frozen
3 ripe apricots, peeled, pitted, and frozen
¾ cup evaporated nonfat milk
¼ cup orange juice concentrate

Nutrition Score per serving: 163 calories, 2 percent fat, 87 percent carbohydrates, 12 percent protein, 167 mg calcium, 41 mcg folic acid, 0.7 mg iron, 1.6 g fiber.

SAUCES

✿ Raspberry Sauce

Ingredients:
2 cups fresh raspberries, rinsed
4 tablespoons lemon juice
½ cup sugar
1 teaspoon orange flavoring

Directions:
Combine all ingredients in a blender and blend until smooth. Use as a syrup for pancakes, ice cream, or angel food cake.

Yield: Makes 4 one-half cup servings.

Nutrition Score per serving: 131 calories, 2 percent fat, 96 percent carbohydrates, 2 percent protein, 15 mg calcium, 18 mcg folic acid, less than 0.5 mg iron, 3 g fiber.

✿ Fruity Spritzer

1 cup cranberry juice cocktail, chilled
1 cup orange juice, chilled
2 cups lemon- or lime-flavored mineral water, chilled
½ lemon, thinly sliced

Mix all the ingredients in a pitcher and serve over ice.

Yield: Makes 4 servings, 1 cup each.

Nutrition Score per serving: 132 calories, 3 percent fat, 94 percent carbohydrates, 3 percent protein, 21 mg calcium, 39 mcg folic acid, 0.5 mg iron, 1 g fiber.

Glossary

ABBOS: Large chunks of protein in milk that enter the bloodstream and possibly trigger an immunological response that results in the initiation of diabetes in susceptible children.

Abortion: Loss of the fetus before it can survive outside the womb.

Abruption: Premature separation of the placenta from the uterine wall, usually associated with pain.

Acid-base balance: The equilibrium between acids and bases (alkalines) in the body.

Acquired Immune Deficiency Syndrome (AIDS): Disease caused by HIV infection and characterized by suppressed immunity.

Aerobic exercise: Slow, steady, nonstop exercise, such as jogging, walking, biking, or swimming, that requires a steady intake of oxygen and that uses large muscle groups.

Aflatoxin: A potent cancer-causing chemical produced by a mold on tainted peanuts, corn, and other grains.

Amenorrhea: Absence or unusual cessation of menstruation.

Amino acids: The building blocks of protein.

Amniocentesis: Penetration of the uterus through the abdominal wall in order to obtain a sample of amniotic fluid for testing the presence or absence of Down's syndrome and other disorders.

Amniotic fluid: The fluid that surrounds and bathes the developing fetus.

Anemia: A change in the size, color, or number of red blood cells that results in reduced oxygen-carrying capacity of the blood.

Anencephaly: Developmental malformation characterized by the absence of nerve tissue in the head.

Antibiotic: A medication used for the treatment of bacterial infections, including tetracycline and erythromycin.

Antioxidant: A compound that reduces or prevents free-radical tissue damage otherwise associated with degenerative diseases, such as heart disease and cancer, and premature aging.

Anorexia nervosa: A disorder characterized by a refusal to eat, extreme weight loss, and low basal metabolism.

Apgar score: A method for determining an infant's condition at birth by scoring the heart rate, respiratory effort, muscle tone, reflex irritability, and skin color.

Areola: Circular pigmented area surrounding the nipple of the breast.

Arrhythmia: Irregular heartbeat.

Aspartame: A nonnutritive sweetener composed of two amino acids—phenylalanine and aspartic acid—and methanol.

Asthma: A condition characterized by bronchospasms of the lungs and difficulty with breathing that alternates with symptom-free periods.

Autonomy: Independent, self-governing, functioning independently of other parts.

Bacteria: A class of microorganisms, some of which are capable of causing infection and disease in the body.

Beriberi: A disease caused by a deficiency of vitamin B_1 and characterized by nerve disorders, weakness, mental disturbances, dermatitis, and heart failure.

Beta carotene: The building block for vitamin A that also functions as an antioxidant independent of its vitamin A activity and is found in dark green or orange fruits and vegetables.

Bilirubin: A pigment produced by the breakdown of hemoglobin and found in the blood.

Binge eating: A large intake of food in a short period of time, usually less than two hours.

Biotin: One of the B vitamins involved in the metabolism of amino acids, carbohydrates, and fats.

Blastocyte: An early stage in the development of the embryo where cells are arranged in a single layer to form a hollow ball.

Body mass index (BMI): A method of converting your height and weight into one value. The higher the number, the greater chance of being overweight.

Bone density: The amount of calcium imbedded into bone. A measure of bone strength and resistance to the development of osteoporosis.

Braxton Hicks: Mild, irregular contractions of the uterus that sometimes are mistaken for labor.

Bronchitis: Inflammation of the bronchi in the lungs.

Bulimia: Food binges followed by purging by vomiting, taking laxatives, and/or using diuretics.

Caffeine: A central nervous system stimulant found in coffee, chocolate, cola drinks, and other foods and beverages.

Calorie: A measurement of energy in food. A calorie is the amount of heat energy required to raise the temperature of 1,000 grams of water 1° centigrade. Protein and carbohydrates in foods supply 4 calories per gram, fat supplies 9 calories per gram, and alcohol supplies approximately 7 calories per gram.

Carbohydrate: The starches and sugars in food.

Cardiovascular disease (CVD): Diseases of the heart and blood vessels.

Cartilage: A white elastic substance attached to bone surfaces and forming parts of the skeleton.

Cell: A fundamental unit that makes up all body tissues and organs.

Cell differentiation: A process whereby a cell changes into a more complex or specialized form.

Cerebral palsy: Partial paralysis and lack of muscle coordination that results from a defect, injury, or disease of the brain and nervous system.

Cervix: The neck or opening of the uterus.

Cesarean: Birth of a baby through a surgical incision in the abdomen.

Chloasma: Excessive skin pigmentation in certain areas of the body.

Cholesterol: A noncaloric fatlike substance (called a sterol) found in foods of animal origin and produced by the liver. High levels of cholesterol in the blood are associated with heart disease.

Chyme: Semidigested food mixed with stomach enzymes that leaves the stomach and enters the small intestine.

Cleft lip: Congenital fissure of the lip.

Cleft palate: Congenital fissure of the palate.

Clinical deficiency: An overt nutrient deficiency that results in classic symptoms, including beriberi (a deficiency of vitamin B_1), scurvy (a deficiency of vitamin C), and xerophthalmia (a deficiency of vitamin A).

Colic: An umbrella term used to describe periods of intense crying that are difficult to soothe in the newborn during the first three months of life.

Collagen: A protein in connective tissue and the organic substance in teeth and bones.

Colostrum: The first liquid excreted from the breast during the first few days after delivery. Colostrum is higher in protein, some nutrients, and immune-stimulating substances and lower in fat and carbohydrate than is mature breast milk.

Complex carbohydrates: The nutrient-rich starches and fibers present in vegetables, some fruits, and cereals.

Conception: The moment when the male sperm fertilizes the female egg, marking the beginning of a new organism.

Congenital: Present at and persisting after the time of birth.

Constipation: A condition characterized by infrequent and difficult evacuation of feces.

Core temperature: Internal body temperature.

Cornea: The exposed and transparent portion of the eyeball.

Cretinism: A fetal deformity that occurs during development in the uterus and is caused by deficient thyroid activity that usually results from insufficient iodine intake during pregnancy. It is characterized by poor physical and mental development, dry skin, and a low metabolic rate.

Critical period: Stages in fetal development when specific organs or tissues are developing.

Cystic fibrosis: A potentially fatal disease in young children characterized by general dysfunction of the exocrine glands, the pancreas, respiratory system, salivary glands, digestive tract, and other systems.

Dehydration: An inadequate amount of water in the tissues.

Diabetes: A disease characterized by an inability to regulate blood sugar levels so that blood and urine levels of glucose rise in the presence of an absolute or relative deficiency of insulin.

Diastolic blood pressure: The lower of two readings that make up a blood pressure test. Diastolic pressure corresponds to the least amount of pressure in the cardiovascular system at any one time and reflects the pressure inherent in the heart and blood vessels when the heart relaxes between beats (contractions).

Dietitian: A registered dietitian (RD) has received at least a bachelor's degree in nutrition or dietetics from an accredited college, has completed the equivalent of a one-year internship in dietetics, has successfully completed a nationally recognized exam, and is expected to maintain the RD credential by completing each year several units of continuing education in a nutrition-related subject.

Dioxin: A by-product of chemical manufacturing most commonly remembered as the contaminant in Agent Orange, the defoliant used in Vietnam.

Diuretic: Medication that promotes fluid loss by increasing urinary secretion.

DNA: Deoxyribonucleic acid. The helix structure that carries the genetic information in the nucleus of all cells.

Down's syndrome: A congenital condition characterized by mental retardation and abnormal facial features, including a flattened nose.

Early fetal period: The first twenty weeks of gestation.

Eclampsia: The combination of edema, high blood pressure, and protein in the urine that can occur in late pregnancy and can progress to convulsions and coma if left untreated.

Ectoderm: The outermost layer of the three primitive cell layers in the embryo.

Ectopic pregnancy: Pregnancy where the fertilized egg becomes implanted outside the uterus.

Eczema: A skin disease with itching and redness.

Efface: A thinning and softening of the cervix in preparation for labor and delivery.

Embryo: The earliest stage of development of the baby.

Embryonic stage: The first seven to nine weeks of pregnancy.

Endoderm: The innermost layer of the three primitive cell layers of the embryo.

Endometriosis: The presence of endometrial tissue in abnormal places, such as outside the uterus in the abdominal cavity.

Endometrium: The lining of the uterus.

Enriched: The addition to processed foods of a few nutrients to bring the level back to the original vitamin or mineral content. Only four nutrients, vitamin B_1, vitamin B_2, niacin, and iron, are added back during enrichment, while many more nutrients are lost in processing.

Enzyme: A compound that acts as a catalyst in starting chemical reactions in the body.

Epidemiologic studies: The investigation of the factors that influence the frequency and distribution of disease in humans by studying disease incidence in various countries.

Epilepsy: A disease of the nervous system characterized by convulsive seizures caused by temporary disturbances in nerve impulses.

Esophagus: The passageway or tube from the throat to the stomach.

Essential hypertension: High blood pressure not caused by a tumor on the kidneys or other diseases.

Estrogen: A family of related female sex hormones, including estradiol, estrone, and estriol, that are produced by maturing follicles in the ovary, placenta, and adrenal cortex. Estrogens are responsible for the development and growth of female sex organs, many of the physiological changes in pregnancy, and calcium metabolism.

Failure to thrive: A term used to describe infants with growth failure usually caused by poor maternal diet, excessive nutrient and calorie losses from excessive vomiting or diarrhea, or unusually high energy requirements.

Fallopian tubes: The channels that the egg travels down on its way from the ovaries to the uterus.

Fatigue: Feelings of physical or mental weariness, tiredness, or weakness.

Fatty acid: Fat fragments. A fat-soluble molecule that consists of a long chain of carbon atoms with hydrogen attached. Three fatty acids linked to a glycerol molecule make up a triglyceride. An example is linoleic acid.

Fetal alcohol syndrome (FAS): A combination of physical deformities in the infant, including facial deformities, that result from exposure to alcohol in utero.

Fetus: The developing baby in the uterus. A term applied especially from the seventh to the ninth week of gestation until birth.

Fiber: The indigestible residue in food, composed of the carbohydrates cellulose, pectin, and hemicellulose; vegetable gums; and the noncarbohydrate lignin.

Fibrous: Composed of fibers.

Flatulence: Intestinal gas.

Flavonoids: A group of more than 200 compounds found in citrus fruits, leafy vegetables, red onions, and soybeans that may have antioxidant capability in protecting against free radical damage to tissues.

Folic acid: A B vitamin essential for cell replication.

Food and Drug Administration (FDA): An agency of the United States government that monitors the safety of foods, drugs, and cosmetics.

Fortification: The addition of vitamins or minerals to a processed food to levels greater than naturally found. Milk is fortified with vitamin D.

Four food groups: Outdated eating plan based on designated servings of grains, fruits and vegetables, meat, and milk products.

Fructose: A sugar found in fruits and honey. Also called fruit sugar.

Gangrene: Death of tissue usually caused by diminished blood supply and followed by bacterial infection.

Gastric: Pertaining to the stomach.

Gestation: The development of a baby within the uterus from conception to birth.

Gestational diabetes: Diabetes that develops in the mother as a result of pregnancy and usually disappears after the baby is born.

Gingivitis: Inflammation of the gums.

Glucose: The carbohydrate that makes up sugar, blood sugar, and the building blocks of starch.

Glucose tolerance: How well the body handles and regulates blood sugar levels.

Glutathione peroxidase: An antioxidant enzyme that includes selenium.

Glycogen: The storage form of glucose in muscles and liver.

Gram (gm): A unit of weight. Twenty-eight grams equal an ounce.

Hair follicle: The organ that surrounds and nourishes the growing hair shaft.

HDL-cholesterol: The high-density lipoprotein that transports cholesterol from the tissues back to the liver. High levels are associated with a low risk for heart disease.

Head circumference: A measurement of the size of an infant's head taken at the forehead.

Heartburn: A burning chest pain caused by overeating, spicy food, or alcohol intake.

Hematocrit: A test for anemia that measures the percent volume of red blood cells in the blood.

Hemoglobin: The iron-rich protein in red blood cells that transports oxygen. A hemoglobin test measures the percentage of hemoglobin in the blood.

Hemorrhoid: An enlarged vein in the mucus membrane inside or just outside the rectum.

Hormone: Chemical substances secreted by an endocrine gland, such as the adrenals, the pancreas, or the pituitary, that travel in the blood to other parts of the body to help regulate function.

Human chorionic gonadotropin: A gonad-simulating substance in human urine during pregnancy, commonly abbreviated HCG.

Glossary

Human immunodeficiency virus (HIV): Virus responsible for the development of AIDS.

Hydrogenated fats: Polyunsaturated vegetable oils that have been treated with hydrogen, a process called hydrogenation, to form more saturated fats and to convert a liquid oil into a solid fat. Examples include margarine and shortening.

Hyperactivity: Excessive activity.

Hyperemesis gravidarum: Severe nausea and vomiting during pregnancy.

Hyperglycemia: High blood sugar.

Hypertension: High blood pressure.

Hypoglycemia: Low blood sugar.

Immune system: The body's intricate defense system, composed of organs, tissues, and cells, that fight against disease and infection.

Infancy: From birth to the first birthday.

Infertility: The inability to conceive after twelve months or more of intercourse.

Insoluble fiber: Fibers in foods that are not soluble in water and that are associated with a reduced risk for colon cancer. An example is wheat bran.

Insomnia: Inability to fall or stay asleep.

Insulin: A hormone secreted by the pancreas that helps regulate blood sugar levels by facilitating sugar into the cells when blood sugar levels rise above normal.

Intelligence quotient (IQ): A number representing a person's level of intelligence. It is the mental age, as assessed by an intelligence test, multiplied by one hundred and divided by the person's chronological age.

International unit (IU): An arbitrary measurement used for the fat-soluble vitamins A, D, and E. These units standardize the potency of the vitamin rather than measure it by weight. IUs can be converted to weight measurements; for example, 3.33 IU of vitamin A are equivalent to 1 mcg.

Intrauterine device (IUD): A small substance implanted within the uterus as a method of birth control.

Intrauterine growth retardation (IUGR): Small-for-gestational-age fetus.

Iron deficiency anemia: Insufficient red blood cell count resulting from inadequate amounts of iron to produce hemoglobin for red blood cells.

Jaundice: Yellowish discoloration of skin caused by excess accumulation of bile pigments in the blood either from a poorly functioning liver or from increased production of the pigments from hemoglobin.

Kegels: Exercises to tone and strengthen the muscles lining the vaginal and urinary tract walls.

Lactase: The digestive enzyme that breaks down milk sugar (lactose) during digestion.

Lactobacillus acidophilus: A bacteria found in some yogurts that might assist in lactose digestion and maintain a healthy environment in the digestive tract and vagina. Also called L. acidophilus or acidophilus.

Lactobacillus bulgarius: Bacteria found in yogurt that assists in lactose digestion.

Lactose: Milk sugar.

Lactose intolerance: The inability to digest the milk sugar lactose. The condition is characterized by abdominal bloating, cramping, intestinal gas, and diarrhea.

Lanugo: A downy coat that covers the developing fetus in the second trimester and that disappears prior to delivery.

Late fetal period: The second twenty weeks of gestation.

Laxative: An agent that acts mildly to promote defecation.

LDL cholesterol: The low-density lipoprotein that transports cholesterol in the blood. High levels are associated with heart disease.

Legumes: Dried beans and peas, such as kidney or black beans, lentils, or split peas.

Lethargy: Tiredness, sluggishness, or fatigue.

Ligaments: A tough band connecting bone or supporting tissues.

Lightening: A term describing the repositioning of the baby into a head-down position at the lower base of the uterus in preparation for delivery.

Linoleic acid: An essential polyunsaturated fatty acid found in safflower oil, soybean oil, and other vegetable oils. A deficiency of this fatty acid results in infantile eczema.

Listeriosis: An infection caused by an organism of the genus Listeria.

Low birth weight: A term describing an infant born weighing less than 2,500 grams (5 pounds, 8 ounces). These infants may be born prematurely or on time but are too small for their gestational age.

Lymphoma: A tumor of the lymph tissue.

Macrocytic anemia: A type of anemia usually caused by a folic acid or vitamin B_{12} deficiency.

Magnesium: A major mineral essential for bone development, muscle relaxation, nerve transmission, and blood sugar regulation.

Manganese: A trace mineral essential for the formation of connective tissue, fat and cholesterol metabolism, bone development, and blood clotting.

Marginal deficiency: The consumption of some, but not enough, of a nutrient so that overt clinical deficiency is avoided, but more subtle physiological processes are curtailed.

Menses: Pertaining to menstruation.

Menstruation: The monthly discharge of the blood-enriched lining of the uterus. Also called menses.

Mesoderm: The middle layer of cells between the endoderm and ectoderm of the embryo.

Metabolic rate: The amount of calories expended by basic body functioning and daily activities.

Metabolism: The sum of all the chemical processes that convert food and its components to the fundamental chemicals that the body uses for energy or for repair, maintenance, and growth of tissues. Metabolism includes all the building-up processes, such as tissue growth, and all the tearing-down processes, such as breaking down glycogen for energy.

Microgram (mcg): A metric unit of weight equivalent to one one-thousandth of a milligram.

Milk ducts: Canals or passageways in the breast that allow the flow of milk to the nipple.

Milligram (mg): A metric unit of weight equivalent to one one-thousandth of a gram.

Mineral: An inorganic fundamental substance found naturally in the soil and taken up by plants and animals that has specific chemical and structural properties. Many minerals are essential nutrients for growth, maintenance, and repair of tissues.

Miscarriage: Spontaneous loss of fetus before the seventh month.

Miso: A fermented soybean product.

Monosodium glutamate (MSG): A food additive that causes in some people an adverse reaction called Chinese Restaurant Syndrome.

Montgomery's glands: Raised white areas in the areola that secrete oil to keep the nipples lubricated.

Morning sickness: The nausea and vomiting that begin in the first trimester and sometimes continue into the second or even third trimester of pregnancy. Also called hyperemesis gravidarum.

Multiple births: Giving birth to more than one infant at a time, including twins, triplets, and quadruplets.

Myoglobin: The iron-rich compound that holds and transports oxygen within the cell.

Neonatal period: The first twenty-eight days following birth.

Nervous system: The brain and nerves that coordinate and control responses to stimuli and that condition behavior and all thinking processes.

Neural tube defects: A type of birth defect in the neural tube that becomes the spinal cord and brain when this tube does not close in the developing embryo. Examples of neural tube defects include spina bifida, anencephaly, and encephalocele. These birth defects result from both genetic and environmental factors, including poor maternal intake of folic acid during pregnancy.

Neurotransmitter: Chemical that transmits messages between nerve cells or between nerve cells and organs or muscles.

Nicotine: A stimulant and addictive drug found in tobacco.

Nitrites: Food additives that are converted to carcinogenic substances, called nitrosamines, in the stomach.

Nutrient: A substance essential to the body that must be obtained from the diet. Essential nutrients include protein, linoleic acid, vitamins, minerals, and water.

Obesity: Body-fat weight more than 20 percent above a desirable body weight. The body weight is excess fat, not muscle or lean tissue.

Omega-3 fatty acids: Polyunsaturated fats in fish oils, including eicosapentaenoic acid (EPA) and docosahexaenoic acid (DHA), that might reduce the risk for developing cardiovascular disease and are suspected to be essential fats in the development of normal vision in infants.

Osteoporosis: A decrease in bone density resulting in brittle, porous bones that are susceptible to fractures.

Otitis media: Inflammation of the middle ear.

Ovary: A glandular organ in the female reproductive system that produces the ovum (egg) and secretes the female hormones estrogen and progesterone. Loss of ovarian function is the deciding factor in menopause.

Over-the-counter medications (OTC): Medications that can be purchased without a prescription.

Ovulation: The maturation and discharge of a mature egg from the ovary.

Ovum: Egg. The female reproductive substance that can develop into a baby if fertilized by the male sperm.

Pallor: Pale. Absence of skin color.

Pancreas: An endocrine gland in the abdomen that secretes a variety of hormones, including blood sugar–regulating hormones such as insulin and glucagon, and digestive enzymes such as pancreatic lipase.

Pantothenic acid: One of the B vitamins involved in the metabolism of amino acids, carbohydrates, and fats.

Pap smear: A routine test for cervical cancer.

Passive smoking: Inhaling other people's cigarette smoke.

Penicillamine: An amino acid derived from penicillin that is used in the treatment of disease associated with excess copper accumulation in the body.

Perinatal period: Includes the late fetal period and the neonatal period, i.e., the time immediately surrounding birth.

Peristalsis: A wavelike motion in the muscles that line the digestive tract that propels food downward.

Pernicious anemia: Anemia caused by an inadequate secretion of a digestive substance called intrinsic factor, necessary for vitamin B_{12} absorption.

Phenylalanine: An amino acid present in many foods.

Phenylketonuria (PKU): A genetically determined metabolic disorder associated with mental retardation.

Phytochemicals: Nonnutritive substances in plants that help in the prevention of disease. Examples include alliin in garlic and bioflavonoids in citrus fruit.

Pica: A desire to eat nonfood substances, such as chalk or dirt.

Placebo: An inactive substance, such as water, used in scientific studies to compare the effects of an experimental drug or nutrient with an inactive substance.

Placenta: The organ that links the blood supply of a mother with the developing fetus.

Placenta previa: A condition wherein the placenta is attached at the lower portion of the uterus, rather than higher up in the uterus.

Polyunsaturated fat: A triglyceride having at least two of its three fatty acids unsaturated (i.e., they have room for the addition of more hydrogen atoms). Vegetable oils and fish oils are polyunsaturated fats.

Postneonatal period: From twenty-eight days after delivery to the first birthday.

Postpartum: After delivery.

Preeclampsia: High blood pressure, protein in the urine, and edema occurring during the latter half of pregnancy. (See *eclampsia* and *pregnancy-induced hypertension.*)

Pregnancy-induced hypertension (PIH): Another term for preeclampsia.

Pregnancy tumors: Benign fingerlike growths of inflamed gum tissue between the teeth.

Prenatal: Preceding birth.

Preterm infant: Infant born under thirty-seven weeks gestation.

Preterm labor: Initiation of labor prior to a woman's due date.

Progesterone: A hormone produced by the ovaries in preparation for the reception and development of a fertilized egg in the uterus. This hormone also is produced by the placenta during pregnancy.

Progestin: A substance that has the ability of the specific hormone of the corpus luteum to prepare the lining of the uterus for implantation of the fertilized egg.

Prolactin: A hormone secreted by the pituitary in the brain, which stimulates milk secretion.

Prostaglandins: A group of hormonelike substances formed from polyunsaturated fatty acids that have a profound effect on the body, including contraction of smooth muscle and dilation or contraction of blood vessels in the regulation of blood pressure.

Protein: Compounds made up of amino acids found in many foods.

Pulse: The impact felt in the blood vessels caused by the blood as it is forced out by a contraction of the heart.

Quickening: The fluttering feeling in the abdomen that a mother experiences in the second or third trimester as a result of movement of the developing fetus.

Recommended Dietary Allowance (RDA): Suggested amounts of most vitamins and minerals needed by healthy individuals to avoid clinical nutrient deficiencies, based on age, gender, and size.

Red blood cells: The iron-rich cells in the blood that are responsible for transporting oxygen to the tissues and removing and transporting carbon dioxide, a waste product from cellular metabolism, back to the lungs for exhalation.

Reference person: A theoretical person with average height, weight, and activity level on which the Recommended Dietary Allowances are based.

Relaxin: A hormone released during pregnancy that helps soften the mother's ligaments in preparation for childbirth.

Rickets: Vitamin D deficiency in infancy and childhood characterized by poorly calcified bones resulting in bowed legs and deformed rib cage.

Rubella: A mild viral infection, characterized by fever and a skin rash, that can be harmful to the developing fetus if a previously unexposed mother contracts the infection during pregnancy.

Saccharin: A nonnutritive sweetener.

Salt: Sodium chloride.

Saturated fat: A triglyceride with the maximum possible number of hydrogen atoms. Saturated fats, such as butter and stick margarine, are typically solid at room temperature and are linked to an increased risk for developing heart disease and possibly breast cancer.

Scurvy: A disease caused by a deficiency of vitamin C and characterized by bleeding gums, loose teeth, small hemorrhages below the skin, and weakness.

Semen: The fluid discharge at ejaculation in the male that consists of sperm capable of fertilizing an egg in a female as the first step in pregnancy.

Serotonin: A nerve chemical in the brain that helps regulate sleep, pain, mood, and appetite.

Serum ferritin: The form of iron in the blood that is a sensitive indicator of tissue iron levels. A value less than 20 mcg/L indicates iron deficiency.

Sidestream smoke: Smoke from the end of a burning cigarette as well as that which is exhaled after a smoker puffs on a cigarette.

Skeletal: Pertaining to the bones.

Small-for-gestational-age infants: Infants born underweight, whatever the gestational age.

Sodium: An electrolyte that combines with chloride to make table salt.

Sphincter: A ringlike muscle that closes a natural opening, such as the passageway from the esophagus to the stomach or from the stomach to the small intestine.

Spina bifida: A congenital deformity of the spine whereby the spinal column fails to close properly.

Spinal cord: The spine or vertebral column that houses the nerve connections between the brain and the body.

Spontaneous abortion: Sudden expulsion of the fetus before it is able to survive outside the womb.

Starch: Complex carbohydrates found in vegetables, some fruits, and cereals.

Stillbirth: A baby that is born dead.

Strict vegetarian: A subgroup of vegetarians who avoid all foods of animal origin.

Sucrose: Table sugar. A simple carbohydrate made up of two molecules, glucose and fructose.

Sudden infant death syndrome (SIDS): Unexplained death in infants less than one year old while sleeping. The third leading cause of infant mortality.

Sugar: A sweet-tasting simple carbohydrate, such as sucrose, glucose, or fructose.

Sulfites: Additives used in wine, dried fruits, and potatoes that cause adverse allergic reactions in some asthmatic people.

Systolic blood pressure: The pressure in the blood vessels when the heart contracts.

Tendon: A fibrous cord of connective tissue continuous with the muscles and that attaches to bone or cartilage.

Teratogen: An agent of disease that causes congenital deformities or other serious disorders during fetal development.

Testosterone: The male hormone responsible for secondary male characteristics.

Tofu: A curd made from soybeans that is high in protein.

Total iron binding capacity (TIBC): A blood test for iron status.

Toxemia: A general term given to disorders of late pregnancy when there is high blood pressure, protein in the urine, and edema. Also called preeclampsia and eclampsia.

Toxoplasma gondii bacteria: A bacteria commonly found in cat feces that causes a potentially serious maternal infection called toxoplasmosis that results in blindness and mental retardation in the fetus.

Trace mineral: An essential mineral found in the body in amounts less than .0005 percent of body weight.

Trans fatty acids (TFA): Polyunsaturated fats formed during hydrogenation of vegetable oils to make margarine or shortening. The shape of these fats is different from other polyunsaturated fats, and it is suspected that they act more like saturated fats in the promotion of heart disease.

Triglyceride: The most common type of calorie-containing fat found in food, a person's fat tissues, and the blood.

Trimester: Pregnancy is characterized by three general periods: the first (weeks one to thirteen), second (weeks fourteen to twenty-seven), and third (weeks twenty-eight to forty) trimesters.

Tryptophan: An amino acid that also is a building block for the nerve chemical serotonin that helps regulate sleep, pain, mood, and appetite.

Tubal pregnancy: A condition wherein the fertilized egg implants in the fallopian tube, rather than in the uterus.

Umbilical cord: The tissue that acts as a passageway in connecting the baby with the placenta and that transfers all nutrients and waste products to and from the baby, respectively.

Urogenital system: The urinary tract and sexual organs.

Uterus: A hollow organ in the female in which the baby develops during gestation.

UV light: Ultraviolet rays from the sun.

Varicose veins: Enlargement of the blood vessels that return blood to the heart from the body.

Vernix caseosa: A waxy protective covering over the fetus that protects the delicate skin from the mineralized amniotic fluid.

Villi: Small protrusions that occur uniformly over a smooth surface and increase surface area.

Vitamin: An essential nutrient that must be obtained from the diet and is required by the body in minute amounts.

Whole grain: An unrefined grain that retains its edible outside layers (the bran) and the highly nutritious inner germ (for example, wheat germ).

Selected References

Introduction

Al M, Smook A, Houwelingen A, et al: Fat intake of women during normal pregnancy: Relationship with maternal and neonatal essential fatty acid status. *J Am Col N* 1996;15:49–55.

Brown J, Kahn E: Maternal nutrition and the outcome of pregnancy. *Clin Perin* 1997;24:433–449.

Emanuel I: An assessment of maternal intergenerational factors in pregnancy outcome. *Am J Epidem* 1997;146:820–825.

King J: Physiology of pregnancy and nutrient metabolism. *Am J Clin N* 2000; 71:1218–1225.

Chapter 1: The Prepregnancy Diet

Allen L: Anemia and iron deficiency: Effects on pregnancy outcome. *Am J Clin N* 2000;71:1280–1284.

Belew C: Herbs and the childbearing woman: Guidelines for midwives. *J Nurse-Mid* 1999;44:231–252.

Bolumar F, Olsen J, Rebagliato M, et al: Body mass index and delayed conception: A European multicenter study on infertility and subfecundity. *Am J Epidem* 2000; 151:1072–1079.

Bunin G: Maternal diet during pregnancy and risk of brain tumors in children. *Int J Canc* 1998;S11:23–25.

Clapp J, Simonian S, Lopez B, et al: The one-year morphometric and neurodevelopmental outcome of the offspring of women who continued to exercise regularly throughout pregnancy. *Am J Obst G* 1998;178:594–599.

Cook J: Defining optimal body iron. *P Nut Soc* 1999;58:489–495.

Czeizel A: Periconceptional folic acid containing multivitamin supplementation. *Eur J Clin N* 1998;78:151–161.

Eskenazi B, Stapleton A, Kharrazi M, et al: Associations between maternal decaffeinated and caffeinated coffee consumption and fetal growth and gestational duration. *Epidemiolog* 1999;10:242–249.

Gale C, Martyn C, Kellinggray S, et al: Intrauterine programming of adult body composition. *J Clin End* 2001;86:267–272.

Godfrey K: Maternal regulation of fetal development and health in adult life. *Eur J Ob Gy* 1998;78:141–150.

Jensen T, Henriksen T, Henrik N, et al: Caffeine intake and fecundability: A follow-up study among 430 Danish couples planning their first pregnancy. *Repro Tox* 1998;12:289–295.

Johnston R, Staples D: Knowledge and use of folic acid by women of childbearing age: United States, 1997. *J Am Med A* 1997;278:892–893.

Kennedy E, Ohls J, Carlson S, et al: The Healthy Eating Index: Design and applications. *J Am Diet A* 1995;95:1103–1108.

Kilbride J, Baker T, Parapia L, et al: Anemia during pregnancy as a risk factor for iron-deficiency anemia in infancy: A case-control study in Jordan. *Int J Epid* 1999; 28:461–468.

Kirchengast S, Hartmann B: Maternal prepregnancy weight status and pregnancy weight gain as major determinants for newborn weight and size. *Ann Hum Bio* 1998;25:17–28.

Kloeblen A: Folate knowledge, intake from fortified grain products, and periconceptional supplementation patterns of a sample of low-income pregnant women according to the Health Belief Model. *J Am Diet A* 1999;99:33–38.

Krebs-Smith S, Cleveland L, Ballard-Barbash R, et al: Characterizing food intake patterns of American adults. *Am J Clin N* 1997;65 (suppl):1264S–1268S.

Kumari A: Pregnancy outcome in women with morbid obesity. *Int J Gyn O* 2001; 73:101–107.

Leger J, Jaquet D, Marchal C, et al: Syndrome X: A consequence of intrauterine malnutrition? *J Ped End M* 2000;13:1257–1259.

Locksmith G, Duff P: Preventing neural tube defects: The importance of periconceptional folic acid supplements. *Obstet Gyn* 1998;91:1027–1034.

Looker A, Dallman P, Carrol M, et al: Prevalence of iron deficiency in the United States. *J Am Med A* 1997;277:973–976.

Lucas A: Programming by early nutrition: An experimental approach. *J Nutr* 1998; 128:S401–S406.

Mancuso S, Palla G: Intrauterine nutrition and development. *Adv Contrac* 1996; 12:285–291.

Mardis A, Kramerler C, Gerrior S, et al: Nutrient intake of pregnant and breast-feeding women: An examination of 9 nutrients of public health concern. *FASEB J* 1999;13:A254 (meeting abstract).

Mastroiacovo P, Mazzone T, Addis A, et al: High vitamin A intake in early pregnancy and major malformations: A multicenter prospective controlled study. *Teratology* 1999;59:7–11.

Mathews F, Neil H: Nutrient intakes during pregnancy in a cohort of nulliparous women. *J Hum Nu Di* 1998;11:151–161.

Menard M: Vitamin and mineral supplement prior to and during pregnancy. *Ob Gyn Clin* 1997;24:479–498.

Mills J, Simpson J, Cunningham G, et al: Vitamin A and birth defects. *Am J Obst G* 1997;177:31–36.

Munger R, Romitti P, West N, et al: Maternal intake of folate, vitamin B$_{12}$, and zinc and risk of orofacial cleft birth defects. *Am J Epidem* 1997;145:117 (meeting abstract).

Nelen W, Blom H, Thomas C, et al: Methylenetetrahydrofolate reductase polymorphism affects the change in homocysteine and folate concentrations resulting from low dose folic acid supplementation in women with unexplained recurrent miscarriages. *J Nutr* 1998;128:1336–1341.

Omu A, Al-Bader A, Dashti H, et al: Magnesium in human semen: Possible role in premature ejaculation. *Arch Androl* 2001;46:59–66.

Putnam J: US food supply providing more food and calories. *Food Rev* 1999; Sept-Oct:2–12.

Rasmussen L, Ovesen L, Biilow I, et al: Folate intake, lifestyle factors, and homocysteine concentrations in younger and older women. *Am J Clin N* 2000;72:1156–1163.

Sayer A, Cooper C, Barker D: Is lifespan determined in utero? *Arch Dis Ch* 1997;77:F162–F164.

Schildkraut J, Demark-Wahnefried W, DeVoto E, et al: Environmental contaminants and body fat distribution. *Canc Epid B* 1999;8:179–183.

Scholl T, Reilly T: Anemia, iron and pregnancy outcome. *J Nutr* 2000;130:S443–S447. USDA. *America's Eating Habits: Changes & Consequences* (Elizabeth Frazao, editor). ERS. Agriculture Information Bulletin Number 750. Washington, D.C., 1999, pp 77,134.

Shaw G, Velie E, Schaffer D: Risk of neural tube defect–affected pregnancies among obese women. *J Am Med A* 1996;275:1093–1096.

Sifakis S, Pharmakides G: Anemia in pregnancy. *Ann NY Acad* 2000;900:125–136.

Signorello L, Harlow B, Wang S, et al: Saturated fat intake and the risk of severe hyperemesis gravidarum. *Epidemiolog* 1998;9:636–640.

Sternfeld B: Physical activity and pregnancy outcome. *Sport Med* 1997;23:33–47.

Tamura T, Goldenberg R, Johnston K, et al: Serum concentrations of zinc, folate, vitamins A and E, and proteins, and their relationships to pregnancy outcome. *Act Obst Sc* 1997;76:63–70.

Van der Put N, van Straaten H, Trijbels F, et al: Folate, homocysteine and neural tube defects: An overview. *Diabet M R* 2001;17:131–136.

Velie E, Block G, Shaw G, et al: Maternal supplemental and dietary zinc intake and the occurrence of neural tube defects in California. *Am J Epidem* 1999;150:605–616.

Waterland R, Garza C: Potential mechanisms of metabolic imprinting that lead to chronic disease. *Am J Clin N* 1999; 69:179–197.

Whincup P: Fetal origins of cardiovascular risk: Evidence from studies on children. *P Nutr Soc* 1998;57:123–127.

Wu T, Buck G, Mendola P: Can regular multivitamin/mineral supplementation modify the relation between maternal smoking and select adverse birth outcomes? *Ann Epidemi* 1998;8:175–183.

Xiong X, Buekens P, Alexander S, et al: Anemia during pregnancy and birth outcome: A meta-analysis. *Am J Perin* 2000;17:137–146.

Chapter 2: The Baby-wise Diet

Dietary guidelines 2000: fruits and vegetables first. *www.5aday.com/meal_comparison.html*

Fox M: Obesity costs U.S. $238 billion a year—survey. Press release/ Frazao E (editor): USDA's *America's Eating Habits: Changes and Consequences*.

Gibbs W: Gaining on fat. *Sci Am* 1996;August:88–94.

Gorsky R, Pamuk E, Williamson D, et al: The 25-year health-care costs of women who remain overweight after 40 years of age. *Am J Prev M* 1996;12:388–394.

Putnam J, Allshouse J: U.S. per capita food supply trends. *Food Review*. USDA Economic Research Service, September-October 1998, pages 2–11.

Subar A, Krebs-Smith S, Cook A, et al: Dietary sources of nutrients among US adults, 1989 to 1991. *J Am Diet A* 1998;98:537–547.

Chapter 3: The Nutrition Primer for Pregnancy

Azais-Braesco V, Pascal G: Vitamin A in pregnancy: Requirements and safety limits. *Am J Clin N* 2000;71(suppl):1325S–1333S.

Baker W: Iron deficiency in pregnancy, obstetrics, and gynecology. *Hemat Oncol* 2000;14:1061–1077.

Brunvand L, Quigstad E, Urdal P, et al: Vitamin D deficiency and fetal growth. *Ear Hum Dev* 1996;45:27–33.

Casanueva E, Vadillo-Ortego F, Pfeffer F, et al: Vitamin C and premature rupture of chorioamniotic membranes. *Nutr Res* 1998;18:241–245.

Caulfield L, Zavaleta N, Shankar A, et al: Potential contribution of maternal zinc supplementation during pregnancy to maternal and child survival. *Am J Clin N* 1998;68:S499–S508.

Dylewski M, Mastro A, Modi C, et al: Maternal selenium nutrition and neonatal immune development. *FASEB J* 2000;14:A239 (meeting abstract).

Glann F, Glenn W, Burdi A: Prenatal fluoride for growth and development. *J Dent Child* 1997;Sept/Oct: 319–321.

Handwerker S, Altura B, Altura B: Serum ionized magnesium and other electrolytes in the antenatal period of human pregnancy. *J Am Col N* 1996;15:36–43.

Hernandez-Avila M, Sanin L, Romeiu I, et al: Higher milk intake during pregnancy is associated with lower maternal and umbilical cord lead levels in postpartum women. *Envir Res* 1997;74:116–117.

Hindmarsh P, Geary M, Rodeck C, et al: Effect of early maternal iron stores on placental weight and structure. *Lancet* 2000;356:719–723.

Jain S, Wise R, Bocchini J: Vitamin E and vitamin E quinone levels in red blood cells and plasma of newborn infants and their mothers. *J Am Col N* 1996;15:44–46.

Keen C, Uriu-Hare J, Hawk S, et al: Effect of copper deficiency on prenatal development and pregnancy outcome. *Am J Clin N* 1998;67:1003–1011.

Kilbride J, Baker T, Parapia L, et al: Anaemia during pregnancy as a risk factor for iron-deficiency anaemia in infancy. *Int J Epid* 1999;28:461–468.

King J: Determinants of maternal zinc status during pregnancy. *Am J Clin N* 2000;71:1334–1343.

Koo W, Walters J, Esterlitz J, et al: Maternal calcium supplementation and fetal bone mineralization. *Obstet Gyn* 1999;94:577–582.

Maden M, Gale E, Zile M: The role of vitamin A in the development of the central nervous system. *J Nutr* 1998;128:S471–S475.

Mathews F: Antioxidant nutrients in pregnancy: A systematic review of the literature. *Nutr Res R* 1996;9:175–195.

Milman N, Bergholt T, Byg K, et al: Iron status and iron balance during pregnancy: A critical reappraisal of iron supplementation. *Act Obst Sc* 1999;78:749–757.

Mock D, Stadler D, Stratton S, et al: Biotin status assessed longitudinally in pregnant women. *J Nutr* 1997;127:710–716.

Msolla M, Kinabo J: Prevalence of anaemia in pregnant women during the last trimester. *Int J F S N* 1997;48:265–270.

Ortega R, Martinez R, Quintas E, et al: Calcium levels in maternal milk: Relationships with calcium intake during the third trimester of pregnancy. *Br J Nutr* 1998;79:501–507.

Prentice A: Maternal calcium metabolism and bone mineral status. *Am J Clin N* 2000;71:1312–1316.

Raju T, Langenberg P, Bhutani V, et al: Vitamin E prophylaxis to reduce retinopathy of prematurity. *J Pediat* 1997;131:844–850.

Ramakrishnan U, Manjrekar R, Rivera J, et al: Micronutrients and pregnancy outcome: A review of the literature. *Nutr Res* 1999;19:103–159.

Scholl T, Johnson W: Folic acid: Influence on the outcome of pregnancy. *Am J Clin N* 2000;71:1295–1303.

Velie E, Block G, Shaw G, et al: Maternal supplemental and dietary zinc intake and the occurrence of neural tube defects in California. *Am J Epidem* 1999;150:605–616.

Villar J, Belizan J: Same nutrient, different hypotheses: Disparities in trials of calcium supplementation during pregnancy. *Am J Clin N* 2000;71:1375–1379.

Xiong X, Buekens P, Alexander S, et al: Anemia during pregnancy and birth outcome: A meta-analysis. *Am J Perin* 2000;17:137–146.

Zile M: Vitamin A and embryonic development: An overview. *J Nutr* 1998;128:S455–S458.

Chapter 4: Your Changing Body: What to Expect

Godfrey K, Barket D, Osmond C: Disproportionate fetal growth and raised IgE concentration in adult life. *Clin Exp Al* 1994;24:641–648.

Hediger M, Overpeck M, Kuczmarski R, et al: Muscularity and fatness of infants and young children born small- or large-for-gestational age. *Pediatrics* 1998;102:360.

Phillips D, Cooper C, Fall C, et al: Fetal growth and autoimmune thyroid disease. *Quart J Med* 1993;86:247–253.

Sorensen H, Sabroe S, Olsen J, et al: Birth weight and cognitive function in young adult life. *Br Med J* 1997;316:401–403.

Strauss R: Adult functional outcome of those born small for gestational age: Twenty-six-year follow-up of the 1970 British Birth Cohort. *J Am Med A* 2000;283:625–632.

Chapter 5: Nutrition during the First Trimester

Badart-Smook A, Houwelingen A, Al M, et al: Fetal growth is associated positively with maternal intake of riboflavin and negatively with maternal intake of linoleic acid. *Hormone Res* 1998;49:28–31.

Bianco A, Smilen S, Davis Y, et al: Pregnancy outcome and weight gain recommendations for the morbidly obese woman. *Obstet Gyn* 1998;91:97–102.

Carmichael S, Abrams B, Selvin S: The pattern of maternal weight gain in women with good pregnancy outcomes. *Am J Pub He* 1997;87:1984–1988.

Caulfield L, Stoltzfus R, Witter F: Implications of the Institute of Medicine weight gain recommendations for preventing adverse pregnancy outcomes in black and white women. *Am J Pub He* 1998;88:1168–1174.

Choi W, Little J, Arslan A: Prenatal vitamin supplementation and pediatric brain tumors: Huge international variation in use and possible reduction in risk. *Child Nerv* 1998;14:551–557.

Conti J, Abraham S, Taylor A: Eating behavior and pregnancy outcome. *J Psychosom* 1998;44:465–477.

Crystal S, Bowen D, Bernstein I: Morning sickness and salt intake, food cravings, and food aversions. *Physl Behav* 1999;67:181–187.

Dawson E, Evans D, Conway M, et al: Vitamin B_{12} and folate bioavailability from two prenatal multivitamin/multimineral supplements. *Am J Perin* 2000;17:193–199.

Emelianova S, Mazzotta P, Einarson A, et al: Prevalence and severity of nausea and vomiting in pregnancy and effect of vitamin supplementation. *Clin Inv M* 1999;22:106–110.

Feig D, Naylor C: Eating for two: Are guidelines for weight gain during pregnancy too liberal? *Lancet* 1998;351:1054–1055.

Flaxman S, Sherman P: Morning sickness: A mechanism for protecting mother and embryo. *Q Rev Biol* 2000;75:113–148.

Houston D, Johnson M: Does vitamin C intake protect against lead toxicity? *Nutr Rev* 2000;58:73–75.

Menard M: Vitamin and mineral supplement prior to and during pregnancy. *Ob Gyn Clin* 1997;24:479–498.

Merialdi M, Caulfield L, Zavaleta N, et al: Adding zinc to prenatal iron and folate tablets improves fetal neurobehavioral development. *Am J Obst G* 1999; 180:483–490.

Muscati S, Gray-Donald K, Koski K: Timing of weight gain during pregnancy: Promoting fetal growth and minimizing maternal weight retention. *Int J Obes* 1996;20:526–532.

Park E, Wagenbichler P, Elmadfa I: Effects of multivitamin/mineral supplementation, at nutritional doses, on plasma antioxidant status and DNA damage estimated by sister chromatid exchanges in lymphocytes in pregnant women. *Int J Vit N* 1999;69:396–402.

Rainville A: Pica practices of pregnant women are associated with lower maternal hemoglobin level at delivery. *J Am Diet A* 1998;98:293–296.

Reynolds R, Phillips D: Long-term consequences of intrauterine growth retardation. *Hormone Res* 1998;49:28–91.

Ross E, Szabo N, Tebbett I: Lead content of calcium supplements. *J Am Med A* 2000;284:1425–1429.

Satter N, Berry C, Greer I: Essential fatty acids in relation to pregnancy complications and fetal development. *Br J Obst G* 1998;105:1248–1255.

Schaefer C, Brown A, Wyatt R, et al: Maternal prepregnant body mass and risk of schizophrenia in adult offspring. *Schizo Bull* 2000;26:275–286.

Schieve L, Cogswell M, Scanlon K, et al: Prepregnancy body mass index and pregnancy weight gain: Associations with preterm delivery. *Obstet Gyn* 2000; 96:194–200.

Siman C, Eriksson U: Vitamin E decreases the occurrence of malformations in the offspring of diabetic rats. *Diabetes* 1997;46:1054–1061.

Snattingius S, Bergstrom R, Lipworth L, et al: Prepregnancy weight and the risk of adverse pregnancy outcomes. *N Eng J Med* 1998;338:147–152.

Wauben I, Wainwright P: The influence of neonatal nutrition on behavioral development: A critical appraisal. *Nutr Rev* 1999;57:35–44.

Zhang J, Savitz D: Exercise during pregnancy among US women. *Ann Epidemi* 1996;6:53–59.

Chapter 6: Nutrition during the Second Trimester

Alcock N, Lederman R, Wilson D, et al: Potential mercury exposure through diet in pregnant women and women of childbearing age. *FASEB J* 1997;11:2351.

Bates J, Young I, Galway L, et al: Antioxidant status and lipid peroxidation in diabetic pregnancy. *Br J Nutr* 1997;78:523–532.

Chappell L, Seed P, Briley A, et al: Effect of antioxidants on the occurrence of preeclampsia in women at increased risk: A randomized trial. *Lancet* 1999; 354:810–816.

Davidson P, Myers G, Cox C, et al: Effects of prenatal and postnatal methylmercury exposure from fish consumption on neurodevelopment. *J Am Med A* 1998; 280:701–707.

Fitzsimons D, Dwyer J, Palmer C, et al: Nutrition and oral health guidelines for pregnant women, infants, and children. *J Am Diet A* 1998;98:182–189.

Hickey C, Cliver S, McNeal S, et al: Prenatal weight gain patterns and birth weight among nonobese black and white women. *Obstet Gyn* 1996;88:490–496.

Hubel C: Oxidative stress in the pathogenesis of preeclampsia. *P Soc Exp M* 1999;222:222–235.

Jovanovic-Peterson L, Peterson C: Exercise and the nutritional management of diabetes during pregnancy. *Ob Gyn Clin* 1996;23:75–85.

Jovanovic-Peterson L, Peterson C: Vitamin and mineral deficiencies which may predispose to glucose intolerance of pregnancy. *J Am Col N* 1996;15:14–20.

Kharb S: Vitamin E and C in preeclampsia. *Eur J Ob Gy* 2000;93:37–39.

Kitzmiller J, Buchanan T, Kjos S, et al: Preconception care of diabetes, congenital malformations, and spontaneous abortions. *Diabet Care* 1996;19:514–541.

Moutquin J, Garner P, Burrows R, et al: Report of the Canadian Hypertension Society Consensus Conference. 2. Nonpharmacologic management and prevention of hypertensive disorders in pregnancy. *Can Med A J* 1997;157:907–919.

Ortega R, Martinez R, Lopez-Sobaler A, et al: Influence of calcium intake on gestational diabetes. *Ann Nutr M* 1999;43:37–46.

Ozan H, Esmer A, Kolsal N, et al: Plasma ascorbic acid level and erythrocyte fragility in preeclampsia and eclampsia. *Eur J Ob Gy* 1997;71:35–40.

Poranen A, Ekblad U, Uotila P, et al: The effect of vitamin C and E on placental lipid peroxidation and antioxidative enzymes in perfused placenta. *Act Obst Sc* 1998;77:372–376.

Ritchie L, King J: Dietary calcium and pregnancy-induced hypertension: Is there a relation? *Am J Clin N* 2000;71(suppl):1371S–1374S.

Sanchez S, Zhang C, Malinow R, et al: Plasma folate, vitamin B_{12}, and homocyst(e)ine concentrations in preeclamptic and normotensive Peruvian women. *Am J Epidem* 2001;153:474–480.

Skarb S: Vitamin E and C in preeclampsia. *Eur J Ob Gy* 2000;93:37–39.

Spinillo A, Capuzzo E, Piazzi G, et al: Risk for spontaneous preterm delivery by combined body mass index and gestational weight gain patterns. *Act Obst Sc* 1998;77:32–36.

Strauss R, Dietz W: Low maternal weight gain in the second or third trimester increases the risk for intrauterine growth retardation. *J Nutr* 1999;129:988–993.

To W, Cheung W: The relationship between weight gain in pregnancy, birth weight and postpartum weight retention. *Aust NZ J O* 1998;38:176–179.

Williams M, King I, Sorensen T, et al: Risk of preeclampsia in relation to elaidic acid (trans fatty acids) in maternal erythrocytes. *Gynecol Obs* 1998;46:84–87.

Yanik F, Amanvermez R, Yanik A, et al: Preeclampsia and eclampsia associated with increased lipid peroxidation and decreased serum vitamin E levels. *Int J Gyn O* 1999;64:27–33.

Zhang J, Zeisler J, Hatch M, et al: Epidemiology of pregnancy-induced hypertension. *Epidemiol R* 1997;19:218–232.

Chapter 7: Nutrition during the Third Trimester

Cardini F, Weixin H: Moxibustion for correction of breech presentation. *J Am Med A* 1998;280:1580–1584.

Carmichael S, Abrams B: A critical review of the relationship between gestational weight gain and preterm delivery. *Obstet Gyn* 1997;89:865–873.

Chen D, Nommsen-Rivers L, Dewey K, et al: Stress during labor and delivery and early lactation performance. *Am J Clin N* 1998;68:335–344.

Koo W, Walters J, Esterlitz J, et al: Maternal calcium supplementation and fetal bone mineralization. *Obstet Gyn* 1999;94:577–582.

Mardones-Santander F, Salazar G, Rosso P, et al: Maternal body composition near term and birth weight. *Obstet Gyn* 1998;91:873–877.

Neufeld L, Pelletier D, Haas J: The timing of maternal weight gain during pregnancy and fetal growth. *Am J Hum B* 1999;11:627–637.

Ortega R, Martinez R, Quintas M, et al: Calcium levels in maternal milk: Relationships with calcium intake during the third trimester of pregnancy. *Br J Nutr* 1998;79:501–507.

Siega-Riz A, Adair L, Hobel C: Maternal underweight status and inadequate rate of weight gain during the third trimester of pregnancy increase the risk of preterm delivery. *J Nutr* 1996;126:146–153.

Chapter 8: Nutrition and High-Risk Pregnancies

Black R: Transmission of HIV-1 in the breast-feeding process. *J Am Diet A* 1996;96: 267–274.

Brown J, Carlson M: Nutrition and multifetal pregnancy. *J Am Diet A* 2000;100: 343–348.

Decarli B, Cavadini C, Grin J, et al: Food and nutrient intakes in a group of 11- to 16-year-old Swiss teenagers. *Int J Vit N* 2000;70:139–147.

Erick M, Yotides E: Do women with triplets eat for three? *J Am Diet A* 1996;96 (suppl):A69.

Friscancho A: Reduction of birth weight among infants born to adolescents: Maternal-fetal growth competition. *Ann NY Acad* 1997;817:272–280.

Harel Z, Riggs S, Vaz R, et al: Adolescents and calcium: What they do and do not know and how much they consume. *J Adoles H* 1998;22:225–228.

Hediger M, Scholl T, Schall J: Implications of the Camden study of adolescent pregnancy: Interactions among maternal growth, nutritional status, and body composition. *Ann NY Acad* 1997;817:281–291.

Jolly M, Sebire N, Harris J, et al: Obstetric risks of pregnancy in women less than 18 years old. *Obstet Gyn* 2000;96:962–966.

Lenders C, Hediger M, Scholl T, et al: Gestational age and infant size at birth are associated with dietary sugar intake among pregnant adolescents. *J Nutr* 1997;127:1113–1117.

Luke B: What is the influence of maternal weight gain on the fetal growth of twins? *Clin O Gyne* 1998;41:57–64.

Luke B, Bigger H, Leurgans S, et al: The cost of prematurity: A case-control study of twins vs singletons. *Am J Pub He* 1996;86:809–814.

Luke B, Gillespie B, Min S, et al: Critical periods of maternal weight gain: Effect on twin birth weight. *Am J Obst G* 1997;177:1055–1062.

Luke B, Leurgans S: Maternal weight gains in ideal twin outcomes. *J Am Diet A* 1996;96:178–181.

Mathews F, Murphy M, Wald N, et al: Twinning and folic acid use. *Lancet* 1999; 353:291–292.

Munoz K, Krebs-Smith S, Ballard-Barbash R, et al: Food intakes of US children and adolescents compared with recommendations. *Pediatrics* 1997;100:323–329.

Rees J: Childbearing adolescents: Demographics, developmental needs, behavior, and outcome. *Ann NY Acad* 1997;817:246–250.

Rees J: Overview: Nutrition and pregnant and childbearing adolescents. *Ann NY Acad* 1997;817:241–245.

Samuelson G, Bratteby L, Berggren K, et al: Dietary iron intake and iron status in adolescents. *Act Paediat* 1996;85:1033–1038.

Siega-Ritz A, Carson T, Popkin B: Three squares or mostly snacks: What do teens really eat? *J Adoles H* 1998;22:29–36.

Ventura S, Mathews T, Curtin S: Teenage births in the United States: State trends, 1991–1996. *Monthly Vital Statistics Report*, 1998, vol 46, no. 11, supp 2.

Chapter 9: Nutrition and Nursing Your Baby

Albers J, Kreis I, Liem A, et al: Factors that influence the level of contamination of human milk with poly-chlorinated organic compounds. *Arch Env C* 1996;30: 285–291.

Anderson J, Johnstone B, Remley D: Breast-feeding and cognitive development: A meta-analysis. *Am J Clin N* 1999;70:525–535.

Birch E, Hoffman D, Uauy R, et al: Visual acuity and the essentiality of docosahexaenoic acid and arachidonic acid in the diet of term infants. *Pediat Res* 1998;44:201–209.

Camargo C, Weiss S, Zhang S, et al: Prospective study of birth weight, breast-feeding, and risk of adult-onset asthma. *Am J Epidem* 1998;147:119 (meeting abstract).

Carey G, Quinn T: Exercise and lactation: Are they compatible? *Can J Ap Ph* 2001;26:55–74.

Clarke L, Cho E, deAssis S, et al: Maternal and prepubertal diet, mammary development and breast cancer risk. *J Nutr* 2001;131:S154–S157.

Cunnane S, Francescutti V, Brenna J, et al: Breast-fed infants achieve a higher rate of brain and whole body docosahexaenoate accumulation than formula-fed infants not consuming dietary docosahexaenoate. *Lipids* 2000;35:105–111.

Davis M: Breast-feeding and chronic diseases in childhood and adolescence. *Ped Clin NA* 2001;48:125–141.

Dewey K: Effects of maternal caloric restriction and exercise during lactation. *J Nutr* 1998;128:S386–S389.

Dietz W: Breast-feeding may help prevent childhood overweight. *J Am Med A* 2001;285:2506–2507.

Gillman M, Rifas-Shiman S, Camargo C, et al: Risk of overweight among adolescents who were breast-fed as infants. *J Am Med A* 2001;285:2461–2467.

Gulson B, Mahaffey K, Jameson C, et al: Mobilization of lead from the skeleton during postnatal period is larger than during pregnancy. *J La Cl Med* 1998;131:324–329.

Gunderson E, Abrams B: Epidemiology of gestational weight gain and body weight changes after pregnancy. *Epidemiol R* 1999;21:261–275.

Harris H, Ellison G: Do the changes in energy balance that occur during pregnancy predispose parous women to obesity? *Nutr Res R* 1997;10:57–81.

Harris H, Ellison G, Clement S: Do the psychosocial and behavioral changes that accompany motherhood influence the impact of pregnancy on long-term weight gain? *J Psych Obs* 1999;20:65–79.

Heinig M, Dewey K: Health effects of breast-feeding for mothers: A critical review. *Nutr Res R* 1997;10:35–56.

Heird W: The role of polyunsaturated fatty acids in term and preterm infants and breast-feeding mothers. *Ped Clin NA* 2001;48:173–188.

Horwood L, Darlow B, Mogridge N: Breast-milk feeding and cognitive ability at 7–8 years. *Arch Dis Ch* 2001;84:F23–F27.

Janney C, Zhang D, Sowers M: Lactation and weight retention. *Am J Clin N* 1997;66:1116–1124.

Jordan M: Should breast-feeding by women with silicone implants be recommended? *Arch Ped Ad* 1996;150:880–881.

Jorgensen M, Hernell O, Hughes E, et al: Is there a relation between docosahexaenoic acid concentration in mother's milk and visual development in term infants? *J Ped Gastr* 2001;32:293–296.

Kalkwarf H, Specker B, Heubi J, et al: Intestinal calcium absorption of women during lactation and after weaning. *Am J Clin N* 1996;63:526–531.

Kolezko B, Agostoni C, Carlson S, et al: Long chain polyunsaturated fatty acids and perinatal development. *Act Pediat* 2001;90:460–464.

Krebs N, Reidinger C, Miller L, et al: Zinc homeostasis in breast-fed infants. *Pediat Res* 1996;39:661–665.

Labbok M: Effects of breast-feeding on the mother. *Ped Clin NA* 2001;48:143–158.

Lonnerdal B: Regulation of mineral and trace elements in human milk: Exogenous and endogenous factors. *Nutr Rev* 2000;58:223–229.

Lopez-Alarcon M, Villalpando S, Farjardo A: Breast-feeding lowers the frequency and duration of acute respiratory infection and diarrhea in infants under six months of age. *J Nutr* 1997;127:436–443.

Lovelady C, Garner K, Moreno K, et al: The effect of weight loss in overweight, lactating women on the growth of their babies. *N Eng J Med* 2000;342:449–453.

Lust K, Brown J, Thomas W: Maternal intake of cruciferous vegetables and other foods and colic symptoms in exclusively breast-fed infants. *J Am Diet A* 1996;96:46–48.

Mackey A, Picciano M: Maternal folate status during extended lactation and the effect of supplemental folic acid. *Am J Clin N* 1999;69:285–292.

Mackey A, Picciano M, Mitchell D, et al: Self-selected diets of lactating women often fail to meet dietary recommendations. *J Am Diet A* 1998;98:297–302.

Malaty H, Logan N, Graham D, et al: Helicobacter pylori infection in preschool and school-aged minority children: Effect of socioeconomic indicators and breast-feeding practices. *Clin Inf D* 2001;32:1387–1392.

McCrory M: Does dieting during lactation put infant growth at risk? *Nutr Rev* 2001;59:18–21.

McCrory M, Rivers L, Mole P, et al: Randomized trial of the short-term effects of dieting compared with dieting plus aerobic exercise on lactation performance. *Am J Clin N* 1999;69:959–967.

Miller J, McVeagh P: Human milk oligosaccharides: 130 reasons to breast-feed. *Br J Nutr* 1999;82:333–335.

Misri S, Sinclair D, Kuan A: Breast-feeding and postpartum depression: Is there a relationship? *Can J Psych* 1997;42:1061–1065.

Ncuba T, Greiner T, Malaba L, et al: Supplementing lactating women with pureed papaya and grated carrots improved vitamin A status in a placebo-controlled trial. *J Nutr* 2001;131:1497–1502.

Quinn T, Carey G: Does exercise intensity or diet influence lactic acid accumulation in breast milk? *Med Sci Spt* 1999;31:105–110.

Patandin S, Kuperus N, deRiddler M, et al: Plasma polychlorinated biphenyl levels in Dutch preschool children either breast-fed or formula-fed during infancy. *Am J Pub He* 1997;87:1711–1714.

Pettitt D, Forman M, Hanson R, et al: Breast-feeding and incidence of non-insulin-dependent diabetes mellitus in Pima indians. *Lancet* 1997;350:166–168.

Piovanetti Y: Breast-feeding beyond 12 months. *Ped Clin NA* 2001;48:199–206.

Prentice A: Calcium in pregnancy and lactation. *Ann R Nutr* 2000;20:249–272.

Raisler J, Alexander C, O'Campo P: Breast-feeding and infant illness: A dose-response relationship? *Am J Pub He* 1999;89:25–30.

Rossowska M, Carvajal W, Joseph F, et al: Postnatal caffeine effects on copper, zinc, and iron concentrations in mammary gland, milk, and plasma of lactating dams and their offspring. *Ann Nutr M* 1997;41:60–65.

Scariati P, Grummer-Strawn L, Fein S: A longitudinal analysis of infant morbidity and the extent of breast-feeding in the United States. *Pediatrics* 1997;99:862.

Slavin J: Phytoestrogens in breast-milk: Another advantage of breast-feeding. *Clin Chem* 1996;42:841–842.

Smit E, Oelen E, Seerat E, et al: Breast milk docosahexaenoic acid (DHA) correlates with DHA status of malnourished infants. *Arch Dis Ch* 2000;82:493–494.

Visness C, Kennedy K, Gross B, et al: Fertility of full breast-feeding women in the early postpartum period. *Obstet Gyn* 1997;89:164–167.

Von Kries R, Koletzko B, Sauerwald T, et al: Breast-feeding and Obesity: Cross sectional study. *Br Med J* 1999;319:147–150.

Wright A: The rise of breast-feeding in the United States. *Ped Clin NA* 2001;1–12.

Wright A, Schanler R: The resurgence of breast-feeding at the end of the second millennium. *J Nutr* 2001;131:S421–S425.

Chapter 10: The Postpregnancy Diet:
Regaining Your Figure and Eating for the Next Baby

Gunderson E, Abrams B, Selvin S: Does the pattern of postpartum weight change differ according to pregravid body size? *Int J Obes* 2001;25:853–862.

Hendricks K, Herbold N: Diet, activity, and other health-related behaviors in college-age women. *Nutr Rev* 1998;56:65–75.

Khan K, Chien P, Khan N: Nutritional stress of reproduction. *Act Obst Sc* 1998;77:395–401.

Metzner H, Lamphiear D, Wheeler N, et al: Relationship between frequency of eating and adiposity in adult men and women in the Tecumseh Community Health Study. *Am J Clin N* 1977;30:712–715.

Poston W, Foreyt J: Obesity is an environmental issue. *Atheroscler* 1999;146:201–209.

Rainey C, Nyquist L: Nuts: Nutrition and health benefits of daily use. *Nutr Today* 1997;32:157–163.

Rosenbaum M, Leibel R, Hirsch J: Obesity. *N Eng J Med* 1997;August 7:396–407.

Index

About the Author

ELIZABETH SOMER, M.A., R.D., is a nationally recognized nutrition expert and award-winning writer. She appears regularly on *The Today Show*, is a former consultant to *Good Morning America*, a contributing editor to *Shape* magazine, and the author of six books, including *The Origin Diet*. She lives with her family in Salem, Oregon. Her Web site can be found at www.elizabethsomer. com.